Essentials for Treating Behavioral Health in Primary Care

Meredith L. C. Williamson, PhD, ABPP ·
Danielle L. Terry, PhD, ABPP
Editors

Essentials for Treating Behavioral Health in Primary Care

A Guide for the Primary Care Provider

Springer

Editors
Meredith L. C. Williamson, PhD, ABPP
Naresh K. Vashisht College of Medicine
Department of Primary Care and Rural Medicine
Texas A&M University
Bryan, TX, USA

Danielle L. Terry, PhD, ABPP
Guthrie Medical Group
Guthrie Family Medicine Residency
Sayre, PA, USA

ISBN 978-3-032-09557-2 ISBN 978-3-032-09558-9 (eBook)
https://doi.org/10.1007/978-3-032-09558-9

This publication was supported by the Health Resources and Services Administration (HRSA) of the U.S. Department of Health and Human Services (HHS) as part of an award totaling $2.4 million with zero percentage financed with non-governmental sources. The contents are those of the author(s) and do not necessarily represent the official views of, nor an endorsement, by HRSA, HHS, or the U.S. Government.

This Springer imprint is published by the registered company Springer Nature Switzerland AG
The registered company address is: Gewerbestrasse 11, 6330 Cham, Switzerland

Acknowledgments

We would like to thank Dylan Hall and Kaytlyn Batson for their generous digital contributions, editing, consultation, and design expertise. We would also like to thank our families for the ways that they inspire us every day to care for those around us. Thank you for championing this publication with us. To our primary care colleagues and patients, thank you for the continuous learning opportunities that allow us to grow as humans, clinicians, and educators.

Contents

Editors and Contributors

About the Editors

Meredith L. C. Williamson, PhD, ABPP is a licensed psychologist and board certified in Clinical Health Psychology. She serves as Clinical Associate Professor and Director of Integrated Behavioral Health for the Department of Primary Care and Rural Medicine in the Naresh K. Vashisht College of Medicine at Texas A&M University. She has a joint appointment in the Department of Psychiatry & Behavioral Sciences. She is also Associate Program Director at the Texas A&M Family Medicine Residency Program. Dr. Williamson has developed innovative integrated behavioral health curriculum and interdisciplinary service delivery for a variety of healthcare disciplines. She has led multiple grant funded initiatives focused on behavioral health education for the primary care workforce. In 2024, the Association of American Medical Colleges awarded Dr. Williamson and her team the Mental and Behavioral Health Training Award for their innovations in integrated behavioral health training. Dr. Williamson has numerous publications and national presentations with an emphasis on behavioral health education. She is a member of the Academy of Distinguished Medical Educations at Texas A&M College of Medicine.

Danielle L. Terry, PhD, ABPP is the Director of Behavioral Science at the Guthrie Family Medicine Residency in Sayre, Pennsylvania, Assistant Professor of Psychiatry in the Neuroscience Institute at Geisinger Commonwealth School of Medicine and is the founder of NeuroKind Consulting LLC, neurokindconsulting.com. She is board certified in health psychology and co-author of the books, *Providing Home Care for Older Adults: A Professional Guide for Mental Health Practitioners and Resilient Caregiving for Neurodivergent Children.*

Contributors

David E. Bauman PsyD Community Health of Central Washington, Yakima, WA, USA

Bridget R. Beachy PsyD Community Health of Central Washington, Yakima, WA, USA

Katherine Bergs PhD John Peter Smith Hospital, Fort Worth, TX, USA

Robert Bonanno MD Prisma Health Family Medicine Residency Program Greenville and University of South Carolina School of Medicine Greenville, Greenville, SC, USA

Rolando Botello MEd Texas A&M University, College Station, TX, USA

Jessica Bracks MD UT Tyler School of Medicine, Tyler, TX, USA

Jay Brieler MD Saint Louis University School of Medicine, St. Louis, MO, USA

Ashley Cipriano DO Guthrie Medical Group, Sayre, PA, USA

Molly Clark PhD, ABPP University of Mississippi Medical Center, Jackson, MS, USA

Rebecca M. Daniel PsyD Wake Forest University School of Medicine, Winston-Salem, NC, USA

Katelin Dias PhD Naresh K. Vashisht College of Medicine, Department of Primary Care and Rural Medicine, Texas A&M University, Bryan, TX, USA

Deepu George PhD, LMFT University of Texas Rio Grande Valley School of Medicine, Edinburg, TX, USA

Adam Guck PhD, ABPP John Peter Smith Hospital, Fort Worth, TX, USA

Rachel Herbst PhD Cincinatti Children's Hospital Medical Center, Cincinnati, OH, USA

Brittany Houston PsyD The University of Texas at Austin Dell Medical School, Austin, TX, USA

Kaylee Jackson PhD Naresh K. Vashisht College of Medicine, Department of Primary Care and Rural Medicine, Texas A&M University, Bryan, TX, USA

Yajaira Johnson-Esparza PhD University of Texas San Antonio, San Antonio, TX, USA

Jessie Kao MD John Peter Smith Hospital, Fort Worth, TX, USA

Lance Kelley PhD The Waco Guide to Psychopharmacology®, Waco Family Medicine, Waco, TX, USA

Nicole L. P. Kroll PhD, APRN, ANP-C, FNP-BC, PMHNP-BC Texas A&M College of Nursing, Bryan, TX, USA

Amy Lacroix MD Children's Physicians University of Nebraska Medical Center, Omaha, NE, USA

Ryan Laschober MD, FAAFP The Waco Guide to Psychopharmacology®, Waco Family Medicine, Waco, TX, USA

Christina L. Lee MD, MPH University of California Davis School of Medicine, Sacramento, CA, USA

Corina Marshall MD, FAAFP Guthrie Medical Group, Sayre, PA, USA

Matthew P. Martin PhD, MS, LMFT Arizona State University College of Health Solutions, Phoenix, AZ, USA

Denise Martinez MPH Department of Primary Care and Rural Medicine, Texas A & M College of Medicine, Bryan, TX, USA

Clare McNutt PA-C Meadows Mental Health Policy Institute, Austin, TX, USA

Giannina Mixco MEd Texas A&M University, College Station, TX, USA

Mariah Montgomery PhD Dell Medical School, University of Texas at Austin, Austin, TX, USA

Taliyah Mosley MEd Texas A&M University, College Station, TX, USA

Michelle Nanda MD, MPH, FAAFP Guthrie Medical Group, Sayre, PA, USA

Jamil Neme MD Saint Louis University School of Medicine, St. Louis, MO, USA

Danielle Porter MS Texas A&M University, College Station, TX, USA

Lisa Ramirez PhD, ABPP The MetroHealth System, Cleveland, OH, USA

Susan Roberman MD, FAAFP Naresh K. Vashisht College of Medicine, Department of Primary Care and Rural Medicine, Texas A&M University, Bryan, TX, USA

Zach Sartor MD, FAAFP The Waco Guide to Psychopharmacology®, Waco Family Medicine, Waco, TX, USA

Morgan Sekula MEd Texas A&M University, College Station, TX, USA

Randi Sokol MD, MPH, MMedEd Tufts Department of Family Medicine, Somerville, MA, USA

Jennifer Swanson MEd Texas A&M University, College Station, TX, USA

Shannon Stark Taylor PhD Prisma Health Family Medicine Residency Program Greenville and University of South Carolina School of Medicine Greenville, Greenville, SC, USA

Danielle L. Terry PhD, ABPP Guthrie Medical Group, Sayre, PA, USA

Brandon Williamson MD, FAAFP Naresh K. Vashisht College of Medicine, Department of Primary Care and Rural Medicine, Texas A&M University, Bryan, TX, USA

Meredith L. C. Williamson PhD, ABPP Naresh K. Vashisht College of Medicine, Department of Primary Care and Rural Medicine, Texas A&M University, Bryan, TX, USA

Eboni Winford PhD, MPH Cherokee Health Systems, Knoxville, TN, USA

Max Zubatsky PhD Saint Louis University School of Medicine, St. Louis, MO, USA

Chapter 1
The Behavioral Health Crisis in Primary Care

Meredith L. C. Williamson PhD, ABPP, Danielle L. Terry PhD, ABPP, Nicole L. P. Kroll PhD, APRN, ANP-C, FNP-BC, PMHNP-BC, Denise Martinez MPH, and Clare McNutt PA-C

An Introduction to the Behavioral Health Crisis

The shortage of assessment and treatment options for individuals suffering from behavioral health (BH) conditions is a significant public health concern in the United States. With screening recommendations for BH conditions on the rise, primary care providers (PCPs) are facing greater demands to provide BH services (Olfson, 2016). There are numerous barriers to accessing BH care, including geographic availability, cost, and stigma. Nearly half of all counties in the United States do not have BH providers and 75% are classified as BH shortage areas (Substance Abuse and Mental Health Services Administration (SAMHSA), 2016). Compared to urban areas, rural areas face even more difficulty with provision of services, especially in regard to availability of outpatient substance use treatment (12.1% versus 43.7%) availability in urban hospitals (Centers for Disease Control and Prevention [CDC],

M. L. C. Williamson PhD, ABPP · D. Martinez MPH
Naresh K. Vashisht College of Medicine, Department of Primary Care and Rural Medicine, Texas A&M University, Bryan, TX, USA
e-mail: meredith.williamson@tamu.edu

D. Martinez MPH
e-mail: denise.martinez@tamu.edu

D. L. Terry PhD, ABPP (✉)
Family Medicine Residency, Guthrie Medical Group, Sayre, PA, USA
e-mail: danielle.terry@guthrie.org

N. L. P. Kroll PhD, APRN, ANP-C, FNP-BC, PMHNP-BC
Texas A&M College of Nursing, Bryan, TX, USA
e-mail: nkroll@exchange.tamu.edu

C. McNutt PA-C
Meadows Mental Health Policy Institute, Austin, TX, USA
e-mail: cmcnutt@mmhpi.org

M. L. C. Williamson and D. L. Terry (eds.), *Essentials for Treating Behavioral Health in Primary Care*, https://doi.org/10.1007/978-3-032-09558-9_1

2018; Substance Abuse and Mental Health Services Administration (SAMHSA), 2016).

With the lack of access to BH care, there are advantages to seeking services in primary care, and most Americans do just that. PCPs are often the only provider available for individuals with these concerns (Faghri et al., 2010). Advantages to seeking BH treatment in primary care include greater anonymity with decreased stigma (Hodgkinson et al., 2017), better access and availability of appointments (Pomerantz et al., 2008), greater financial coverage by insurance (Cummings et al., 2009; Monson et al., 2012), and patient preference to receive BH care within their medical home (Ogbeide et al., 2018).

It is estimated that over 25% of *presenting* concerns within primary care include BH concerns (Beck et al., 2019). Nearly three quarters of primary care visits have a BH component (American Academy of Family Physicians (AAFP), 2018; Hunter et al., 2009). In addition, antidepressants are among the most commonly prescribed medications within outpatient care (Rui et al., 2014).

As front-line providers, primary care physicians and advanced practice providers often diagnose and manage numerous BH conditions (Adams & Vanderhoef, 2021; Beck et al., 2019). Most often, they diagnose depression, anxiety, and substance use disorders (36%, 31%, and 25%, respectively; Beck et al., 2019). They may also diagnose bipolar disorder and ADHD. Diagnosis and management of severe mental illness like schizophrenia occurs, but is less common, and physicians report a lack of confidence in assessment and treatment of these conditions (Beck et al., 2019). See Chap. 3 for a full discussion of conditions commonly seen in primary care.

While many individuals present to their PCP for BH care, these treatment opportunities are not always optimized. An estimated 70% of individuals with BH conditions such as depression go undetected within primary care (Martin et al., 2005). Approximately 50% of people who die by suicide have seen their PCP within the previous month (Luoma et al., 2002). Thus, finding ways to detect and treat routine and acute BH conditions in settings that serve as a "touch point" is paramount.

It is well established that there is a duality between the body and the mind. As highlighted in Engel's (1977) biopsychosocial model, there is an interaction between BH conditions and physical health outcomes. Consistent with this model, individuals with chronic diseases such as heart disease and cancer have an increased risk of depression (Frasure-Smith & Lespérance, 2006). In addition, childhood trauma has been associated with early mortality (Grummitt et al., 2021). Comorbid BH conditions negatively impact outcomes of other chronic health conditions, including respiratory and heart diseases (American Psychological Association [APA], 2014). Comprehensive treatment of chronic health conditions requires that providers address BH concerns. It is imperative that PCPs obtain competence in the treatment of BH conditions to improve overall health and wellbeing of those that they serve.

A National Call for BH in Primary Care

National recommendations exist for universal screening for both anxiety and depression within primary care settings (Hunter et al., 2022; U.S. Preventive Services Task Force [USPSTF], 2023a, 2023b). The U.S. Preventive Services Task Force (USPSTF) recognizes that PCPs are on the front lines of the BH crisis in America. In recent years, the USPSTF has recommended PCPs initiate routine screening for depression, anxiety, and substance use in addition to screening for other medical concerns within adult populations (U.S. Preventive Services Task Force [USPSTF], 2020, 2022a, 2023b). The taskforce has included screening for anxiety and depression in pediatric populations to increase early identification of undiagnosed BH conditions (U.S. Preventive Services Task Force [USPSTF], 2022a, 2022b).

Over the last decade there has been significant advancement with integrating BH services into primary care. Currently, there are multiple, evidence-based models for BH integration to assist PCPs on the front lines. The most prominent include the Collaborative Care Model and the Primary Care Behavioral Health Model (Hunter et al., 2022; University of Washington, 2023). These models will be reviewed in Chap. 12. United States federal agencies including the Health Services & Research Administration (HSRA), Substance Use and Mental Health Service Administration (SAMHSA), and National Institutes of Mental Health (NIMH) have supported research, training, and clinical service advancement for BH integration within primary care through national funding opportunities. In 2022, American President Joe Biden outlined a strategy to expand access to resources by integrating BH in primary care (U.S. Department of Health and Human Services, 2022). In 2024, Centers for Medicaid and Medicare Services announced the Innovation in Behavioral Model, which aims to improve quality of care and outcomes, for individuals with BH conditions via use of interprofessional care teams (Centers for Medicare and Medicaid Services, 2024).

While there are existing models and initiatives that aim to increase integrated BH access in primary care, there are still significant limitations in the ability to access and use these services due to financial barriers and workforce limitations. Lack of implementation of these services is even greater in rural and underserved areas and results in a significant need for BH intervention in primary care. PCPs continue to be the sole medical provider for BH concerns. Global and national recommendations continue to highlight the need for support of BH assessment and treatment within primary care (World Health Organization [WHO], 2022). Despite these calls to action, there has been minimal advancement in medical education to prepare the healthcare workforce to integrate BH into primary care settings (Choi et al., 2019). There are limited opportunities for learners in undergraduate and graduate medical education to learn about integrated BH, and most specialties do not specify or mandate BH curriculum.

Undergraduate Medical Education While the majority of medical schools require BH exposure via psychiatry clerkships, there are limited curricular recommendations or examples for training medical students to assess and treat BH conditions within primary care settings (Choi et al., 2019). Dubé and Verduin (2015) identified that the majority of BH clinical exposure occurs within primary care rotations without expertise from psychiatric specialties. A survey of American and Canadian medical schools found that less than 50% of medical students across all institutions are exposed to BH support for primary care physicians within family medicine clerkships (Choi et al., 2019). While the reality is that primary care is the predominant home for BH assessment and treatment, regardless of specialty, medical students graduate without a consistent understanding of the duality of behavioral and physical health conditions that they will face for their entire career.

Graduate Medical Education

Graduate medical education for primary care specialties have made inconsistent strides in preparing PCPs to be the predominant member of the clinical care team caring for those with BH conditions. Aside from psychiatry, the BH educational requirements specified for family medicine residencies are arguably the most extensive in contrast with other primary care training programs and specialties. Guidelines outlined by the Accreditation Council for Graduate Medical Education (ACGME) specify that family medicine residencies "must incorporate BH into all aspects of patient care, including experience in integrated interprofessional BH care in the family medicine practice" (Accreditation Council for Graduate Medical Education [ACGME], 2023b). Further, it specifies that:

1. Residents must have a dedicated experience in the diagnosis and management of common mental illness, including interprofessional training in cognitive behavioral therapy, motivational interviewing, and psychopharmacology (Accreditation Council for Graduate Medical Education [ACGME], 2023c).
2. This experience should include identification and treatment of substance use disorders, including alcohol use disorder and Opioid Use Disorder. Treatment should include pharmacologic and nonpharmacologic methods and an interprofessional team.

Current guidelines also specify that there must be at least one faculty member who is dedicated to providing BH training (Accreditation Council for Graduate Medical Education [ACGME], 2023a).

Like family medicine, graduating pediatric residents must demonstrate basic competency in the management of BH conditions, but the ACGME does not dictate specific training requirements or what defines competency (Accreditation Council for Graduate Medical Education [ACGME], 2022). Other primary care specialties, including internal medicine and obstetrics and gynecology (OB/GYN), have few (if any) mandatory requirements. Internal medicine residency programs are required to provide clinical experiences in addiction medicine (Accreditation Council for Graduate Medical Education [ACGME], 2023a). To date, OB/GYN does not require any educational experiences and/or clinical training in BH (Accreditation Council for Graduate Medical Education [ACGME], 2023b).

Additional Primary Care Provider Training

Physician assistants (PAs) and nurse practitioners (NPs), many of whom are on the front lines of primary care, have some exposure to BH training, but quantity and modality is often not specified (Accreditation Review Commission on Education for the Physician Assistant [ARC-PA], 2024; Morreale et al., 2020). For PAs, didactics and lecture curriculum "must include instruction in psychiatric/behavioral conditions." It further dictates that the training curriculum should include instruction in death, dying, and loss, human sexuality, normal and abnormal development across the lifespan, patient response to illness or injury, patient response to stress, substance use disorders, and violence identification and prevention. PA education in BH is most commonly related to the area of specialty that the PA enters upon employment post-graduation.

Undergraduate Nursing Education Undergraduate nursing students are most often exposed to BH conditions through simulation, pedagogies of critical thinking, and clinical experiences (Goh et al., 2021). BH concepts are included on the National Council Licensure Examination (NCLEX), a test to determine if recently graduated nursing students meet the minimum requirement to practice. Nursing schools in the United States provide exposure to signs and symptoms of acute and chronic mental illnesses including schizophrenia, depression, anxiety, and bipolar disorder. Graduate registered nurses are expected to apply knowledge of BH concepts, provide care and education for patients with psychiatric issues that will assist them in adherence to a treatment plan (National Council of State Boards of Nursing [NCSBN], 2023).

Graduate Nursing Education NP education focuses more on exposure to specific populations but is less defined regarding academic content. Primary care NP education builds on a baccalaureate nursing education foundation and many programs require professional nursing experience for admission (Bednar et al., 2007; Dugan & Altmiller, 2023). While academic institutions vary in the way they deliver educational content, most credentialed programs follow the American Association of Colleges of Nursing (AACN) Essentials: Core Competencies for Professional Nursing Practice and align the content with the National Organization of Nurse Practitioner Faculties (NONPF) core competencies and the National Task Force Standards for Quality Nurse Practitioner Education. The AACN core competencies and essentials do not specifically list BH conditions as a core training requirement, however, they do address person-centered care which encompasses health problems/status, emotional support, and diagnostic reasoning (Dugan & Altmiller, 2023). Didactic content and clinical experiences for NPs cover BH and the NP certifying bodies American Nurses Credentialing Center (ANCC) and the American Academy of Nurse Practitioners (AANP) examination blueprints both include psychiatric/psychological content (American Academy of Nurse Practitioners [AANP] Certification Board, 2024; American Nurses Credentialing Center [ANCC], 2022). Currently, all states with the exception of New York and California require board certification to practice (Fitzgerald, 2024).

Realities of Behavioral Health in Primary Care

Fewer medical students are seeking and matching into primary care specialties despite record numbers of available training and post-training positions (American Academy of Family Physicians (AAFP), 2018; Knight, 2019). With this strain, it is important to find ways to provide efficient and streamlined care. While the general consensus is to increase access to BH services in the nation, numerous barriers currently circumvent this lofty goal. Until the nation is able to "catch up" and implement sustainable solutions to the BH crisis, primary care providers will continue to be the solution for serving the BH needs of our communities. Unfortunately, these front-line providers often lack specialized training in providing these services personally or collaborating with integrated BH providers working within primary care settings. While integrating BH services into primary care has been associated with decreased PCP burnout (Zubatsky et al., 2018), these collaborative services are often unavailable in underserved settings due to workforce shortages and financial barriers.

Nevertheless, primary care will likely continue to be the preferable place to seek BH care due to ease of access and decreased stigma (Flynn et al., 2020; Ogbeide et al., 2018; Pomerantz et al., 2008, 2010). Integrated BH teams alongside PCPs have demonstrated success with pharmacologic and nonpharmacologic treatment. Currently due to BH workforce shortages, PCPs will likely continue to be the main support for BH across the nation and the globe.

Notably, public health initiatives have steadily recognized the importance of integrating BH in primary care settings to address mental health disparities (Halkitis, 2020; Monson et al., 2012). Additionally, the public health field advocates for the acknowledgment and integration of social workers and community health workers (CHWs) to aid BH and integrated care workforce shortages (Noel et al., 2022; Petruzzi et al., 2024). In general, this collective integration may help reduce barriers to access, and aid in the promotion of early detection and intervention for BH concerns. Hopefully as integrated BH teams expand and potentially incorporate other workforces, additional literature and guidance on their integration could provide valuable support for navigating implementation in primary care settings.

Text Overview

This seminal text has been developed to equip and support PCPs in the assessment and treatment of BH concerns within their clinical encounters. This is not an exhaustive tutorial for BH assessment and treatment within primary care. Rather, it serves to provide practical guidelines and best practices to empower PCPs to efficiently and effectively handle basic BH concerns. This book is divided into three sections. First, we will provide an overview of BH care within the primary care setting, including essentials of communication, basic recommendations for screening, risk assessment, and assessment of cognitive impairment. Second, we will provide guidance for common presenting conditions, and behavioral treatments that might be utilized by the PCP during the clinical encounter including use of psychotropic medications, brief behavioral interventions, addressing concerns with addiction, and special considerations for pediatric and peripartum populations. The final portion of the book will highlight leading models of integrated BH in primary care and how to maximize use of the medical team.

Primary care is the heart and soul of medicine—it is the place where families come to seek safe harbor and solutions for their health. As the home for all medical care, it is imperative that PCPs have support and training to meet not only the medical needs, but also the BH needs of their communities. This book provides a short-hand resource to better equip PCPs to address the BH needs of the community at large, needs they may not envision as part of their practice, but care they have been tasked to provide.

References

Accreditation Council for Graduate Medical Education [ACGME]. (2022). *ACGME program requirements for graduate medical education in pediatrics.* https://www.acgme.org/globalassets/pfassets/programrequirements/320_pediatrics_2022.pdf&sa=D&source=docs&ust=1728401087115830&usg=AOvVaw0Xav5rGK1HR75BpZEuJapn

Accreditation Council for Graduate Medical Education [ACGME]. (2023a). *ACGME program requirements for graduate medical education in internal medicine.* https://www.acgme.org/globalassets/pfassets/programrequirements/140_internalmedicine_2023.pdf

Accreditation Council for Graduate Medical Education [ACGME]. (2023b). *ACGME program requirements for graduate medical education in obstetrics and gynecology.* https://www.acgme.org/globalassets/pfassets/programrequirements/220_obstetricsandgynecology_2023.pdf

Accreditation Council for Graduate Medical Education [ACGME]. (2023c). *ACGME program requirements for graduate medical education in family medicine.* https://www.acgme.org/globalassets/pfassets/programrequirements/120_familymedicine_2023.pdf

Accreditation Review Commission on Education for the Physician Assistant [ARC-PA]. (2024). *About ARC-PA.* ARC-PA. https://www.arc-pa.org/about/

Adams, S. M., & Vanderhoef, D. M. (2021). The critical role of primary care providers in meeting mental health care needs in 2021. *The Journal for Nurse Practitioners, 17*(1), 3–4. https://doi.org/10.1016/j.nurpra.2020.12.014

American Academy of Family Physicians (AAFP). (2018). *Mental health care services by family physicians (position paper).* https://www.aafp.org/about/policies/all/mental-health-services.html

American Academy of Nurse Practitioners [AANP] Certification Board. (2024). *Family nurse practitioner*. Retrieved November 4, 2024, from https://www.aanpcert.org/certs/fnp

American Nurses Credentialing Center [ANCC]. (2022). *Nursing certifications.* ANA. https://www.nursingworld.org/our-certifications/

American Psychological Association [APA]. (2014). *Briefing series on the role of psychology in health care.* https://www.apa.org/health/briefs/primary-care.pdf

Beck, A. J., Page, C., Buche, J., Schoebel, V., & Wayment, C. (2019). *Behavioral service provision by primary care physicians.* University of Michigan Behavioral Health Workforce Research Center. https://www.behavioralhealthworkforce.org/wp-content/uploads/2019/12/Y4-P10-BH-Capacityof-PC-Phys_Full.pdf

Bednar, S., Atwater, A., & Keough, V. (2007). Educational preparation of nurse practitioners and physician assistants: An exploratory review. *Advanced Emergency Nursing Journal, 29*(2), 158–171. https://doi.org/10.1097/01.TME.0000270339.19380.16

Centers for Disease Control and Prevention [CDC]. (2018). *Mental health-related physician office visits by adults aged 18 and over: United States 2012–2014*. https://www.cdc.gov/nchs/products/databriefs/db311.htm

Centers for Medicare and Medicaid Services. (2024). *CMS announces new model to advance integration in behavioral health*. https://www.cms.gov/newsroom/press-releases/cms-announces-new-model-advance-integration-behavioral-health

Choi, R. J., Betancourt, R. M., DeMarco, M. P., & Bream, K. D. W. (2019). Medical student exposure to integrated Behavioral health. *Academic Psychiatry, 43*(2), 191–195. https://doi.org/10.1007/s40596-018-0936-0

Cummings, N. A., O'Donohue, W. T., & Cummings, J. L. (2009). The financial dimension of integrated behavioral/primary care. *Journal of Clinical Psychology in Medical Settings, 16*(1), 31–39. https://doi.org/10.1007/s10880-008-9139-2

Dubé, B., & Verduin, M. L. (2015). A brief examination of integrated care in undergraduate medical education. *Academic Psychiatry, 39*(4), 457–460. https://doi.org/10.1007/s40596-015-0332-y

Dugan, M. A., & Altmiller, G. (2023). AACN essentials and nurse practitioner education: Competency-based case studies grounded in authentic practice. *Journal of Professional Nursing, 46*, 59–64. https://doi.org/10.1016/j.profnurs.2023.02.003

Engel, G. L. (1977). The need for a new medical model: A challenge for biomedicine. *Science, 196*(4286), 129–136. https://doi.org/10.1126/science.847460

Faghri, N. M. A., Boisvert, C. M., & Faghri, S. (2010). Understanding the expanding role of primary care physicians (PCPs) to primary psychiatric care physicians (PPCPs): Enhancing the assessment and treatment of psychiatric conditions. *Mental Health in Family Medicine, 7*(1), 17–25.

Fitzgerald, M. A. (2024). *State licensure and certification: Myths and realities*. https://www.fhea.com/certification-qa/state-licensure-and-certification-myths-and-realities/

Flynn, A., Gonzalez, V., Mata, M., Salinas, L. A., & Atkins, A. (2020). Integrated care improves mental health in a medically underserved U.S.-Mexico border population. *Families, Systems & Health, 38*(2), 105–115. https://doi.org/10.1037/fsh0000490

Frasure-Smith, N., & Lespérance, F. (2006). Recent evidence linking coronary heart disease and depression. *The Canadian Journal of Psychiatry, 51*(12), 730–737. https://doi.org/10.1177/070674370605101202

Goh, Y.-S., Owyong, J. Q. Y., Seetoh, Y.-T. M., Hu, Y., Chng, M.-L., & Li, Z. (2021). Exploring pedagogies used in undergraduate mental health nursing curriculum: An integrative literature review. *International Journal of Mental Health Nursing, 30*(1), 47–61. https://doi.org/10.1111/inm.12816

Grummitt, L. R., Kreski, N. T., Kim, S. G., Platt, J., Keyes, K. M., & McLaughlin, K. A. (2021). Association of childhood adversity with morbidity and mortality in us adults: A systematic review. *JAMA Pediatrics, 175*(12), 1269–1278. https://doi.org/10.1001/jamapediatrics.2021.2320

Halkitis, P. N. (2020). A new public health psychology to mend the chasm between public health and clinical care. *American Psychologist, 75*(9), 1289–1296. https://doi.org/10.1037/amp0000743

Hodgkinson, S., Godoy, L., Beers, L. S., & Lewin, A. (2017). Improving mental health access for low-income children and families in the primary care setting. *Pediatrics, 139*(1), e20151175. https://doi.org/10.1542/peds.2015-1175

Hunter, C. L., Goodie, J. L., Oordt, M. S., & Dobmeyer, A. C. (2009). *Integrated behavioral health in primary care: Step-by-step guidance for assessment and intervention (first)*. American Psychological Association. https://doi.org/10.1037/11871-000

Hunter, C. L., Goodie, J. L., Oordt, M. S., & Dobmeyer, A. C. (2022). *Integrated behavioral health in primary care: Step-by-step guidance for assessment and intervention (second)*. American Psychological Association.

Knight, V. (2019). *American medical students less likely to choose to become primary care doctors.* Kaiser Health News. https://health.wusf.usf.edu/npr-health/2019-07-03/american-medical-students-less-likely-to-choose-to-become-primary-care-doctors

Luoma, J. B., Martin, C. E., & Pearson, J. L. (2002). Contact with mental health and primary care providers before suicide: A review of the evidence. *American Journal of Psychiatry, 159*(6), 909–916. https://doi.org/10.1176/appi.ajp.159.6.909

Martin, L. R., Williams, S. L., Haskard, K. B., & DiMatteo, M. R. (2005). The challenge of patient adherence. *Therapeutics and Clinical Risk Management, 1*(3), 189–199. https://doi.org/10.2147/tcrm.s12160382

Monson, S. P., Sheldon, J. C., Ivey, L. C., Kinman, C. R., & Beacham, A. O. (2012). Working toward financial sustainability of integrated behavioral health services in a public health care system. *Families, Systems & Health, 30*(2), 181–186. https://doi.org/10.1037/a0028177

Morreale, M. K., Balon, R., Coverdale, J., Louie, A. K., Beresin, E., Guerrero, A. P. S., Aggarwal, R., & Brenner, A. M. (2020). Supporting the education of nurse practitioners and physician assistants in meeting shortages in mental health care. *Academic Psychiatry, 44*(4), 377–379. https://doi.org/10.1007/s40596-020-01256-3

National Council of State Boards of Nursing [NCSBN]. (2023). *NCLEX-RN test plan.* https://www.nursingworld.org/-/media/CNANews/NursingWorld/ANCC/ANCC-NCLEX-RN-Test-Plan.pdf

Noel, L., Chen, Q., Petruzzi, L. J., Phillips, F., Garay, R., Valdez, C., Aranda, M. P., & Jones, B. (2022). Interprofessional collaboration between social workers and community health workers to address health and mental health in the United States: A systematised review. *Health & Social Care in the Community, 30*(6), e6240–e6254. https://doi.org/10.1111/hsc.14061

Ogbeide, S. A., Landoll, R. R., Nielsen, M. K., & Kanzler, K. E. (2018). To go or not go: Patient preference in seeking specialty mental health versus behavioral consultation within the primary care behavioral health consultation model. *Families, Systems & Health, 36*(4), 513–517. https://doi.org/10.1037/fsh0000374

Olfson, M. (2016). The rise of primary care physicians in the provision of US mental health care. *Journal of Health Politics, Policy and Law, 41*(4), 559–583. https://doi.org/10.1215/03616878-3620821

Petruzzi, L., Milano, N., Chen, Q., Noel, L., Golden, R., & Jones, B. (2024). Social workers are key to addressing social determinants of health in integrated care settings. *Social Work in Health Care, 63*(2), 89–101. https://doi.org/10.1080/00981389.2023.2292565

Pomerantz, A. S., Cole, B. H., Watts, B. V., & Weeks, W. B. (2008). Improving efficiency and access to mental health care: Combining integrated care and advanced access. *General Hospital Psychiatry, 30*(6), 546–551. https://doi.org/10.1016/j.genhosppsych.2008.09.004

Pomerantz, A. S., Shiner, B., Watts, B. V., Detzer, M. J., Kutter, C., Street, B., & Scott, D. (2010). The White River model of colocated collaborative care: A platform for mental and behavioral health care in the medical home. *Families, Systems & Health, 28*(2), 114–129. https://doi.org/10.1037/a0020261

Rui, P., Hing, E., & Okeyode, T. (2014). *National Ambulatory Medical Care Survey: 2014 state and national summary tables.* Centers for Disease Control and Prevention (CDC). http://www.cdc.gov/nchs/ahcd/ahcd_products.htm

Substance Abuse and Mental Health Services Administration (SAMHSA). (2016). *Rural behavioral health: Telehealth challenges and opportunities.* https://store.samhsa.gov/sites/default/files/d7/priv/sma16-4989.pdf

U.S. Department of Health and Human Services. (2022). *HHS roadmap for behavioral health integration.* https://www.hhs.gov/about/news/2022/12/02/hhs-roadmap-for-behavioral-health-integration-fact-sheet.html

U.S. Preventive Services Task Force [USPSTF]. (2020). *Unhealthy drug use: Screening.* https://www.uspreventiveservicestaskforce.org/uspstf/recommendation/drug-use-illicit-screening

U.S. Preventive Services Task Force [USPSTF]. (2022a). *Anxiety in children and adolescents: Screening.* https://www.uspreventiveservicestaskforce.org/uspstf/recommendation/screening-anxiety-children-adolescents

U.S. Preventive Services Task Force [USPSTF]. (2022b). *Depression and suicide risk in children and adolescents: Screening.* https://www.uspreventiveservicestaskforce.org/uspstf/recommendation/screening-depression-suicide-risk-children-adolescents

U.S. Preventive Services Task Force [USPSTF]. (2023a). *Anxiety disorders in adults: Screening.* https://www.uspreventiveservicestaskforce.org/uspstf/recommendation/anxiety-adults-screening

U.S. Preventive Services Task Force [USPSTF]. (2023b). *Depression and suicide risk in adults: Screening.* https://www.uspreventiveservicestaskforce.org/uspstf/recommendation/screening-depression-suicide-risk-adults#fullrecommendationstart

University of Washington. (2023). *Principles of collaborative care—AIMS Center*. https://aims.uw.edu/principles-of-collaborative-care/.

World Health Organization [WHO]. (2022). *World mental health report: Transforming mental health for all.* World health Organization. https://iris.who.int/handle/10665/356119

Zubatsky, M., Pettinelli, D., Salas, J., & Davis, D. (2018). Associations between integrated care practice and burnout factors of primary care physicians. *Family Medicine, 50*(10), 770–774. https://doi.org/10.22454/FamMed.2018.655711

Chapter 2
Essential Communication Skills Needed for High-Quality Primary Care

David E. Bauman PsyD, Bridget R. Beachy PsyD, and Brittany Houston PsyD

The Guiding Philosophies of Patient-Centered Care

While recent reports and training guidelines have promoted the importance of primary care provider (PCP) communication skills to effectively work in the primary care system, many clinicians have been aware of this reality for some time. Effective communication is essential. The majority of patients prefer patient-centered communication over a purely bio-medical approach (Swenson et al., 2004). In comparison with the bio-medical model, the patient-centered approach incorporates patients' values, preferences, and needs to guide medical decisions and evaluate evidence-based treatment options (Committee on Quality of Health Care in America, 2001).

Primary care visits are often single encounters spread out over a lifetime. Further, most primary care visits have a behavioral health (BH) component (Hunter et al., 2017) requiring an understanding of the patient's biopsychosocial life context (biological, social/cultural, and psychological considerations) to intervene effectively. Patient-provider communication can best be understood through the lenses of single-session approaches (Schleider, 2023; Talmon, 1990) and Functional Contextualism (Hayes & Fryling, 2019).

D. E. Bauman PsyD (✉) · B. R. Beachy PsyD
Community Health of Central Washington, Yakima, WA, USA
e-mail: davidbauman4@gmail.com

B. R. Beachy PsyD
e-mail: bridgetbeachy@gmail.com

B. Houston PsyD
The University of Texas at Austin Dell Medical School, Austin, TX, USA
e-mail: brittany.houston@ascension.org

M. L. C. Williamson and D. L. Terry (eds.), *Essentials for Treating Behavioral Health in Primary Care*, https://doi.org/10.1007/978-3-032-09558-9_2

A Single Encounter Approach Single-Session Approaches (SSAs; Schleider, 2023; Talmon, 1990) align harmoniously with the goals of primary care. A single-encounter approach highlights care that is in the moment and strives to see the individual within the context they are coming from. This approach seeks to increase hope and agency among patients at every visit due to the reality that they may never return for follow-up or only seek treatment sporadically over time.

A Functional Contextual Approach Functional Contextualism (Hayes & Fryling, 2019) encourages PCPs to view all behaviors within the context they arise. Instead of focusing solely on dissecting a presenting concern and implementing an algorithm to eradicate the identified pathology, we encourage providers to assume the presenting problem makes sense from the context that it is arising from. For example, a patient presenting with uncontrolled blood sugars may be instructed to start a medication, improve their diet, and increase their physical activity indiscriminately from the context surrounding them. From a Functional Contextualism perspective, the provider would first be curious about the individual's context and why it would make *sense* that the individual would be struggling with their blood sugars. Potentially there may be food insecurities, demands that require the individual's health to be placed as a lesser priority, or an unsupportive social environment, all of which may make such lifestyle changes difficult to enact. When applied, a Functional Contextualist perspective requires the PCP to be constantly curious of the human they are working with, often eliciting the very collaborative, patient-centered stance being called for by National Academies of Sciences, Engineering, and Medicine (2021) and the Accreditation Council for Graduate Medical Education.

Components of Patient-Centered Communication in Primary Care

Applying a patient-centered approach is beneficial and potentially crucial to patient outcomes. However, true barriers exist that often prevent PCPs from delivering such care. For example, many PCPs identify limited time as a major barrier to exercising these practices during visits (Mauksch et al., 2008). Confirming this reality, Tai-Seale et al. (2007) reported the median time for primary care visits lasts approximately 15 min and often encompasses multiple concerns with varied complexity. Further, our experience has illuminated the lack of training medical residents receive in medical school regarding patient-centered communication. It often seems there is an assumption that patient-centered and effective communication is about simply being "nice" to patients. Combining potential barriers with lack of training, the feat of accomplishing a patient-centered visit by addressing the patient's most pressing needs must be deliberately and intentionally trained to allow successful negotiation through transparent and attentive communication. The key components in a

Table 2.1 Common acronyms and meanings

Acronym	Meaning
AIDET	Acknowledge, Introduce, Duration, Explain, Thank You
EEE Empathetic Interruption Technique	Excuse, Empathize, Explain
5 A's Model of Behavior Change	Assess, Advise, Agree, Assist, Arrange
CI	Contextual Interviewing
LWPHb	Love, Work, Play, Health Behaviors
ACCESS-V	Adverse Childhood Experiences, Cultural Consideration, Context Internal, Context External, Social and Structural Determinants of Health, Stages of Change, Values
CV	Internal Context and Values

patient-centered visit include: (1) eliciting and negotiating the visit agenda, (2) understanding the patient's perspective, (3) expressing empathy, (4) revealing the diagnosis, assessing the patient's prior knowledge of the diagnosis, and understanding their current emotional response, and (5) engaging in shared decision-making for treatment recommendations (Hashim, 2017).

The following will include an overview of patient-centered communication principles and techniques, including AIDET principles, setting an agenda, utilizing the Five A's, and Contextual Interviewing to encourage collaboration during patient visits. To assist the reader that may be unfamiliar with specific acronyms, we have provided a table (see Table 2.1) that includes a list of the specific acronyms used regularly throughout the chapter.

AIDET Principles

A physician begins to set a healing context designed to effectively navigate patient-provider communication in the first 1–2 min of a patient encounter. Implementing communication skills at the beginning of the visit can lead to effectively using these skills throughout the encounter and reduce the likelihood of inefficient skill use later in the visit (Cegala & Lenzmeier Broz, 2002).

The communication tool AIDET (Acknowledge, Introduce, Duration, Explain, Thank you) is a format that promotes beginning the visit with empathy while setting up the expected structure of the appointment. Research confirms that patients desire transparency in their provider-patient communication. Moreover, a lack of clarity or misalignment in expectations can lead to a lack of motivation to engage in treatment plans that promote patient health (Huron Consulting Group Inc, n.d.; Scott, 2012).

The first step using the AIDET tool happens when the physician first walks into the room. The PCP Acknowledges the patient and their support network in the room with a greeting. Next, the PCP Introduces themselves and their role in the patient care team. The PCP then talks about the expected Duration of the visit and offers an Explanation of each step of the visit (i.e. Agenda setting, Patient Medical history, etc.). This enables the PCP and patient to negotiate what is important to address in the allotted time frame. Communication skills such as shared decision-making and empathetic interruptions mentioned previously will be important to utilize in this section to focus the visit. Finally, the visit is closed by the PCP Thanking the patient and their support network for choosing their facility, communicating their needs, and/or engaging in their health care. Below is a provider script for implementing AIDET at the beginning of their visit.

> Provider (Acknowledge and Introduce): "Good morning, Cher, I am Dr. Johns. It is
> nice to meet you."
> Patient: "Good morning, nice to meet you as well."
> Provider: "Who do you have with you today?"
> Patient: "This is my mother, Mary; she helps me with all my medical appointments."
> Provider: "Mary, it is good to have you here."
> Provider: "I am going to start with just telling you a little bit about my role in your
> health care. As your primary care provider, I am here to help you with your overall health
> including your physical health and behavioral health."
> Provider (Duration and Explanation): "In order to do this we will spend the next 10
> minutes getting a list of your concerns, talking about your medical history and other
> areas of your life that impact your health and do a quick physical exam. We may not be
> able to get to all your concerns today and we will make the decision together on what is
> most important to address in today's visit."
> Provider (Thank you): "Thank you for coming to see us at [Organization Name] today,
> I'll have my Medical Assistant come in and schedule a follow-up visit in 2 weeks so we
> can talk more about that knee pain. Take care."

Establishing an Agenda

Amplifying the AIDET approach is delivering and developing a patient-centered agenda. Due to patients typically reporting three to six concerns per visit and often not stating their most important concern first (Beasley et al., 2004; Braddock III et al.,

1999), it behooves providers to establish a collaborative agenda for the proceeding visit. If providers prematurely begin to investigate a patient's concerns before understanding all of the patient's worries, they will frequently be met with unvoiced concerns at the end of the visit (Beckman & Frankel, 1984; Marvel et al., 1999). Additionally, if providers fail to elicit all the patient's concerns and clearly define the goals for the visit, other concerns may arise throughout the interview and result in a lengthy and dysfunctional appointment (Andersson & Mattsson, 1994). Inviting the patient to share the responsibility of setting the agenda allows the patient to feel respected as a valuable part of their care team.

Baker et al. (2005) outlined the following five questions for the provider to consider while setting the agenda for the visit: (1) What are the patient's main concerns for today?, (2) What are the clinician's concerns about the patient?, (3) What are the patient's specific requests?, (4) How much of the patient's or clinician's concerns need to be addressed today, and which ones or part of ones can be deferred to a subsequent contact?, (5) What disagreements about priorities exist, and how will they be negotiated? In pursuit of an agreed-upon agenda, providers need to stay in tune with patient cues that signify an emotionally charged concern, in which patients may need to tell their story before moving forward with the appointment. Often patients do not take more than 2 min to detail their experience before they can return to agenda-setting (Langewitz et al., 2002).

Empathetic Interruption Technique

However, if patients begin to talk at length about their concerns, the Empathetic Interruption Technique (Excuse, Empathize, Explain; EEE), may be helpful to employ to negotiate with the patient if exploring the current concern in depth for the rest of their visit is their preference (Mauksch, 2017). When using the EEE technique, the provider first Excuses themselves by acknowledging and apologizing for the interruptions. Then the provider Empathizes with the patient about the current unfinished concern. The provider finishes with Explaining why the interruption is necessary. This technique can be used during planning the agenda phase, closing an important topic, or stopping the interview to explore an important patient cue that the provider noticed. The following script outlines agenda setting and the empathic interruption technique.

> Provider (intuiting the agenda): "....... From what I understand you are here to talk about your rash today, is that correct?"
> Patient: "Yes, I have had this rash for about 3 weeks, and it just won't go away. It has really been bothering me Doc. I cannot sleep because I am just so itchy, and my mom keeps yelling at me to stop scratching it, but I just can't stop. It hurts so bad............"

Provider: "Excuse me Cher. I am sorry to interrupt you (EXCUSE). It sounds like this rash has been horrible for you in so many different ways (EMPATHIZE). I just want to make sure I understand all your concerns for today, so we can pick what is most important to address in our visit. Was there something else besides your rash that you wanted to talk about today?" (EXPLAIN).
Patient: "Yes, I need a refill on my metformin".
Provider (Eliciting list of patient concerns): "Ok, we will put that on our list to address. Is there something more important for us to discuss today?"
Patient: "Not more important, but I have had this knee pain for about 2 years now."
Provider (negotiating and confirming agenda): "Ok, so most important for us after we grab general information is your rash and getting your refill. Then we can bring you back soon to discuss your knee pain. Is there something else we should put on our agenda to address at our next visit?"
Patient: "Not that I can think of."

The Five A's of Collaborative Visits

After solidifying the collaborative agenda for the visit, the next step is sequentially gathering information to help develop an informed intervention and treatment plan. A helpful format for assessment and intervention is Whitlock et al. (2002) 5 A's Model of Behavioral Change in Primary Care: Assess, Advise, Agree, Assist, and Arrange. The 5 A's Model applies to any patient with any presenting concern. Additionally, it provides a structure for incorporating patient-centered communication skills.

The physician first Assesses the history of the primary concern, and subsequent concerns, by eliciting the patient's perspective on biopsychosocial factors (i.e., context) that may have initiated, exacerbated, alleviated, and maintained the concern. Contextual factors such as patient behaviors, environment, thoughts, and emotions are then integrated into the physician's conceptualization of the problem. This phase aims to uncover variables related to the patient's symptoms, understand how it is impacting their functioning, and help develop an individualized treatment plan based on the patient's values and resources. Additionally, it may be important for the physician to assess the patient's current knowledge and understanding of the concern (i.e. What do you know about diabetes?). This can allow the physician to effectively tailor their advice in the next phase.

In the Advise phase, the physician empathetically summarizes their biopsychosocial findings then delivers the diagnosis, and presents viable treatment options and expected outcomes.

The patient considers the options presented by the provider in the Agree phase. The patient may choose one option, come up with another option, choose no option, or decide to delay deciding at this time to consult with their support network or other members of their care team. If the provider notices ambivalence or resistance, it may be helpful for the provider to employ motivational interviewing (MI) strategies and assess the patient's stage of change.

Motivational interviewing is a strategy designed to help patients acknowledge problems and resolve ambivalence impeding health behavior change (Rollnick et al., 2022). Instead of reacting to resistance with confrontation, providers using MI seek to elicit motivational statements for change from the patient. Numerous MI strategies can be useful for addressing barriers and enhancing patient motivation. Additionally, MI can be valuable when engaging in shared decision-making. For more information about MI reference Rollnick et al. (2022).

Shared decision-making is a collaborative process between provider and patient, in which they examine the evidence for treatment options and consider the patient's values, beliefs, and preferences in the final decision (National Institute for Health and Care Excellence, 2023). This allows the patient to develop an understanding of the cost and benefits of different treatment options and make the best-informed decision based on their personal context. For additional information and strategies on shared decision-making visit the National Institute for Health and Care Excellence (2023) website.

Next is the Assist phase, where the provider helps the patient outline an individualized plan informed by the previous phases. The provider may need to give the patient new information, teach a new skill, or help problem-solve internal and external barriers to plan follow-through. A helpful acronym to remember during this phase is the SMART GOAL (Doran, 1981). The provider assists the patient in setting a goal that is Specific, Measurable, Achievable, Relevant, and Time-Bound. More specific goals generated by the patient and the provider are more likely to be successful (e.g. reduce your sweets vs limit your desserts to two times a week) (Hunter et al., 2024).

Lastly, in the Arrange phase, the provider and patient designate when follow-up will occur, with whom, and the agenda items to be discussed at that next visit.

Contextual Interviewing: Love-Work-Play and ACCESS-V

In addition to the skills and approaches discussed previously, we would like to end with a strategy and skillset to elicit a patient's context in an efficient, primary care relevant manner. Specifically, the Contextual Interview (CI; See Table 2.2), also known as the Love-Work-Play-Health Behaviors (LWPHb) interview, was first proposed by two psychologists and a family physician (Robinson et al., 2011) as an interview that attempts to help PCPs learn about patients' contexts. Bauman et al. (2018) described a specific CI structure to the LWPHb categories, as they found clinicians from all guilds were hungry to learn an efficient and effective way of gathering and organizing pertinent patient information. Cahill et al. (2024) provided a table containing the most up to date version of the CI, which is provided below.

As described in Cahill et al. (2024), the CI is more than a set of questions or a checklist. Instead, the CI provides a framework for eliciting and organizing information

Table 2.2 Contextual interview

Contextual interview
• Love (identify the patient's social relationships) – Living situation – Relationship status – Family – Friends – Spiritual life
• Work (identify the patient's work and financial situation) – Work – Source of income
• Play (identify meaningful activities to patient) – Hobbies – Fun activities
• Health risk and behaviors – Caffeine use – Tobacco/nicotine use – Alcohol use – Marijuana use – Substance use – Diet/supplements – Exercise – Sleep – Sexual activity

about the key factors that are important in one's life, which can help clinicians (and patients) put their overall health into context. If done with open curiosity, it can also double as a value clarification exercise, again, for both the clinician and the patient. The goal is for clinicians to become so proficient in the CI that it can be used conversationally while promoting genuine connection within the clinician-patient relationship (Cahill et al., 2024).

The original intent of the CI was to get a quick snapshot for busy PCPs to help promote health behavior change. Although subsequent iterations helped delineate more specific questions and gave more structure for training and learning purposes, in our experience, it can become unwieldy for PCPs to become fixated on getting every CI question answered, especially given time constraints and task overload. Therefore, we propose PCPs become efficient with the "CI Lite," which is structured to give providers key insight related to a patient's social relationships, financial status and meaningful activities (see Table 2.3).

Having a conceptualization or working model of patients' LWPHb, whether through the full CI or the CI Lite, is key to providing care that is patient-centered, collaborative, and compassionate. The CI Lite can be particularly helpful in the context of more acute (versus chronic) concerns, providing care for another PCP, or when patients have multiple chief complaints. In fact, knowing a patient's LWP via the CI Lite may provide crucial information that allows for more expedient and informed medical visits. The full CI might be better utilized in situations where a patient is assigned to a PCP's panel and can be supplemented and synthesized via

Table 2.3 Contextual interview (CI) lite

Contextual interview (CI) lite
• Love (identify the patient's social relationships) – Living situation – Relationship status – Inner circle Family Friends
• Work/school/income
• Fun/passions/areas of interest.

electronic health record (EHR) information, information from other team members, and gathered over the longitudinal relationship. We encourage PCPs to utilize the full CI or CI Lite whenever behavioral plans are being generated to address chronic conditions and/or lifestyle changes. Further, if PCPs perceive resistance from a patient in setting goals or adhering to treatment, the CI is encouraged to be utilized to gather why the perceived resistance may make sense. Lastly, the CI or the CI Lite can be utilized when there are unclear presentations of patient problems. Essentially, if the dots are not connecting clinically, that is another key time to revisit whether the PCP is aware of a patients' LWPHb.

To get the most out of the CI, another mnemonic was created to help clinicians to "know what they are looking for" as they are gathering information.

If PCPs are going to ask about an individual's context, they should utilize it to provide high-quality health care. As outlined in Cahill et al. (2024), the ACCESS-V (See Table 2.4) framework provides PCPs key elements of a patient's context that may influence their ability to make behavioral change or adhere to treatment recommendations. ACCESS-V may be best utilized as a framework to improve communication across the continuity of care as it can often take multiple patient encounters and significant patient-provider trust.

The "A" stands for Adverse Childhood Events, which are a set of ten categories of negative experiences that children can experience that have been shown to negatively impact a person's overall physical and mental health. The first "C" is for Cultural Considerations, such as someone's traditions, beliefs, identity.

The second "C" is for Context (Internal), which encourages PCPs to consider how the patient and the PCP may understand the patient's internal thoughts, emotions, and behaviors (Hayes et al., 2011). The "E" stands for Context (External) which aims to help clinicians imagine the realities of a patient's everyday life. What would it be like to walk a day in the patient's shoes? What current realities exist for this patient?

The first "S" stands for Social and Structural Determinants of Health. The Office of Disease Prevention and Health Promotion explains that social determinants of health (SDoH) "are the conditions in the environments where people are born, live, learn, work, play, worship, and age that affect a wide range of health, functioning, and quality of life outcomes and risks" (Committee on Quality of Health Care in America, 2001). Clinicians should also be aware of structural inequities related to

Table 2.4 ACCESS-V

ACCESS-V
• **A**CEs – Adverse childhood experiences • **C**ultural considerations – Traditions, beliefs, identity, etc. • **C**ontext, internal – How patients see themselves, others and the world – Patients' thoughts, emotions, associations, memories and sensations (TEAMS) • **C**ontext, external – Key situations, circumstances, relationships, etc. that impact patients' health • **S**ocial determinants of health – Conditions related to where patients live, learn and work • **S**tages of change – Patients' readiness and ability to change • **V**alues – Who and what is important to patients

patients' race, ethnicity, gender identity, sexual orientation, etc., and how this affects their healthcare.

The next "S" stands for Stage of Change, which describes health behavior change progressing through five stages of change: Precontemplation, Contemplation, Preparation, Action, and Maintenance (See Chap. 9 for an additional description). Considering the patient's stage of change is crucial in matching the intervention to the patient's context. Lastly, the "V" stands for Values which refers to who and what a patient finds meaningful. Values are critical to motivation as well as understanding patients' perspectives. PCPs can utilize the "CV" in most patient encounters to improve patient-provider communication by understanding the patient's context (see Table 2.5).

We propose that if a PCP can learn a patient's CI Lite and listen for their internal and external context and values, the PCP is going to be well on their way to providing care that is patient-centered, contextual, and compassionate, rendering a higher probability of high-quality care being delivered.

Undoubtedly, time will always be a factor within primary care visits. Below is an example visit outline that includes AIDET, Agenda Setting, the Five A's, and the CI Lite (See Table 2.6). Each one of these techniques must be practiced with intention in the same way that procedural skills such as suturing must be developed. Meaning,

Table 2.5 CV from ACCESS-V

"CV" from ACCESS-V
• **C**ontext, internal – How do patients see themselves, others and the world? – What's it like to walk a mile in their shoes? • **V**alues – Who and what is important to patients?

Table 2.6 Visit outline

Component of visit	Expected time (min)
Acknowledge, introduce, duration, explain	1–2
Agenda setting	1–2
Assess: CI Lite	5–10
Advise, agreed, assist, arrange, thank you	2–5

not only does it take repetitious practice, it also requires a methodical approach to practice.

Final Considerations

PCPs working within primary care must deliver services that are person-centered, contextual, and compassionate. There are a variety of ways PCPs can influence the interactions within their communities to answer the call of delivering high-quality primary care. This includes understanding the importance of providing care from a curious perspective with a focus on the patient's environment and contextual realities, setting agendas, and structuring visits to promote collaboration that supports patient autonomy. Reflecting on patient-provider communication and the relationship opportunities in medicine often rejuvenates and fortifies the primary care mission and values.

Key Points

- PCPs must effectively communicate with patients in order deliver services that answer the call of high-quality primary care.
- Underlying philosophies which facilitate effective communication include patient-centered approaches, single-session approaches, and Functional Contextualism.
- Patient-centered strategies include AIDET, agenda setting, the 5A's of a collaborative visit.
- Additional contextual strategies include the use of the abbreviated Love-Work-Play or contextual interview (CI) also known as the CI Lite, and the knowledge of the ACCESS-V pneumonic and utilizing understanding how patients see themselves, the world and others as well as who and what matters to them.

References

Andersson, S.-O., & Mattsson, B. (1994). Features of good consultation in general practice: Is time important? *Scandinavian Journal of Primary Health Care, 12*(4), 227–232. https://doi.org/10.3109/02813439409029245

Baker, L. H., O'Connell, D., & Platt, F. W. (2005). "What else?" setting the agenda for the clinical interview. *Annals of Internal Medicine, 143*(10), 766–770. https://doi.org/10.7326/0003-4819-143-10-200511150-00033

Bauman, D., Beachy, B., & Ogbeide, S. A. (2018). Stepped care and behavioral approaches for diabetes management in integrated primary care. In *Principle-based stepped care and brief psychotherapy for integrated care settings*. Springer Science, Business Media, LLC.

Beasley, L. J., Hackett, A. F., & Maxwell, S. M. (2004). The dietary and health behaviour of young people aged 18–25 years living independently or in the family home in Liverpool, UK. *International Journal of Consumer Studies, 28*(4), 355–363. https://doi.org/10.1111/j.1470-6431.2004.00394.x

Beckman, H. B., & Frankel, R. M. (1984). The effect of physician behavior on the collection of data. *Annals of Internal Medicine, 101*(5), 692–696. https://doi.org/10.7326/0003-4819-101-5-692

Braddock, C. H., III, Edwards, K. A., Hasenberg, N. M., Laidley, T. L., & Levinson, W. (1999). Informed decision making in outpatient practice: Time to get back to basics. *JAMA, 282*(24), 2313–2320. https://doi.org/10.1001/jama.282.24.2313

Cahill, A., Martin, M., Beachy, B., Bauman, D., & Howard-Young, J. (2024). The contextual interview: A cross-cutting patient-interviewing approach for social context. *Medical Education Online, 29*(1), 2295049. https://doi.org/10.1080/10872981.2023.2295049

Cegala, D. J., & Lenzmeier Broz, S. (2002). Physician communication skills training: A review of theoretical backgrounds, objectives and skills. *Medical Education, 36*(11), 1004–1016. https://doi.org/10.1046/j.1365-2923.2002.01331.x

Committee on Quality of Health Care in America. (2001). *Crossing the quality chasm: A new health system for the 21st century*. National Academies Press.

Doran, G. T. (1981). There's a S.M.A.R.T. way to write managements's goals and objectives. *Management Review, 70*(11), 35.

Hashim, M. J. (2017). Patient-centered communication: Basic skills. *American Family Physician, 95*(1), 29–34.

Hayes, L. J., & Fryling, M. J. (2019). Functional and descriptive contextualism. *Journal of Contextual Behavioral Science, 14*, 119–126. https://doi.org/10.1016/j.jcbs.2019.09.002

Hayes, S. C., Strosahl, K. D., & Wilson, K. G. (2011). *Acceptance and commitment therapy: The process and practice of mindful change*. Guilford Press.

Hunter, C. L., Goodie, J. L., Oordt, M. S., & Dobmeyer, A. C. (2017). *Integrated behavioral health in primary care: Step-by-step guidance for assessment and intervention* (2nd ed.). American Psychological Association. https://doi.org/10.1037/0000017-000

Hunter, C. L., Goodie, J. L., Oordt, M. S., & Dobmeyer, A. C. (2024). *Integrated behavioral health in primary care: Step-by-step guidance for assessment and intervention* (3rd ed.). American Psychological Association.

Huron Consulting Group Inc. (n.d.). *The AIDET® Communication Framework—Huron*. https://www.huronconsultinggroup.com/insights/aidet-communication-framework

Langewitz, W., Denz, M., Keller, A., Kiss, A., Rütimann, S., & Wössmer, B. (2002). Spontaneous talking time at start of consultation in outpatient clinic: Cohort study. *BMJ, 325*(7366), 682–683. https://doi.org/10.1136/bmj.325.7366.682

Marvel, M. K., Epstein, R. M., Flowers, K., & Beckman, H. B. (1999). Soliciting the patient's agenda: Have we improved? *JAMA, 281*(3), 283–287. https://doi.org/10.1001/jama.281.3.283

Mauksch, L. B. (2017). Questioning a taboo: Physicians' interruptions during interactions with patients. *JAMA, 317*(10), 1021–1022. https://doi.org/10.1001/jama.2016.16068

Mauksch, L. B., Dugdale, D. C., Dodson, S., & Epstein, R. (2008). Relationship, communication, and efficiency in the medical encounter: Creating a clinical model from a literature review.

Archives of Internal Medicine, 168(13), 1387–1395. https://doi.org/10.1001/archinte.168.13.1387

National Academies of Sciences, Engineering, and Medicine. (2021). *Implementing high-quality primary care: Rebuilding the foundation of health care.* The National Academies Press. https://doi.org/10.17226/25983

National Institute for Health and Care Excellence. (2023). *Shared decision making.* NICE. https://www.nice.org.uk/about/what-we-do/our-programmes/nice-guidance/nice-guidelines/shared-decision-making

Robinson, P., Gould, D., & Strosahl, K. (2011). *Real behavior change in primary care: Improving patient outcomes and increasing job satisfaction.* New Harbinger Publications.

Rollnick, S., Miller, W. R., & Butler, C. C. (2022). *Motivational interviewing in health care: Helping patients change behavior* (2nd ed.). Guilford Press.

Schleider, J. (2023). Little treatments, big effects: How to build meaningful moments that can transform your mental health..

Scott, J. (2012). Utilizing AIDET and other tools to increase patient satisfaction scores. *Radiology Management, 34*(3), 29–35.

Swenson, S. L., Buell, S., Zettler, P., White, M., Ruston, D. C., & Lo, B. (2004). Patient-centered communication. *Journal of General Internal Medicine, 19*(11), 1069–1079. https://doi.org/10.1111/j.1525-1497.2004.30384.x

Tai-Seale, M., McGuire, T. G., & Zhang, W. (2007). Time allocation in primary care office visits. *Health Services Research, 42*(5), 1871–1894. https://doi.org/10.1111/j.1475-6773.2006.00689.x

Talmon, M. (1990). *Single-session therapy: Maximizing the effect of the first (and often only) therapeutic encounter* (p. 146). Jossey-Bass.

Whitlock, E. P., Orleans, C. T., Pender, N., & Allan, J. (2002). Evaluating primary care behavioral counseling interventions: An evidence-based approach. *American Journal of Preventive Medicine, 22*(4), 267–284. https://doi.org/10.1016/S0749-3797(02)00415-4

Chapter 3
Understanding Behavioral Health Conditions in Primary Care

Robert Bonanno MD and Shannon Stark Taylor PhD

About 47.6 million US adults experience a diagnosable behavioral health (BH) condition, and of these, more than 24 million do not receive any treatment (Mental Health America (MHA), 2019; Substance Abuse and Mental Health Services Administration (SAMHSA), 2019). For those who do, half of all care received for BH conditions is provided by primary care providers (PCPs) due to limited access to specialty BH support (Mental Health America (MHA), 2019; National Institute of Mental Health (NIMH), 2017). A high prevalence of BH conditions in addition to ongoing shortages of BH providers have contributed to the increasing role for PCPs in treating concerns (Rotenstein et al., 2023).

Anxiety and depression are two of the most common overall complaints in primary care for developed countries. Today more than ever, BH is a foundational component of competent primary care practice. PCPs, through their continuity relationships and long-term perspective on health, are uniquely situated to provide whole person care. Involving both physical and BH in the context of each patient's unique social context will lead to the best outcomes for patient health and well-being.

R. Bonanno MD (✉) · S. S. Taylor PhD
Prisma Health Family Medicine Residency Program Greenville and University of South Carolina School of Medicine Greenville, Greenville, SC, USA
e-mail: Robert.Bonanno@prismahealth.org

S. S. Taylor PhD
e-mail: Shannon.Taylor2@prismahealth.org

M. L. C. Williamson and D. L. Terry (eds.), *Essentials for Treating Behavioral Health in Primary Care*, https://doi.org/10.1007/978-3-032-09558-9_3

Diagnostic Approach to Behavioral Health Conditions in Primary Care

By virtue of their unique position in the healthcare landscape, PCPs often serve as the point of first contact for patients struggling with a myriad of BH conditions. For the PCP, diagnosing these conditions is made even more challenging due to the complex and often competing social and medical needs of the patients they serve. This chapter highlights the critical role of building rapport in the context of BH assessment, outlines a systematic approach to managing common BH concerns, and introduces diagnostic resources available to PCPs when approaching these patients.

Building Rapport: A Foundation for Effective Assessment

Establishing rapport is a foundational component of providing effective and holistic care. This is most evident when approaching BH concerns, as some patients may readily articulate these concerns, while others require more time and patience. PCPs should recognize there are a wide range of possibilities that might deter a patient from sharing concerns related to their BH: embarrassment, lack of insight, societal/cultural/familial stigmatization, mistrust in the healthcare system, etc. This distress may be expressed through subtle verbal and nonverbal cues, necessitating astute observation and empathetic inquiry from the PCP to prompt further investigation into a possible BH condition. Recognizing these nuances, PCPs must be intentional about cultivating an environment of trust and openness where patients feel comfortable divulging their concerns. Steps to facilitate positive rapport include utilizing active listening strategies alongside both verbal and nonverbal expressions of empathy, concern, and understanding to ensure that the patient feels heard and respected. Legitimizing the patient's concerns and emphasizing the existence of a partnership between patient and provider help to build a strong foundation for a lasting therapeutic relationship. A review article by English et al. published in the journal, *Patient Education and Counseling*, provides greater insight regarding how rapport is defined and characterized within healthcare settings (English et al., 2022). Practical strategies to facilitate rapport building and positive communication can also be found in greater detail in Chap. 2 of *Bates' Guide to Physical Examination and History Taking* (Bickley et al., 2020).

The Diagnostic Approach

Once a BH concern is recognized, PCPs should employ a systematic yet adaptable approach to evaluation which integrates clinical assessment, diagnostic criteria, and evidence-based practice. Here we will outline a structure for identifying and diagnosing BH conditions commonly encountered by PCPs. For a comprehensive guide to the psychiatric interview, including recommendations for interviewing unique patient populations, consider the American Psychiatric Association's publication, *The Psychiatric Interview in Clinical Practice Third Edition* (MacKinnon et al., 2015).

Conduct a Comprehensive Clinical Assessment

Gather information about the patient's presenting symptom(s) including context and level of functional impairment while considering their medical history (See Table 3.1) and psychosocial (i.e., contextual) circumstances. See Chap. 2 for more information on contextual interviewing. The assessment should also include a focused mental status exam. Key components of this assessment include:

- *Frequency, duration, and course of symptoms:* Many BH conditions require a specified duration and/or frequency of symptoms to be present to meet criteria for diagnosis. Furthermore, changes in severity or pattern of symptoms over time can be helpful in the diagnostic evaluation.
- *Triggers and alleviating factors:* Identify factors that exacerbate and/or alleviate symptoms to better understand the patient's condition as well as their coping strategies or prior response to treatment. Understanding situational and environmental influences provides valuable context for diagnosis and treatment planning.
- *Medical history*: Assess whether the patient has ever received a BH diagnosis or has ever been under the care of a psychiatrist or other BH provider. Later in this section we will review common medical and pharmacologic causes of BH symptoms.
- *Psychosocial assessment:* Factors such as substance use, trauma/abuse, interpersonal conflicts, life changes, inadequate sleep or financial/occupational stressors should be considered as all might manifest as BH concerns for patients.
- *Level of impairment*: To what degree are the patient's quality of life, relationships, occupation, or social functioning being impacted by their symptoms?
- *Mental status exam:* A mental status exam should be performed after a thorough history is taken. An excellent comprehensive review of the components and nuances of a mental status exam can be found in Chap. 9 of *Bates' Guide to Physical Examination and History Taking* (Bickley et al., 2020). Key areas for assessment as outlined by this text include:

Table 3.1 Alternative etiologies for behavioral health symptoms to consider during assessment

Condition
Medication effects (intended or adverse)
Obstructive sleep apnea
Hepatic encephalopathy
Hypoxia/hypercapnia
Vitamin B12 deficiency
Parkinson's disease
Intracranial hemorrhage or mass
Stroke/TIA
Hydrocephalus
Multiple sclerosis
Neurocognitive disorders (e.g. Alzheimer's/vascular/frontotemporal dementia)
Infection (e.g. urinary tract infection, pneumonia, neurosyphilis, encephalitis)
Metabolic/electrolyte derangements (e.g. sodium, calcium, glucose)
Endocrine disorders (e.g. Cushing disease, hyperparathyroidism, thyroid disease, menopause)

- Appearance/behavior—observe for alertness, affect, facial expressions, body movements, grooming, and hygiene
- Speech—note quantity, rate, volume, articulation, and fluency
- Mood
- Thoughts and perceptions—Assess thought process/content as well as sensory awareness
- Insight and Judgment
- Cognitive function—assessment includes orientation and attention as well as higher cognitive function. There are numerous tools that may be used in the primary care setting to screen for cognitive impairment including but not limited to the Saint Louis University Mental Status Exam (SLUMS) (Tariq et al., 2006) and the Montreal Cognitive Assessment (MoCA) (Nasreddine et al., 2005), both freely available online.

Apply Diagnostic Criteria

Reference standardized diagnostic criteria, such as those outlined in the *Diagnostic and Statistical Manual of Mental Disorders* (Current edition DSM-5-TR; American Psychiatric Association (APA), 2022), to guide the diagnostic evaluation. Diagnostic criteria provide a framework for identifying and categorizing specific BH conditions based on symptomatology and level of functional impairment. Familiarity with the diagnostic criteria for common BH conditions encountered in primary care will aid in organizing a differential diagnosis and guiding further assessment.

Incorporate Screening Tools and Rating Scales Supplementing the clinical assessment with validated screening tools and rating scales can aid in assessing symptom severity, screening for specific conditions, and monitoring symptoms over time. Examples include the Patient Health Questionnaire-9 (PHQ-9) (Kroenke et al., 2001) for Major Depressive Disorder, Generalized Anxiety Disorder Scale (GAD-7) (Spitzer et al., 2006), and the Alcohol Use Disorders Identification Test (AUDIT-C) (Bush et al., 1998). Refer to Chap. 4 for a more comprehensive overview of screening tools and rating scales.

Additional Diagnostic Considerations

(BH) assessment in the primary care setting requires a nuanced approach as it entails navigating complex clinical presentations, potential comorbidities, and diagnostic uncertainties set within the context of limited encounter times and competing visit priorities. This section explores key considerations and potential pitfalls encountered by PCPs when assessing and diagnosing BH conditions.

Diagnostic Clarity vs. Treatment Initiation When diagnosing BH conditions, it is important to differentiate between when it is necessary to rule out specific diagnoses prior to initiating treatment versus when starting empiric treatment is safe and appropriate. There are validated screeners that can be used to guide clinical decision-making. For example, it is essential to rule out bipolar disorder in a patient with mood changes prior to prescribing an antidepressant to avoid precipitating a manic episode. However, in clinical scenarios with low risk of harm and symptoms which would be expected to respond to treatment, empiric therapy may be appropriate while working towards a definitive diagnosis.

Flexibility in Diagnostic Approach Diagnosing BH conditions is often an iterative process requiring trust, rapport, and a longitudinal approach. PCPs should embrace a flexible diagnostic process, as symptoms may evolve over time and evidence supporting a diagnosis may converge across several visits.

Utilizing Unspecified Diagnosis Codes In cases where established diagnostic criteria are not fully met for a specific condition, it may be prudent to employ unspecified diagnosis codes, such as "Unspecified mood [affective] disorder" or "Other anxiety disorders". Unspecified codes allow for diagnostic flexibility while further evaluation is undertaken, especially in cases where symptoms do not neatly align with established diagnostic frameworks.

Behavioral Health Comorbidities PCPs should recognize that BH conditions often exist concurrently, a reality that has the potential to complicate the diagnostic evaluation (Andrews et al., 2002; Bijl et al., 1998; Kessler et al., 2005; Plana-Ripoll et al.,

2019). Multiple studies have estimated the prevalence of BH comorbidities to range from 30–50% (Andrews et al., 2002; Bijl et al., 1998; Kessler et al., 2005; Plana-Ripoll et al., 2019). There may be significant overlap in symptoms between two discrete BH conditions, such as may be observed in the setting of a patient with both major depressive disorder as well as attention-deficit/hyperactivity disorder struggling with difficulty concentrating. Recognizing and avoiding cognitive biases such as premature closure and/or anchoring bias is helpful in these circumstances with some strategies outlined below.

Cultural Considerations

PCPs should understand that an individual's culture can impact their experience, expression, and willingness to seek help for mental distress, thus it should be considered as a part of a holistic assessment. The U.S. Department of Health and Human Services (HHS) Office of Minority Health, through their "Think Cultural Health" initiative, has compiled numerous resources that healthcare providers can utilize to enhance their cultural competency and communication with patients from diverse backgrounds and walks of life (Office of Minority Health, U.S. Department of Health, & Human Services, 2024). Additionally, Chap. 2 of the supplement to *Mental Health: A Report of the Surgeon General* entitled "Culture Counts: The Influence of Culture and Society on Mental Health" provides excellent insight into the impact that culture and society have on BH, both from the perspective of the patient as well as the clinician (Satcher, 2001).

Common Pitfalls

Guarding Against Over-Diagnosis PCPs should be careful to avoid over-diagnosing BH conditions in the context of typical "human" responses to life stressors such as grief or worry. Mislabeling typical reactions as clinical disorders can lead to unnecessary treatment and psychological harm to patients. *Tip: Before assigning a specific BH diagnosis to a patient, ensure they meet all symptomatic as well as time-based criteria to warrant that diagnosis. Otherwise, consider a less specific diagnostic label until enough information is available to assign a formal diagnosis.*

Premature Labeling The risk of making an inaccurate premature BH diagnosis for a patient is that, once documented and propagated within the medical record, it can become difficult to remove or amend. This is especially true in the modern era of electronic medical records. Patients may also anchor onto a diagnosis which could make it difficult to change course with treatment plans or set appropriate expectations.

Recognizing Medical Mimics There are many medical conditions as well as medication reactions (both intended and adverse) that mimic BH symptoms. We have outlined a number of these examples later in the chapter and their inclusion underscores the importance of conducting a comprehensive medical assessment to rule out organic causes when evaluating BH concerns.

Cognitive Biases and Objectivity Awareness of cognitive biases (including, but not limited to confirmation, recency, premature closure, and anchoring biases) is essential to remaining objective during diagnostic assessment. Intentional self-reflection, curiosity, and adherence to evidence-based practices can help to mitigate the effects of cognitive biases during evaluations. Further strategies to minimize the impact of cognitive biases include education and mindfulness of the types of biases to increase awareness and insight, minimizing time pressures/competing tasks when conducting assessments, intentionally maintaining a broad differential during evaluation of undifferentiated concerns, or seeking feedback through direct observation, simulation, or debriefing after encounters.

Addressing Time Constraints and Discomfort PCPs may feel reluctant to address BH concerns in their practice due to time constraints and/or lack of comfort with addressing these concerns. This may stem from a lack of familiarity with diagnostic criteria, management options or communication strategies. We hope that this book will help fill some of those gaps and lead to greater confidence amongst PCPs in addressing this crucial need within their patient populations.

Common Mental Health Concerns in Primary Care

This section will provide a brief overview of important notes for medical providers regarding common mental health conditions seen in primary care. Please refer to Chap. 9 for information regarding BH interventions in primary care.

Depression Depressed mood is a common complaint in primary care. Estimated lifetime prevalence of depression is 29% in the US (Witters, 2023). Risk factors for depression include internal factors (female sex, history of anxiety, low self-esteem, neuroticism), external factors (conduct disorder, substance use), and adverse life events (Maurer et al., 2018). Many patients with depression will present with complaints of sleep difficulties or low energy (Maurer et al., 2018). Depression may present differently in women and men, with women more likely to complain of physical symptoms like headaches, myalgias, or gastrointestinal problems and men more likely to complain of acts of aggression, anger, substance use, and risky behavior (Dekker et al., 2008; Martin et al., 2013). For those reporting depressed mood, attention to the symptom number, intensity, interference criteria in the DSM-5-TR (American Psychiatric Association (APA), 2022) can help distinguish between a major depressive episode and normal sadness or Adjustment Disorder with Depressed Mood in those who have recently experienced a significant stressor. The DSM-5-TR (American Psychiatric Association (APA), 2022) provides helpful guidance regarding distinguishing normal grief from major depression. Broad routine screening for all primary care patients (the general adult population, adolescents aged 12–18, and postpartum women) to help detect depression in those who do not report depressed mood is also critical (refer to Chap. 4 for guidance on screening). The most important rule out diagnosis for those who meet criteria for a major depressive episode is bipolar disorder because use of antidepressants without concurrent treatment with a mood stabilizer is associated with increased risk of manic symptoms (Park & Zarate, 2019). Suicide assessment is critical for anyone reporting depressed mood or found to meet criteria for depression. See Chap. 5 for a complete discussion on risk assessment in primary care.

Bipolar and Related Disorders Bipolar disorders affect more than 1% of the world's population and have no race, sex, ethnicity, or socioeconomic risk factors (Grande et al., 2016). One fourth of primary care patients presenting with depression or anxiety have been diagnosed with bipolar disorder (American Psychiatric Association (APA), 2022). These disorders involve recurrent episodes of elevated mood and depression. Hypomania may occur in bipolar I and II disorders, but mania only occurs in bipolar I (American Psychiatric Association (APA), 2022). Patients with bipolar disorder usually present with depression, anxiety, or mixed features (concurrent mania and depression) (American Psychiatric Association (APA), 2022; Judd et al., 2002). Because depressive episodes in bipolar disorder are difficult to differentiate from major depressive disorder, bipolar disorders are often misdiagnosed (Yatham et al., 2018). Thus, as mentioned previously, any patient presenting with depressive symptoms should also be screened for manic symptoms. Screening tools like the Mood Disorder Questionnaire can help with this effort (Wang et al., 2015) (Chap. 4 for more information on screening). Manic symptoms are often not a presenting concern because they are seen as desirable by the patient (Rainone & Mancini, 2018). Bipolar disorders are multifactorial with a strong genetic component and are often triggered by acute significant life stressors (Kerner, 2015; Yatham et al., 2018). Three quarters of patients with bipolar disorder have three or more additional BH conditions, most commonly anxiety disorders, impulse control and attention-deficit/hyperactivity disorders, and substance use disorders, which are associated with worse outcomes (Goodwin et al., 2016; Merikangas et al., 2007). This population also experiences high rates of psychosocial problems including concerns about housing/homelessness, and lack of social support (Cerimele et al., 2014). Individuals with bipolar disorder are at high risk for suicide; one-third will attempt suicide in their lifetime (Schaffer et al., 2015; Yatham et al., 2018). As such, suicide screening is of high importance in this population.

Anxiety About 12.7% of Americans and 20% of primary care patients meet criteria for an anxiety disorder, but correct detection of anxiety diagnoses is estimated to be only 44.5% (Kroenke et al., 2007; Olariu et al., 2015; Olfson et al., 2019). Rate of detection improves with screening (see Chap. 4 for evidence-based anxiety disorder screening suggestions). Many patients in primary care with high levels of anxiety do not express their concerns directly, but they often show physical signs of anxiety (sweating, flushing, trembling, fidgeting), speak rapidly, make more requests, ask more questions, and share more psychosocial information than less anxious patients (Bensing et al., 2008; Chaturvedi, 2008). They may also present with somatic complaints like headaches, muscle tension, gastrointestinal symptoms, back pain, and insomnia (Stein & Sareen, 2015). Anxiety is a normal part of the human experience and does not warrant diagnosis or intervention if the symptoms do not meet severity, frequency, persistence of co-occurring symptoms aspects of DSM-5-TR criteria or if they do not cause significant psychological distress or life impairment. Common anxiety diagnoses include generalized anxiety disorder (6.2% lifetime prevalence), social anxiety disorder (13% lifetime prevalence), and panic disorder (5.2% lifetime prevalence) (Kessler et al., 2012). The focus of excessive, difficult to control worries in generalized anxiety disorder is on multiple topics, whereas the focus in social anxiety disorder is social and performance situations to the point where they are avoided or endured with intense distress (American Psychiatric Association (APA), 2022). Panic attacks, unexpected, rapid-onset, discrete episodes of intense fear with accompanying physical symptoms, are common and may occur without the individual meeting criteria for a DSM-5-TR diagnosis. They may also occur secondary to other anxiety disorders. For an individual to meet criteria for panic disorder, they must persistently fear panic attacks, worry about the consequences of panic attacks, and have changed behavior due to panic attacks, e.g., avoid potential triggers (American Psychiatric Association (APA), 2002).

Trauma Post-traumatic stress disorder (PTSD) is another common BH condition, with a lifetime prevalence of 6% (Goldstein et al., 2016). It often goes undetected in primary care (Spoont et al., 2015). PTSD can develop a month after a traumatic event which involved actual or threatened death, serious injury, or sexual violence (e.g., witnessing a death, being the victim of a sexual assault or violent attack, learning that a violent or accidental actual or threatened death to a loved one, or experiencing repeated or extreme exposure to aversive details of a traumatic event). Symptoms that have been present less than 1 month would be considered Acute Stress Disorder (American Psychiatric Association (APA), 2022). PTSD symptom categories include: reexperiencing the event through nightmares, flashbacks, or memories; avoidance of reminders of the event, negative alterations in cognitions and/or mood, and increased arousal and reactivity.

Over one half of adults have experienced a traumatic event and less than 10% develop PTSD (Kessler et al., 2013; Yehuda et al., 2015). Even for those without PTSD, trauma can significantly impact individuals' lives and emotional and physical well-being. Because many traumas involve violations of bodily integrity, medical visits can be particularly stressful and trauma survivors often avoid visits, procedures, or disclosing information to providers (Raja et al., 2015; Reeves, 2015). Familiarizing yourself with trauma-informed care can help to optimize patient health while minimizing risk of retraumatization. The core principles of trauma-informed care are described by the 4 R's: (1) realizing the widespread impact of trauma, (2) recognizing signs and symptoms of trauma in patients, their families, and clinical staff,

(3) responding by integrating knowledge about trauma into policies, procedures, and practices, and (4) seeking actively to avoid retraumatization (Substance Abuse and Mental Health Services Administration (SAMHSA), 2014). Many helpful resources exist for learning more about trauma-informed care including those provided by the National Center for Trauma-Informed Care, National Child Traumatic Stress Network, National Council for Behavioral Health, and the U.S. Department of Veterans Affairs National Center for PTSD (Ravi & Little, 2017).

Attention-Deficit/Hyperactivity Disorder and Autism Spectrum Disorder Attention-deficit/hyperactivity disorder (ADHD) affects an estimated 7.2–8.4% of children, 4–5% of adults in the United States (Danielson et al., 2018; Kessler et al., 2006; Thomas et al., 2015). Three key features of ADHD are inattention (inability to focus, disorganization) and/or hyperactivity (excessive motor activity, restlessness) and impulsivity (hasty actions without much forethought) (American Psychiatric Association (APA), 2002). Patients and/or their parents often present to primary care with complaints of having trouble at school/work, difficulty focusing, trouble completing tasks, and fidgeting. Clinical evaluation for ADHD should focus on (1) assessing current symptoms and ensuring a pediatric/adolescent history of symptoms, (2) establishing that these symptoms cause impairment across multiple settings, and (3) excluding medical, psychiatric, or other causes of inattention or hyperactivity/impulsivity (Huang et al., 2020). Most children and adults with ADHD also meet criteria for another behavior, psychiatric, and/or substance use disorder which can mask, be masked by, or co-occur with ADHD symptoms (Caye et al., 2016; Moffitt et al., 2015; Wolraich et al., 2019).

Autism spectrum disorder (ASD) is a neurodevelopmental disorder which affects one in 59 children in the United States (Hyman et al., 2020). Diagnostic criteria include three social communication issues and two to four restrictive or repetitive behaviors (American Psychiatric Association (APA), 2022). Nearly one-third of children with ASD meet criteria for an intellectual disability or have minimal verbal ability (Hyman et al., 2020). Although the U.S. Preventative Services Task Force (USPSTF) found insufficient evidence for ASD screening, the American Academy of Pediatrics (AAP) recommends a combination of developmental surveillance and standardized autism screening tests at 18 and 24 months as earlier intervention leads to better outcomes (Hyman et al., 2020). Early symptoms for surveillance include not responding to name by 12 months, not pointing to items of interest by 14 months, avoiding eye contact, repetitive movements, unusual reactions to sensations and echolalia. The Modified Checklist for Autism in Toddlers (M-CHAT) should be used for initial screening in children up to 30 months of age (Hyman et al., 2020; Robins et al., 2014). After diagnosis, referrals should be made for formal cognitive, language, occupational therapy, physical therapy, audiology, and visual assessments in addition to early intervention school services (Hyman et al., 2020). Because the symptom severity of this disorder is, by definition, on a "spectrum", and due to historical lack of awareness leading to non-diagnosis or misdiagnosis, adults may also seek ASD diagnosis (Nicolaidis et al., 2014). Adult diagnosis can be challenging due to adaptations individuals make to their symptoms over time, thus may look different than symptoms in children. Providers should consider potential risks and benefits of obtaining an ASD diagnosis in adults; see Nicolaidis et al. (2014) for a thoughtful list. Adults with ASD often struggle to find primary care providers who feel comfortable providing care. PCPs should work to educate themselves on the unique needs of this population including common medical comorbidities. A number of toolkits for PCPs exist through Vanderbilt Kennedy Center for Research on Human Development and the Academic Autistic Spectrum Partnership in Research and Education (Nicolaidis et al., 2016; Vanderbilt Kennedy Center (VKC), 2024).

Gender Dysphoria Individuals whose experienced or expressed gender differs from their sex assigned at birth may identify as transgender or gender-diverse (encompassing a number of alternative identities). In the United States, approximately 300,000 youth and 1.3 million adults identify as transgender (Herman et al., 2022). Gender dysphoria refers to distress or functional challenges that may be experienced by transgender or gender diverse persons and should be used to describe distressing symptoms rather than to pathologize the experience. Gender identity is distinct from sexual orientation, sex development, and external gender expression; each construct varies by culture and exists along continuums. PCPs should utilize published guidelines (published by the World Professional Association for Transgender Health; Coleman et al., 2022) in relating to this population and treating this condition. This population experiences extreme disparities in mental and physical health, due in part to the ostracism and discrimination they experience regularly in their communities and in healthcare (Daniel & Butkus, 2015; Dawson et al., 2021; Frost et al., 2015). As such, PCPs should take extra care to learn and provide staff training in care specific to this population, ways to create a welcoming and affirming environment, and assessing personal biases (Klein et al., 2018). Depending on comfort level and local subspecialist availability, PCPs can evaluate gender dysphoria and manage hormone therapy, or monitor well-being and provide primary care and potentially life-saving referrals (Chen & Loshak, 2020). Gender-affirming hormone therapy is generally safe, but partially irreversible. Affirming surgical referrals may improve outcomes (Swan et al., 2023). PCPs should identify and treat BH conditions in the transgender population, avoiding the assumption that these conditions are related to gender identity.

Eating Disorders Eating disorders have a lifetime prevalence of 8% in women, and 2% in men (Galmiche et al., 2019). They are associated with serious medical complications including risk of death and high rates of suicide. Despite this, research and education on this topic is lacking. The US Preventive Services Task Force in 2022 issued an I Statement rather than a recommendation for or against screening “asymptomatic” non-help-seeking individuals due to insufficient evidence (U.S. Preventive Services Task Force (USPSTF), 2022). Many organizations do recommend regular confidential psychosocial screening for adults and adolescents including questions about eating behaviors, body image, and mood (Klein et al., 2021). Early detection of eating disorders can decrease the risk of long-term pathology and disability. Monitoring height, weight, body mass index trends and growth curves can be helpful information to guide identification and is often compatible with basic health monitoring and well-visits completed in primary care. PCPs should be aware that an individual's motivation to change can be impacted by perceived benefits of the disorder, malnutrition, lack of self-awareness, or fear, especially among those with restrictive eating patterns (Klein et al., 2021). Using empathetic, nonjudgmental Motivational Interviewing techniques can help overcome barriers and resistance (Klein et al., 2021). Clinicians should engage a multidisciplinary team for treatment of eating disorders and refer for escalation of care based on health status, co-occurring conditions, suicidality, weight patterns, outpatient options, and social support. In general, clinicians should focus communication with all patients on health and positive body image rather than weight and dieting to avoid unintentionally reinforcing disordered eating (Kennedy et al., 2022).

Psychosis Psychosis is a group of symptoms that may include hallucinations, delusions, and disorganized speech or behavior (American Psychiatric Association (APA), 2022). It can be caused by a number of psychiatric disorders (primary psychosis), or medical conditions (secondary psychosis) (American Psychiatric Association (APA), 2022). Whereas those with primary psychosis are more likely to have auditory hallucinations, prominent cognitive disorders, and complicated delusions, those with secondary psychosis may show cognitive changes, abnormal vital signs, and visual hallucinations (Griswold et al., 2015). Recreational drug use is the most common cause of acute secondary psychosis. A thorough history, examination, labs, and testing can help determine etiology.

Personality Disorders Individuals with personality disorders often do not personally seek treatment for their condition but may seek care for comorbid BH conditions. Understanding personality disorders can help PCPs learn helpful strategies to maintain therapeutic rapport and support patients in their health goals.

Insomnia Insomnia affects about 30% of Americans, 5–15% of whom meet criteria for chronic insomnia (Grandner & Perlis, 2015; Ohayon, 2002; Trauer et al., 2015). Individuals experiencing insomnia have impairment in the initiation, duration, consolidation, or quality of sleep despite adequate opportunity for sleep. To meet criteria for insomnia, patients must experience daytime impairment (Sateia et al., 2017). Trouble with sleep and subsequent impact on quality of life are common motivators for patients to present to their primary care provider. Individuals can experience insomnia secondary to a number of physical (e.g., hypertension, asthma, chronic obstructive pulmonary disease, benign prostatic hyperplasia, chronic pain, gastroesophageal reflux disease) and behavioral (e.g., depression, anxiety, PTSD, substance use disorders) health concerns (Bhaskar et al., 2016). It is important to assess for and treat the primary condition, but also consider insomnia as a comorbid diagnosis rather than a symptom, as insomnia does not always remit following successful treatment for conditions like PTSD and depression (Lichstein, 2006). Neglecting insomnia can worsen the prognosis for comorbid conditions (Gehrman et al., 2013).

Substance Use Disorders When assessing any patient for a BH condition, substance use should always be included in the differential, as many BH symptoms can be brought on by substances and/or withdrawal from substances. The DSM-5-TR makes clear in all criteria that the symptoms of any given condition must not be secondary to substance use (American Psychiatric Association (APA), 2022). Substance use is commonly comorbid with BH conditions as well; substances serve as a way to manage BH symptoms.

Substance use disorders (SUDs) are common; in 2022 17.3% of Americans over age 12 met criteria for a SUD in the past year (Substance Abuse and Mental Health Services Administration (SAMHSA), 2022). They are also a leading cause of preventable death. Despite this, only a small percentage of this population receives treatment, and even fewer receive evidence-based care. Due to stigma, or ambivalence about change, patients may not present requesting help for substance use. See Chap. 10 for a complete discussion of the management of substance use disorder in primary care.

Somatic Symptom Disorders Somatic symptom disorders will present, by definition, as physical health concerns, which are the manifestation of mental distress. Patients with multiple persistent physical symptoms that are not otherwise medically explained are common in the primary care setting (Rosendal et al., 2013). An estimated 5–7% of the general population meets criteria for somatic symptom disorder, which can cause significant disability and distress (Harris et al., 2009). Screening tools can help establish an appropriate diagnosis, which is important for minimizing risk of harm due to unnecessary testing and treatment (Kurlansik & Maffei, 2016). For patients with somatic symptom disorder, PCPs should establish a strong therapeutic rapport, schedule regular visits, and legitimize the patient's symptoms.

Sexual Disorders Sexual dysfunction is common across all sexual identities and can lead to distress and issues with medication adherence (Faubion & Rullo, 2015). An estimated 50–98% of women report at least one sexual health concern, including hypoactive sexual drive disorder, female sexual arousal disorder, female orgasmic disorder, and sexual pain disorders, e.g., vaginismus and dyspareunia (Braxton et al., 2005; Nusbaum et al., 2000). Around 40% of men report at least one sexual health concern, most commonly erectile dysfunction or premature ejaculation (Read et al., 1997). Despite this, many find it challenging to bring up these issues to their PCP (Savoy et al., 2020). Including proactive, integrated, comprehensive sexual history taking for all patients is good practice and can help uncover these concerns. Intentionally creating safe spaces for all patients (including those with trauma history and gender-diverse individuals) is essential in order to deliver positive, affirming, nonjudgmental sexual health care. Sexual dysfunction is often multifactorial, involving biological, psychological, sociocultural, and relational factors; thus, treatment must encompass these factors as well (Savoy et al., 2020). PCPs can be instrumental in the treatment of sexual dysfunction by providing education and counseling, prescribing appropriate medications and/or adjusting medications that can cause dysfunction, and making appropriate BH and/or subspecialty and/or community resource referrals (Savoy et al., 2020). Communication strategies like the Ex-PLISSIT model can help providers develop helpful language for sexual health conversations (Annon, 1976; Faubion & Rullo, 2015).

Other Conditions A full description of all DSM-5 TR condition categories is beyond the scope of this book; however, physicians should be generally aware of criteria for conditions like Obsessive Compulsive Disorder and categories including neurocognitive, dissociative, and paraphilic disorders.

Special Populations

Children and adolescents experience many of the conditions described above, but treatment recommendations can differ. It is important to understand unique considerations for this population. Parents/guardians play a key role in describing symptoms and implementing treatment. Clinicians should also be aware of conditions unique to pediatrics populations including enuresis/encopresis and behavior issues which often necessitates behavioral interventions including the child and parent/guardian.

Clinicians should also be aware of unique BH needs for individuals during and after pregnancy. Prescription medications should be adjusted using established guidelines and shared decision-making. Individuals should be regularly screened for BH concerns including mood and anxiety during pregnancy and post-partum. See Chap. 11 for further discussion on peripartum concerns.

Key Points

- PCPs are uniquely positioned to build the type of positive rapport that is a crucial component of effectively eliciting BH concerns from patients.
- Behavioral health concerns in primary care are most effectively addressed through employing a holistic, culturally sensitive, and systemic approach which may span the course of multiple visits.
- It is not always necessary to have a formal diagnosis prior to initiating treatment when safe and appropriate, in fact, prematurely assigning an incorrect diagnosis to a patient may cause additional harm or complications.
- Recognize that comorbidities amongst BH conditions is common and that primary medical conditions may present with BH symptoms.
- Recognizing and taking action to minimize the effects of cognitive biases during BH assessments will improve diagnostic accuracy and treatment planning.

References

American Psychiatric Association (APA). (2002). Practice guideline for the treatment of patients with bipolar disorder (revision). *The American Journal of Psychiatry, 159*(4 Suppl), 1–50.

American Psychiatric Association (APA). (2022). *Diagnostic and statistical manual of mental disorders* (5th ed.). American Psychiatric Publishing. https://doi.org/10.1176/appi.books.9780890425787

Andrews, G., Slade, T., & Issakidis, C. (2002). Deconstructing current comorbidity: Data from the Australian National Survey of mental health and Well-being. *The British Journal of Psychiatry, 181*(4), 306–314. https://doi.org/10.1192/bjp.181.4.306

Annon, J. S. (1976). The PLISSIT model: A proposed conceptual scheme for the behavioral treatment of sexual problems. *Journal of Sex Education Therapy, 2*(1), 1–15.

Bensing, J. M., Verheul, W., & van Dulmen, A. M. (2008). Patient anxiety in the medical encounter. *Health Education, 108*(5), 373–383. https://doi.org/10.1108/09654280810899993

Bhaskar, S., Hemavathy, D., & Prasad, S. (2016). Prevalence of chronic insomnia in adult patients and its correlation with medical comorbidities. *Journal of Family Medicine and Primary Care, 5*(4), 780. https://doi.org/10.4103/2249-4863.201153

Bickley, L. S., Szilagyi, P. G., Hoffman, R. M., & Soriano, R. P. (2020). *Bates' pocket guide to physical examination and history taking* (9th ed.). Lippincott Williams & Wilkins.

Bijl, R. V., Ravelli, A., & van Zessen, G. (1998). Prevalence of psychiatric disorder in the general population: Results of The Netherlands mental health survey and incidence study (NEMESIS). *Social Psychiatry and Psychiatric Epidemiology, 33*, 587–595. https://doi.org/10.1007/s001270050098

Braxton, L., Nusbaum, M. R., & Strayhorn, G. (2005). The sexual concerns of African American, Asian American, and white women seeking routine gynecological care. *The Journal of the American Board of Family Practice, 18*(3), 173–179. https://doi.org/10.3122/jabfm.18.3.173

Bush, K., Kivlahan, D. R., McDonell, M. B., Fihn, S. D., & Bradley, K. A. (1998). The AUDIT alcohol consumption questions (AUDIT-C): An effective brief screening test for problem drinking. Ambulatory care quality improvement project (ACQUIP). Alcohol use disorders identification test. *Archives of Internal Medicine, 158*(16), 1789–1795. https://doi.org/10.1001/archinte.158.16.1789

Caye, A., Rocha, T. B.-M., Anselmi, L., Murray, J., Menezes, A. M. B., Barros, F. C., Gonçalves, H., Wehrmeister, F., Jensen, C. M., Steinhausen, H.-C., Swanson, J. M., Kieling, C., & Rohde, L. A. (2016). Attention-deficit/hyperactivity disorder trajectories from childhood to young adulthood: Evidence from a birth cohort supporting a late-onset syndrome. *JAMA Psychiatry, 73*(7), 705–712. https://doi.org/10.1001/jamapsychiatry.2016.0383

Cerimele, J. M., Chan, Y.-F., Chwastiak, L. A., Avery, M., Katon, W., & Unützer, J. (2014). Bipolar disorder in primary care: Clinical characteristics of 740 primary care patients with bipolar disorder. *Psychiatric Services, 65*(8), 1041–1046.

Chaturvedi, A. (2008). Communicating with anxious or angry patient. In *Medicine* (Vol. 18). Elsevier.

Chen, S., & Loshak, H. (2020). *Primary care initiated gender-affirming therapy for gender dysphoria: A review of evidence based guidelines*. National Institutes of Health.

Coleman, E., Radix, A. E., Bouman, W. P., Brown, G. R., de Vries, A. L. C., Deutsch, M. B., Ettner, R., Fraser, L., Goodman, M., Green, J., Hancock, A. B., Johnson, T. W., Karasic, D. H., Knudson, G. A., Leibowitz, S. F., Meyer-Bahlburg, H. F. L., Monstrey, S. J., Motmans, J., Nahata, L., & Arcelus, J. (2022). Standards of care for the health of transgender and gender diverse people, version 8. *International Journal of Transgender Health, 23*(S1), S1–S259. https://doi.org/10.1080/26895269.2022.2100644

Daniel, H., & Butkus, R. (2015). Lesbian, gay, bisexual, and transgender health disparities: Executive summary of a policy position paper from the American College of Physicians. *Annals of Internal Medicine, 163*(2), 135–137. https://doi.org/10.7326/M14-2482

Danielson, M. L., Bitsko, R. H., Ghandour, R. M., Holbrook, J. R., Kogan, M. D., & Blumberg, S. J. (2018). Prevalence of parent-reported ADHD diagnosis and associated treatment among U.S. children and adolescents, 2016. *Journal of Clinical Child & Adolescent Psychology, 47*(2), 199–212. https://doi.org/10.1080/15374416.2017.1417860

Dawson, L., Frederiksen, B., Long, M., Ranji, U., & Kates, J. (2021). *LGBT+ people's health and experiences accessing care*. https://www.kff.org/report-section/lgbt-peoples-health-and-experiences-accessing-care-report/

Dekker, J., Koelen, J. A., Peen, J., Schoevers, R. A., & Gijsbers-Van Wijk, C. (2008). Gender differences in clinical features of depressed outpatients: Preliminary evidence for subtyping of depression? *Women & Health, 46*(4), 19–38. https://doi.org/10.1300/J013v46n04_02

English, W., Gott, M., & Robinson, J. (2022). The meaning of rapport for patients, families, and healthcare professionals: A scoping review. *Patient Education and Counseling, 105*(1), 2–14. https://doi.org/10.1016/j.pec.2021.06.003

Faubion, S. S., & Rullo, J. E. (2015). Sexual dysfunction in women: A practical approach. *American Family Physician, 92*(4), 281–288.

Frost, D. M., Lehavot, K., & Meyer, I. H. (2015). Minority stress and physical health among sexual minority individuals. *Journal of Behavioral Medicine, 38*, 1–8.

Galmiche, M., Déchelotte, P., Lambert, G., & Tavolacci, M. P. (2019). Prevalence of eating disorders over the 2000–2018 period: A systematic literature review. *The American Journal of Clinical Nutrition, 109*(5), 1402–1413. https://doi.org/10.1093/ajcn/nqy342

Gehrman, P., Seelig, A. D., Jacobson, I. G., Boyko, E. J., Hooper, T. I., Gackstetter, G. D., Ulmer, C. S., & Smith, T. C. (2013). Predeployment sleep duration and insomnia symptoms as risk factors for new-onset mental health disorders following military deployment. *Sleep, 36*(7), 1009–1018. https://doi.org/10.5665/sleep.2798

Goldstein, R. B., Smith, S. M., Chou, S. P., Saha, T. D., Jung, J., Zhang, H., Pickering, R. P., Ruan, W. J., Huang, B., & Grant, B. F. (2016). The epidemiology of DSM-5 posttraumatic stress disorder in the United States: Results from the National Epidemiologic Survey on alcohol and related conditions-III. *Social Psychiatry and Psychiatric Epidemiology, 51*(8), 1137–1148. https://doi.org/10.1007/s00127-016-1208-5

Goodwin, G., Haddad, P., Ferrier, I., Aronson, J., Barnes, T., Cipriani, A., Coghill, D. R., Fazel, S., Geddes, J. R., Grunze, H., Holmes, E. A., Howes, O., Hudson, S., Hunt, N., Jones, I., Macmillan, I. C., McAllister-Williams, H., Miklowitz, D. R., Morriss, R., & Young, A. H. (2016). Evidence-based guidelines for treating bipolar disorder: Revised third edition recommendations from the British Association for Psychopharmacology. *Journal of Psychopharmacology, 30*(6), 495–553. https://doi.org/10.1177/0269881116636545

Grande, I., Berk, M., Birmaher, B., & Vieta, E. (2016). Bipolar disorder. *The Lancet, 387*(10027), 1561–1572. https://doi.org/10.1016/S0140-6736(15)00241-X

Grandner, M. A., & Perlis, M. L. (2015). Treating insomnia disorder in the context of medical and psychiatric comorbidities. *JAMA Internal Medicine, 175*(9), 1472–1473. https://doi.org/10.1001/jamainternmed.2015.3015

Griswold, K. S., Del Regno, P. A., & Berger, R. C. (2015). Recognition and differential diagnosis of psychosis in primary care. *American Family Physician, 91*(12), 856–863.

Harris, A. M., Orav, E. J., Bates, D. W., & Barsky, A. J. (2009). Somatization increases disability independent of comorbidity. *Journal of General Internal Medicine, 24*, 155–161. https://doi.org/10.1007/s11606-008-0845-0

Herman, J. L., Flores, A. R., & O'Neill, K. K. (2022). *How many adults and youth identify as transgender in the United States?* The Williams Institute, UCLA. https://escholarship.org/uc/item/4xs990ws

Huang, H., Huang, H., Spottswood, M., & Ghaemi, N. (2020). Approach to evaluating and managing adult attention-deficit/hyperactivity disorder in primary care. *Harvard Review of Psychiatry, 28*(2), 100. https://doi.org/10.1097/HRP.0000000000000248

Hyman, S. L., Levy, S. E., Myers, S. M., Kuo, D. Z., Apkon, S., Davidson, L. F., Ellerbeck, K. A., Foster, J. E. A., Noritz, G. H., Leppert, M. O., Saunders, B. S., Stille, C., Yin, L., Weitzman, C. C., Childers, D. O., Jr., Levine, J. M., Peralta-Carcelen, A. M., Poon, J. K., & Bridgemohan, C. (2020). Identification, evaluation, and management of children with autism spectrum disorder. *Pediatrics, 145*(1), e20193447. https://doi.org/10.1542/peds.2019-3447

Judd, L. L., Akiskal, H. S., Schettler, P. J., Endicott, J., Maser, J., Solomon, D. A., Leon, A. C., Rice, J. A., & Keller, M. B. (2002). The long-term natural history of the weekly symptomatic status of bipolar I disorder. *Archives of General Psychiatry, 59*(6), 530–537. https://doi.org/10.1001/archpsyc.59.6.530

Kennedy, A. B., Taylor, S. S., Lavie, C. J., & Blair, S. N. (2022). Ending the stigma: Improving care for patients who are overweight or obese. *Family Practice Management, 29*(2), 21–25.

Kerner, B. (2015). Toward a deeper understanding of the genetics of bipolar disorder. *Frontiers in Psychiatry, 6*, 105. https://doi.org/10.3389/fpsyt.2015.00105

Kessler, R. C., Adler, L., Barkley, R., Biederman, J., Conners, C. K., Demler, O., Faraone, S. V., Greenhill, L. L., Howes, M. J., Secnik, K., Spencer, T., Ustun, T. B., Walters, E. E., & Zaslavsky, A. M. (2006). The prevalence and correlates of adult ADHD in the United States: Results from the National Comorbidity Survey Replication. *American Journal of Psychiatry, 163*(4), 716–723. https://doi.org/10.1176/ajp.2006.163.4.716

Kessler, R. C., Chiu, W. T., Demler, O., & Walters, E. E. (2005). Prevalence, severity, and comorbidity of 12-month DSM-IV disorders in the National Comorbidity Survey Replication. *Archives of General Psychiatry, 62*(6), 617–627. https://doi.org/10.1001/archpsyc.62.6.617

Kessler, R. C., Petukhova, M., Sampson, N. A., Zaslavsky, A. M., & Wittchen, H.-U. (2012). Twelve-month and lifetime prevalence and lifetime morbid risk of anxiety and mood disorders in the United States. *International Journal of Methods in Psychiatric Research, 21*(3), 169–184. https://doi.org/10.1002/mpr.1359

Kessler, R. C., Sonnega, A., Bromet, E., Hughes, M., & Nelson, C. B. (2013). Posttraumatic stress disorder in the national comorbidity survey. In *Fear and anxiety*. Routledge.

Klein, D. A., Paradise, S. L., & Goodwin, E. T. (2018). Caring for transgender and gender-diverse persons: What clinicians should know. *American Family Physician, 98*(11), 645–653.

Klein, D. A., Sylvester, J. E., & Schvey, N. A. (2021). Eating disorders in primary care: Diagnosis and management. *American Family Physician, 103*(1), 22–32.

Kroenke, K., Spitzer, R. L., & Williams, J. B. W. (2001). The PHQ-9 validity of a brief depression severity measure. *Journal of General Internal Medicine, 16*(9), 606–613. https://doi.org/10.1046/j.1525-1497.2001.016009606.x

Kroenke, K., Spitzer, R. L., Williams, J. B. W., Monahan, P. O., & Löwe, B. (2007). Anxiety disorders in primary care: Prevalence, impairment, comorbidity, and detection. *Annals of Internal Medicine, 146*(5), 317–325. https://doi.org/10.7326/0003-4819-146-5-200703060-00004

Kurlansik, S. L., & Maffei, M. S. (2016). Somatic symptom disorder. *American Family Physician, 93*(1), 49–54A.

Lichstein, K. L. (2006). Secondary insomnia: A myth dismissed. *Sleep Medicine Reviews, 10*(1), 3–5. https://doi.org/10.1016/j.smrv.2005.10.001

MacKinnon, R. A., Michels, R., & Buckley, P. J. (2015). *The psychiatric interview in clinical practice*. American Psychiatric Publication.

Martin, L. A., Neighbors, H. W., & Griffith, D. M. (2013). The experience of symptoms of depression in men vs women: Analysis of the National Comorbidity Survey Replication. *JAMA Psychiatry, 70*(10), 1100–1106. https://doi.org/10.1001/jamapsychiatry.2013.1985

Maurer, D. M., Raymond, T. J., & Davis, B. N. (2018). Depression: Screening and diagnosis. *American Family Physician, 98*(8), 508–515.

Mental Health America (MHA). (2019). *Mental health in America-adult data*. https://mhanational.org/issues/state-mental-health-america

Merikangas, K. R., Akiskal, H. S., Angst, J., Greenberg, P. E., Hirschfeld, R. M. A., Petukhova, M., & Kessler, R. C. (2007). Lifetime and 12-month prevalence of bipolar spectrum disorder in the National Comorbidity Survey Replication. *Archives of General Psychiatry, 64*(5), 543–552. https://doi.org/10.1001/archpsyc.64.5.543

Moffitt, T. E., Houts, R., Asherson, P., Belsky, D. W., Corcoran, D. L., Hammerle, M., Harrington, H., Hogan, S., Meier, M. H., Polanczyk, G. V., Poulton, R., Ramrakha, S., Sugden, K., Williams, B., Rohde, L. A., & Caspi, A. (2015). Is adult ADHD a childhood-onset neurodevelopmental disorder? Evidence from a four-decade longitudinal cohort study. *American Journal of Psychiatry, 172*(10), 967–977. https://doi.org/10.1176/appi.ajp.2015.14101266

Nasreddine, Z. S., Phillips, N. A., Bédirian, V., Charbonneau, S., Whitehead, V., Collin, I., Cummings, J. L., & Chertkow, H. (2005). The Montreal cognitive assessment, MoCA: A brief screening tool for mild cognitive impairment. *Journal of the American Geriatrics Society, 53*(4), 695–699. https://doi.org/10.1111/j.1532-5415.2005.53221.x

National Institute of Mental Health (NIMH). (2017). *Integrated care.* https://www.nimh.nih.gov/health/topics/integrated-care/index.shtml

Nicolaidis, C., Kripke, C. C., & Raymaker, D. (2014). Primary care for adults on the autism spectrum. *Medical Clinics, 98*(5), 1169–1191. https://doi.org/10.1016/j.mcna.2014.06.011

Nicolaidis, C., Raymaker, D., McDonald, K., Kapp, S., Weiner, M., Ashkenazy, E., Gerrity, M., Kripke, C., Platt, L., & Baggs, A. (2016). The development and evaluation of an online healthcare toolkit for autistic adults and their primary care providers. *Journal of General Internal Medicine, 31*(10), 1180–1189. https://doi.org/10.1007/s11606-016-3763-6

Nusbaum, M. R. H., Gamble, G., Skinner, B., & Heiman, J. (2000). The high prevalence of sexual concerns among women seeking routine gynecological care. *Journal of Family Practice, 49*(3), 229–232.

Office of Minority Health, U.S. Department of Health & Human Services. (2024). *Think cultural health.* https://thinkculturalhealth.hhs.gov/

Ohayon, M. M. (2002). Epidemiology of insomnia: What we know and what we still need to learn. *Sleep Medicine Reviews, 6*(2), 97–111. https://doi.org/10.1053/smrv.2002.0186

Olariu, E., Forero, C. G., Castro-Rodriguez, J. I., Rodrigo-Calvo, M. T., Álvarez, P., Martín-López, L. M., Sánchez-Toto, A., Adroher, N. D., Blasco-Cubedo, M. J., Vilagut, G., Fullana, M. A., & Alonso, J. (2015). Detection of anxiety disorders in primary care: A meta-analysis of assisted and unassisted diagnoses. *Depression and Anxiety, 32*(7), 471–484. https://doi.org/10.1002/da.22360

Olfson, M., Blanco, C., Wall, M. M., Liu, S.-M., & Grant, B. F. (2019). Treatment of common mental disorders in the United States: Results from the National Epidemiologic Survey on alcohol and related conditions-III. *The Journal of Clinical Psychiatry, 80*(3), 21534. https://doi.org/10.4088/JCP.18m12532

Park, L. T., & Zarate, C. A. (2019). Depression in the primary care setting. *New England Journal of Medicine, 380*(6), 559–568. https://doi.org/10.1056/NEJMcp1712493

Plana-Ripoll, O., Pedersen, C. B., Holtz, Y., Benros, M. E., Dalsgaard, S., de Jonge, P., Fan, C. C., Degenhardt, L., Ganna, A., Greve, A. N., Gunn, J., Iburg, K. M., Kessing, L. V., Lee, B. K., Lim, C. C. W., Mors, O., Nordentoft, M., Prior, A., Roest, A. M., & McGrath, J. J. (2019). Exploring comorbidity within mental disorders among a Danish national population. *JAMA Psychiatry, 76*(3), 259–270. https://doi.org/10.1001/jamapsychiatry.2018.3658

Rainone, A., & Mancini, F. (2018). When positive emotions lead to feeling bad. The role of secondary evaluation and affect as information in hypomania and mania. *Rivista di Psichiatria, 53*(6), 317–323.

Raja, S., Hasnain, M., Hoersch, M., Gove-Yin, S., & Rajagopalan, C. (2015). Trauma informed care in medicine: Current knowledge and future research directions. *Family & Community Health, 38*(3), 216. https://doi.org/10.1097/FCH.0000000000000071

Ravi, A., & Little, V. (2017). Providing trauma-informed care. *American Family Physician, 95*(10), 655–657.

Read, S., King, M., & Watson, J. (1997). Sexual dysfunction in primary medical care: Prevalence, characteristics and detection by the general practitioner. *Journal of Public Health, 19*(4), 387–391. https://doi.org/10.1093/oxfordjournals.pubmed.a024665

Reeves, E. (2015). A synthesis of the literature on trauma-informed care. *Issues in Mental Health Nursing, 36*(9), 698–709. https://doi.org/10.3109/01612840.2015.1025319

Robins, D. L., Casagrande, K., Barton, M., Chen, C.-M. A., Dumont-Mathieu, T., & Fein, D. (2014). Validation of the modified checklist for autism in toddlers, revised with follow-up (M-CHAT-R/F). *Pediatrics, 133*(1), 37–45. https://doi.org/10.1542/peds.2013-1813

Rosendal, M., Blankenstein, A. H., Morriss, R., Fink, P., Sharpe, M., & Burton, C. (2013). Enhanced care by generalists for functional somatic symptoms and disorders in primary care. *Cochrane Database of Systematic Reviews.* https://doi.org/10.1002/14651858.CD008142.pub2

Rotenstein, L. S., Edwards, S. T., & Landon, B. E. (2023). Adult primary care physician visits increasingly address mental health concerns: Study examines primary care physician visits for mental health concerns. *Health Affairs, 42*(2), 163–171. https://doi.org/10.1377/hlthaff.2022.00705

Satcher, D. (2001). *Mental health: Culture, race, and ethnicity—A supplement to mental health: A report of the surgeon general.* U.S. Department of Health and Human Services. https://doi.org/10.13016/jela-ckxw

Sateia, M. J., Buysse, D. J., Krystal, A. D., Neubauer, D. N., & Heald, J. L. (2017). Clinical practice guideline for the pharmacologic treatment of chronic insomnia in adults: An American Academy of sleep medicine clinical practice guideline. *Journal of Clinical Sleep Medicine, 13*(02), 307–349. https://doi.org/10.5664/jcsm.6470

Savoy, M., O'Gurek, D., & Brown-James, A. (2020). Sexual health history: Techniques and tips. *American Family Physician, 101*(5), 286–293.

Schaffer, A., Isometsä, E. T., Azorin, J.-M., Cassidy, F., Goldstein, T., Rihmer, Z., Sinyor, M., Tondo, L., Moreno, D. H., Turecki, G., Reis, C., Kessing, L. V., Ha, K., Weizman, A., Beautrais, A., Chou, Y.-H., Diazgranados, N., Levitt, A. J., Zarate, C. A., & Yatham, L. (2015). A review of factors associated with greater likelihood of suicide attempts and suicide deaths in bipolar disorder: Part II of a report of the International Society for Bipolar Disorders Task Force on suicide in bipolar disorder. *The Australian and New Zealand Journal of Psychiatry, 49*(11), 1006–1020. https://doi.org/10.1177/0004867415594428

Spitzer, R. L., Kroenke, K., Williams, J. B. W., & Löwe, B. (2006). A brief measure for assessing generalized anxiety disorder: The GAD-7. *Archives of Internal Medicine, 166*(10), 1092–1097. https://doi.org/10.1001/archinte.166.10.1092

Spoont, M. R., Williams, J. W., Jr., Kehle-Forbes, S., Nieuwsma, J. A., Mann-Wrobel, M. C., & Gross, R. (2015). Does this patient have posttraumatic stress disorder? Rational clinical examination systematic review. *JAMA, 314*(5), 501–510. https://doi.org/10.1001/jama.2015.7877

Stein, M. B., & Sareen, J. (2015). Generalized anxiety disorder. *New England Journal of Medicine, 373*(21), 2059–2068. https://doi.org/10.1056/NEJMcp1502514

Substance Abuse and Mental Health Services Administration (SAMHSA). (2014). *SAMHSA's concept of trauma and guidance for a trauma-informed approach.* https://store.samhsa.gov/sites/default/files/sma14-4884.pdf

Substance Abuse and Mental Health Services Administration (SAMHSA). (2019). *Results from the 2018 National Survey on Drug Use and Health: Detailed tables.* https://www.samhsa.gov/data/report%20/2018-nsduh-detailed-tables

Substance Abuse and Mental Health Services Administration (SAMHSA). (2022). *2022 National Survey on Drug Use and Health (NSDUH) releases.* https://www.samhsa.gov/data/release/2022-national-survey-drug-use-and-health-nsduh-releases

Swan, J., Phillips, T. M., Sanders, T., Mullens, A. B., Debattista, J., & Brömdal, A. (2023). Mental health and quality of life outcomes of gender-affirming surgery: A systematic literature review. *Journal of Gay & Lesbian Mental Health, 27*(1), 2–45. https://doi.org/10.1080/19359705.2021.2016537

Tariq, S. H., Tumosa, N., Chibnall, J. T., Perry, M. H., & Morley, J. E. (2006). Comparison of the Saint Louis university mental status examination and the mini-mental state examination for detecting dementia and mild neurocognitive disorder—A pilot study. *The American Journal of Geriatric Psychiatry, 14*(11), 900–910. https://doi.org/10.1097/01.JGP.0000221510.33817.86

Thomas, R., Sanders, S., Doust, J., Beller, E., & Glasziou, P. (2015). Prevalence of attention-deficit/hyperactivity disorder: A systematic review and meta-analysis. *Pediatrics, 135*(4), e994–e1001. https://doi.org/10.1542/peds.2014-3482

Trauer, J. M., Qian, M. Y., Doyle, J. S., Rajaratnam, S. M. W., & Cunnington, D. (2015). Cognitive behavioral therapy for chronic insomnia: A systematic review and meta-analysis. *Annals of Internal Medicine, 163*(3), 191–204. https://doi.org/10.7326/M14-2841

U.S. Preventive Services Task Force (USPSTF). (2022). Screening for eating disorders in adolescents and adults: US preventive services task force recommendation statement. *JAMA, 327*(11), 1061–1067. https://doi.org/10.1001/jama.2022.1806

Vanderbilt Kennedy Center (VKC). (2024). *Health care for adults with intellectual and developmental disabilities*. https://iddtoolkit.vkcsites.org/

Wang, H. R., Woo, Y. S., Ahn, H. S., Ahn, I. M., Kim, H. J., & Bahk, W.-M. (2015). The validity of the mood disorder questionnaire for screening bipolar disorder: A meta-analysis. *Depression and Anxiety, 32*(7), 527–538. https://doi.org/10.1002/da.22374

Witters, D. (2023). *U.S. depression rates reach new highs*. Gallup. https://news.gallup.com/poll/505745/depression-rates-reach-new-highs.aspx

Wolraich, M. L., Hagan, J. F., Jr., Allan, C., Chan, E., Davison, D., Earls, M., Evans, S. W., Flinn, S. K., Froehlich, T., Frost, J., Holbrook, J. R., Lehmann, C. U., Lessin, H. R., Okechukwu, K., Pierce, K. L., Winner, J. D., & Zurhellen, W. (2019). Clinical practice guideline for the diagnosis, evaluation, and treatment of attention-deficit/hyperactivity disorder in children and adolescents. *Pediatrics, 144*(4), e20192528. https://doi.org/10.1542/peds.2019-2528

Yatham, L. N., Kennedy, S. H., Parikh, S. V., Schaffer, A., Bond, D. J., Frey, B. N., Sharma, V., Goldstein, B. I., Rej, S., Beaulieu, S., Alda, M., MacQueen, G., Milev, R. V., Ravindran, A., O'Donovan, C., McIntosh, D., Lam, R. W., Vazquez, G., Kapczinski, F., & Berk, M. (2018). Canadian network for mood and anxiety treatments (CANMAT) and International Society for Bipolar Disorders (ISBD) 2018 guidelines for the management of patients with bipolar disorder. *Bipolar Disorders, 20*(2), 97–170. https://doi.org/10.1111/bdi.12609

Yehuda, R., Hoge, C. W., McFarlane, A. C., Vermetten, E., Lanius, R. A., Nievergelt, C. M., Hobfoll, S. E., Koenen, K. C., Neylan, T. C., & Hyman, S. E. (2015). Post-traumatic stress disorder. *Nature Reviews Disease Primers, 1*(1), 1–22. https://doi.org/10.1038/nrdp.2015.57

Chapter 4
Screening Recommendations for Common Behavioral Health Conditions in Primary Care

Rebecca M. Daniel PsyD and Jessica Bracks MD

Screening Recommendations for Common Behavioral Health Conditions

In 2021, one in five adults and one in six youth experienced some type of mental illness. The average time between symptom onset and initiating treatment is 11 years (National Alliance on Mental Illness, 2023; Salinas et al., 2023). Although there continues to be a shortage of mental health services, primary care providers (PCPs) can help close the gap and initiate screening and treatment before symptoms lead to negative outcomes. The most frequently presenting behavioral health (BH) conditions in the primary care office for adults include depression, anxiety, substance abuse, insomnia, and suicidal ideation (Ashman et al., 2019; Rogers et al., 2021; Sayre et al., 2020; Sun et al., 2021). Similarly, for children and adolescents, common concerns include depression, anxiety, suicidal ideation, and neurodevelopmental concerns (e.g., attention-deficit/hyperactivity disorder [ADHD], autism spectrum disorder [ASD], specific learning disorders; [Biel et al., 2020; Ogundele & Morton, 2022]). While these concerns are certainly not exhaustive of all potential BH concerns a patient may have, screening for these conditions can provide the PCP with critical information that can help guide necessary interventions (i.e., referral for an in-depth psychological evaluation for diagnostic clarification, medication management, psychotherapy, or ruling in or out comorbid conditions).

R. M. Daniel PsyD (✉)
Wake Forest University School of Medicine, Winston-Salem, NC, USA
e-mail: rebecca.daniel@wfusm.edu

J. Bracks MD
UT Tyler School of Medicine, Tyler, TX, USA

M. L. C. Williamson and D. L. Terry (eds.), *Essentials for Treating Behavioral Health in Primary Care*, https://doi.org/10.1007/978-3-032-09558-9_4

Considerations for Behavioral Health Screening in Primary Care

Rationale and Implementation of Screening There are several reasons why a PCP may initiate screening for any given BH condition. Of import, BH conditions often coexist with chronic physical conditions, such as diabetes, hypertension, even concern for patient noncompliance. Routine screening in primary care helps normalize conversations about mental health. In so doing, it reduces the stigma associated with behavioral health. Addressing BH can lead to better adherence to treatment plans for other physical conditions. When a person's mental state is addressed, they are more likely to follow medical advice and maintain healthier lifestyles. In addition to a patient's overall well-being, certain insurance payors may require depression screening over a certain period of time (Mulvaney-Day et al., 2018). Different specialties (e.g., AAFP, ACOG, AAP, etc.) also have BH screening guidelines to improve best practices. Some clinics and hospital systems mandate certain screeners for certain visit types (e.g., Medicare Annual Wellness Visits, annual physicals, etc.). PCPs might suspect that a patient is experiencing emerging symptoms of a BH condition and wish to provide a screener to help guide clinical decision making. Screeners may also be used to track a patient's symptom presentation over time to monitor treatment progress.

There are multiple factors for the PCP to consider in screening:

- Mode of administration (e.g., paper vs electronic).
- Timing of administration (e.g., pre-visit, post-visit, during rooming).
- Frequency of administration (e.g., yearly, monthly, quarterly).
- Brevity of the screener and impact on clinic flow.
- Choosing between a combined or single-disorder screener.
- Potential cost associated with screeners.
- Reading level of the patient population.
- Language of the patient and available screeners.
- Psychometric properties (e.g., sensitivity, specificity, reliability, validity).

There is not a universal or required protocol for screening that is consistent across organizations, which means that PCPs and their clinics can consider what types of screening practices best fit their patient population and would be most efficient for their clinic flow. Of note, *screening alone does not improve outcomes.* Rather, the combination of screening, identification of early concerns, education, and initiation of treatment and/or diagnostic follow-up provides the greatest impact (Mulvaney-Day et al., 2018). As such, for clinics that do not already have a streamlined process for screening and subsequent steps in place, the American Medical

Association (AMA) created a toolkit designed to help PCPs consider how to integrate behavioral health services into their clinics (Drake & Valenstein, 2021). See Chap. 12 for more detail regarding different models of integrated behavioral health (e.g., CoCM, PCBH). Below are five steps to consider when integrating behavioral health (including screening) into a clinic (Drake & Valenstein, 2021):

1. Assess your current needs and resources.
2. Choose a team-based model.
3. Train members of the primary care team on how to implement the screener.
4. Implement the model.
5. Evaluate and improve.

Time-Saving Screening Practices One of the major barriers to implementing BH screening is the time demands already placed on PCPs (Drake & Valenstein, 2021; Salinas et al., 2023). Below are some time-saving practices that may help to reduce barriers to administration:

- Automatically include screeners as part of the patient check-in process, to be completed in the waiting room or exam room prior to the patient being seen by the physician. During the rooming process, clinical staff can score the measures and notify the PCP of any relevant findings prior to the visit. For clinics with advanced electronic capabilities (e.g., tablets), there are often automatic scoring programs that can be used.
- Utilize the electronic health record (EHR) to automatically send patients BH screeners to complete prior to their visit may also be advantageous, if this functionality is available.
- If a BH concern arises unexpectedly (i.e., during an office visit), the patient can complete a BH screener while the PCP steps out of the patient's room before returning to discuss results.
- For patients whose symptoms are being tracked over time for treatment monitoring, administering screeners after a visit may also be appropriate.
- Pre-charting and creating quick-phrases or templates within the EHR for frequently used screeners can save time with documentation.
- Having pre-printed handouts for commonly presenting concerns (e.g., depression, anxiety, insomnia) available at the nurses' station to provide patient upon presentation can also save time.

Screening Vs. Diagnostic Ability When deciding to screen a patient for BH concerns, the PCP should consider that screeners are meant to guide clinical discussion, not necessarily provide an official diagnosis for the patient. For patients who screen positive for any given behavioral health concern, a more in-depth discussion regarding history, symptoms, coinciding conditions, impairment, and other relevant factors should be considered, which may require additional follow-up visits.

Additionally, there are scenarios where patients would benefit from a referral to a specialist for additional testing to provide diagnostic clarification (e.g., neurocognitive concerns). The significance of an accurate diagnosis cannot be overstated, as diagnoses are crucial in determining best practices for a patient's well-being, whether it be medication, use of community supports, psychotherapy, or higher levels of care. As such, it is essential to carefully consider how screening results are recorded in the patient's chart.

Sharing Results with Patients When a patient screens positive for a behavioral health condition, it is important to share this information with them in a way that is clear and useful. Some patients are more familiar with various BH conditions than others, so it is important to meet the patient at the point of their understanding—we are to meet people where they are. Remind the patient that a positive screen does not necessarily indicate diagnostic certainty, only that the condition should be further explored, is important. After the screening results have been shared and the patient has been given the opportunity to provide their insight, the PCP now has a rich opportunity to discuss pt's readiness for change, openness to intervention, and next best steps (see Chap. 4 for more guidance on motivational interviewing and important communication skills).

Disorder-Specific Screeners

Tables 4.1 and 4.2 include brief, freely available, psychometrically valid, and widely used screeners for the most commonly presenting BH concerns for adults and children and are often recommended by major medical organizations. Most of the screeners below are also available in multiple languages. While this list is not exhaustive, it can be used as a starting point to help develop a battery of screeners that fit the culture and workflow of the PCPs clinic. Unless otherwise noted, questionnaires noted below are open access and can be found using the references included in the table, or by conducting a simple internet search.

Table 4.1 Common behavioral health screeners for adults

Diagnosis	Name	Target population	Length/time frame	Special considerations	References
Anxiety and PTSD	Generalized anxiety disorder scale (GAD-7)	Individuals age 11+	7 items/past 2 weeks	Self-report scale. This measure assesses panic disorder, social anxiety disorder, and posttraumatic stress disorder. Widely used in primary care clinics. The GAD-2 can also be used to screen for generalized anxiety disorder (i.e., the first two items of the GAD-7) available in multiple languages	Kroenke et al. (2007), Spitzer et al. (2006)
	Geriatric anxiety scale (GAS-10)	Adults 60+	10 items/ past week	Self-report or nurse administered scale. Assesses somatic, cognitive, and affective symptoms. Available in multiple languages	Mueller et al. (2015), Segal et al. (2010)
	Primary care PTSD screen for DSM-5 (PC-PTSD-5)	Adults 18+	5 items; past month	Self-report scale. Item #1 is the initial screening item that can quickly determine whether the five following questions need to be administered. Available in multiple languages	Prins et al. (2016)
Depression	Center for Epidemiologic Studies Depression Scale (CES-D)	Adults 18+	20 items/ past week	This self-report scale does not include an explicit item assessing suicidal ideation. Includes several reverse-scored items. Available in multiple languages	Radloff (1977)

(continued)

Table 4.1 (continued)

Diagnosis	Name	Target population	Length/time frame	Special considerations	References
	Edinburgh postnatal depression scale (EPDS)	Pregnant and postpartum adults (18+)	10 items/ past week	Self-report scale. Item #10 explicitly asks about self-harm. Available in multiple languages	Cox et al. (1987)
	Geriatric depression scale (GDS short-form)	Adults (55+)	15 items/ past week	This self-report scale does not explicitly assess suicidal ideation. The GDS can be used with patients post-stroke and with mild cognitive impairment or aphasia. Available in multiple languages	Sheikh and Yesavage (1986)
	Mood disorder questionnaire (MDQ)	Adults 18+	5 items	Self-report scale. This scale assesses for likelihood of bipolar disorder I disorder (it is not as sensitive to bipolar II disorder). While developed for adults, it has been useful with adolescents age 12+. Available in multiple languages	Hirschfeld (2002)
	Patient health questionnaire (PHQ-9)	Adolescents and adults (12+)	9 items/past 2 weeks	Self-report scale. Item #9 explicitly assesses suicidal ideation. The first two items of the PHQ-9 (i.e., the PHQ-2) is also an appropriate screener. Available in multiple languages. This is the most used depression screener in primary care	Kroenke et al. (1999)

(continued)

Table 4.1 (continued)

Diagnosis	Name	Target population	Length/time frame	Special considerations	References
Interpersonal violence	Extended-hurt, insult, threaten, scream (E-HITS)	Women of childbearing age through age 64	5 items/past 12 months	Self-report scale. Assesses the frequency of emotional, physical, and sexual violence	Iverson et al. (2015)
	Humiliation, afraid, rape, kick (HARK)	Women of childbearing age through age 64	4 items/past year	Self-report scale. Assesses history emotional, physical, and sexual violence	Sohal et al. (2007)
Insomnia	Insomnia severity index (ISI)	Individuals age 17+	7 items/past 2 weeks	Assesses daytime and nighttime sleepiness. Items two and three of the ISI (i.e., the ISI-2) can also be used as a screener. Available in multiple languages	Bastien et al. (2001), Kraepelien et al. (2021)
Substance use (see Chap. 13)	Alcohol, smoking, and substance involvement screening test (ASSIST)	Adults 18+	8 items/historical and past 3 months	Clinician administered. Can help with determining if further diagnostic assessment is needed due to risk severity. Can be administered via paper or electronically	Humeniuk et al. (2010)
	Alcohol use identification test (AUDIT)	Individuals age 14+	10 items/past 12 months	Self-report scale. This is the most widely used screener for detecting risky drinking patterns. Can be administered via paper or electronically	Saunders et al. (1993)

(continued)

Table 4.1 (continued)

Diagnosis	Name	Target population	Length/time frame	Special considerations	References
	National Institute on Drug Abuse (NIDA) quick screen	Age 18+	4-items; past 3 months	Clinician administered. Feasible in busy primary care clinics due to brevity; if patient screens positive, there is the option for further assessment of risk included (i.e., NIDA-modified ASSIST)	National Institute on Drug Abuse (NIDA) (n.d.)
	Prenatal risk overview (PRO): Cigarette, alcohol, and drug use domains	Pregnant individuals age 18+	4, 8, and 3 items, respectively/ varying time frames	Self-report scale. For use with identifying substance abuse or dependence in pregnant individuals. This is part of a larger screener for various psychosocial factors that includes 13 total domains	Harrison and Sidebottom (2008)
	Tobacco, alcohol, prescription medication, and other substance use (TAPS-1)	Age 12+	4-items/past year	Self- or clinician administered. Feasible in busy primary care clinics due to brevity; if patient screens positive, there is the option for further assessment of risk included (i.e., TAPS-2)	McNeely et al. (2016)
	Tolerance, worried, eye-opener, amnesia, Kut down (TWEAK)	Pregnant individuals age 18+	5-items/ historical use	Self- or clinician administered. Can be administered via paper or computer. Available in English and Spanish	Russell (1994)

(continued)

Table 4.1 (continued)

Diagnosis	Name	Target population	Length/time frame	Special considerations	References
Suicidal ideation (see Chap. 7)	Ask suicide screening questions (ASQ)	Individuals age 10+	4 items	Clinician administered; includes a straightforward worksheet that yields a recommendation for immediate clinical action. Available in multiple languages	Horowitz et al. (2020)
	Columbia suicide severity rating scale—Screen version (C-SSRS)	Individuals age 6+	5 items/last month	Clinician administered; assesses suicidal ideation over past several months. Scoring yields recommendation for clinical action. Available in multiple languages	Posner et al. (2011)
	SAD PERSONS scale	Adults 18+	10 items/ historical events	Clinician administered; explores 10 significant risk factors for suicide. Scoring yields a recommendation for immediate clinical action	Patterson et al. (1983)

Table 4.2 Common behavioral health screeners for children

Diagnosis	Name	Target population	Length/time frame	Special considerations	References
Common screeners for children (see Chap. 12)					
Anxiety	Screen for child anxiety related disorders—Child & Parent Report (SCARED-C & SCARED-P)	Children ages 8–18	41 items/last 3 months (for both reports)	It is recommended that parents read the child report aloud to children ages 8–11. Older children can complete independently. Can differentiate between panic disorder, significant somatic symptoms, generalized anxiety disorder, social anxiety disorder, separation anxiety disorder, and school avoidance. Available in multiple languages	Birmaher et al. (1997)
	5-item screen for child anxiety related disorders (5-item SCARED-P)	Children ages 8–18	5 items/last 3 months	Includes items 41, 28, 36, 24, and 25 of the SCARED-P	Birmaher et al. (1999)

(continued)

Table 4.2 (continued)

Diagnosis	Name	Target population	Length/time frame	Special considerations	References
Attention-deficit/hyperactivity disorder (ADHD)	Vanderbilt attention deficit/hyperactive disorder—Parent & Teacher Report (VADPRS +& VADTRS)—Third edition	Children ages 5–12	VADPRS (56 items plus additional questions about impairment and comorbid conditions)/last 6 months. VADTRS (36 questions plus additional questions about impairment)	Cost associated with purchasing these measures (via AAP). Parent version includes subscales for depression/anxiety, oppositional defiant disorder, and conduct disorder. Teacher version includes subscales for oppositional defiant disorder and depression/anxiety. Available in multiple languages	Wolraich et al. (2003)
Autism Spectrum disorder (ASD)	Modified checklist for autism in toddlers, revised (M-CHAT-R)	Children ages 16mos-30mos	20 items/present focus	Parent report. Can be completed via paper or computer. Available in multiple languages	Robins et al. (2018)
	Social challenges screening questionnaire	Children ages 5–18	15 questions/present focus	Can be completed via paper or computer by a parent, teacher, or others. Designed to help screen for autism spectrum disorder (level 1 ASD; formerly known as Asperger's syndrome)	Smith et al. (2015)

(continued)

Table 4.2 (continued)

Diagnosis	Name	Target population	Length/time frame	Special considerations	References
Depression	Center for Epidemiologic Studies Depression Scale for children (CES-DC)	Children and adolescents (6–17)	20 items/past week	Parent or self-report. Does not include explicit item related to suicidal ideation. Includes several reverse-scored items. Available in multiple languages	Faulstich et al. (1986)
	Patient health questionnaire modified (PHQ-9A)	Adolescents (11–17)	9-items/past two weeks	Self-report scale. Item #9 explicitly assesses suicidal ideation	Aggarwal et al. (2017)
	Pediatric symptom checklist (PSC-17)	Children ages 4–17	35 items/ present focus	Parent or self-report (for children over age 13). Assesses cognitive, emotional, and behavioral problems. There is also a 35-item version (PCS) that is available in multiple languages. PSC can also be administered via computer	Gardner et al. (1999)
	SAD PERSONS scale (adapted)	Adolescents 15+	10 items/ historical events	Clinician administered; explores 10 significant risk factors for suicide. Scoring yields a recommendation for immediate clinical action	Juhnke (1996)

(continued)

Table 4.2 (continued)

Diagnosis	Name	Target population	Length/time frame	Special considerations	References
Sleep	Bedtime, excessive sleepiness, awakenings, regularity, sleep disordered breathing (BEARS)	Ages 2–5; 6–12; 13–18	5 items/ present focus	Clinician administered. Interview can be directed toward the parent or child (if over age 13). Available in multiple languages	Owens and Dalzell (2005)
Social determinants of health	Protocol for responding to and assessing patients' assets, risks, and experiences (PRAPARE)	Parents, caregivers	21 questions/ historical focus	Self-report questionnaire that includes items referencing domestic violence, social connectedness, refugee status, stress levels. Available in multiple languages	National Association of Community Health Centers (2016)
	Well-child care, evaluation, community resources, advocacy, referral, education survey instrument (WE CARE)	Parents, caregivers	6 items/ historical focus	Self-report questionnaire. Ideal for busy primary care clinics. Available in multiple languages	Garg et al. (2015)
Substance use	Alcohol, smoking, and substance involvement screening test for youth (ASSIST-Y)	Ages 10–17	6 items for age 10–14; 7 items for age 15–17/ historical and past 3 months	Clinician administered. Can help with determining if further diagnostic assessment is needed due to risk severity	Humeniuk et al. (2016)
	Alcohol use identification test (AUDIT)	Individuals age 14+	10 items/past 12 months	Self-report scale. This is the most widely used screener for detecting risky drinking patterns. Can be administered via paper or electronically	Saunders et al. (1993)

(continued)

Table 4.2 (continued)

Diagnosis	Name	Target population	Length/time frame	Special considerations	References
	Car, relax, alone, forget, family, friends, trouble (CRAFFT 2.1 + N)	Ages 12–21	4 item screener; past 12 months	Clinician administered or self-report. Focus is on alcohol, drugs, and nicotine. Additional follow-up questions provided with a positive screen. Can be administered via paper or virtually. Available in multiple languages	Knight et al. (1999)
	NIAAA two question screener	Ages 9–11; 11–14; 14–18	2 item screener/past year and historical	Clinician administered. Three separate age groups dictate the questions asked. Results yield an action plan for clinician. Available in multiple languages	National Institute on Alcohol Abuse and Alcoholism (NIAAA) (n.d.)
	Tobacco, alcohol, prescription medication, and other substance use (TAPS-1)	Age 12+	4-items/past year and past 3 months	Self- or clinician administered. Feasible in busy primary care clinics due to brevity; if patient screens positive, there is the option for further assessment of risk included (TAPS-2)	McNeely et al. (2016)

(continued)

Table 4.2 (continued)

Diagnosis	Name	Target population	Length/time frame	Special considerations	References
Suicide risk	Columbia suicide severity rating scale—Screen version (C-SSRS)	Individuals age 6+	5 items/last month	Clinician administered; assesses suicidal ideation over past several months. Scoring yields recommendation for clinical action. Available in multiple languages	Posner et al. (2011)
	Columbia suicide severity rating scale for very young children	Preschoolers (4–5)	5 items/last month	Clinician administered. This can be used with people who are cognitively impaired. Scoring yields recommendation for clinical action	Posner et al. (2011)
Trauma	Child and adolescent trauma screen (CATS)	Children ages 3–17	15 items assessing historical traumatic events; 20 items assessing DSM-5 PTSD criteria; 5 items assessing psychosocial functioning in the past 2 weeks	Caregiver reports for children ages 3–6 and 7–17; self-report for children ages 7–17. Available in multiple languages	Sachser et al. (2017)

Organization-Specific Screening Practices

United States Preventive Services Task Force (USPSTF) and American Academy of Family Physicians (AAFP) The USPSTF originally convened in 1984 and has since aimed to provide comprehensive and evidence-based recommendations for various screening measures, preventative medications, and behavioral counseling for PCPs (United States Preventive Services Task Force, n.d.). USPSTF recommendations for screening are based upon systematic reviews of evidence related to various conditions in order to make conclusions about the benefits and/or harms of different preventative services (United States Preventive Services Task Force, n.d.). For any given disorder, the USPSTF assigns a letter grade (A, B, C, D, or I) to describe the strength of the screening recommendation (see United States Preventive Services Task Force (2018) for grade definitions). For our purposes, we include screening recommendations for BH conditions that are either Strongly Recommended (Grade A) or Recommended (Grade B); related screening recommendations that are rated as Insufficient are included as well (Grade I). Notably, most other major medical organizations typically follow screening guidelines made by the USPSTF (i.e., AAFP, ACOG, AAP). In fact, the AAFP is almost entirely aligned with the USPSTF, except for screening for unhealthy drug use. Organization-specific exceptions to USPSTF guidelines will be noted below in Table 4.3.

Table 4.3 USPSTF & AAFP screening guidelines for adults

Condition	Screening recommendation	Special considerations	References
Alcohol use	All adults aged 18+ including pregnant and postpartum persons (grade B).	No specific guidelines for screening intervals. Do not avoid screening with adolescents if there are current or suspected diagnoses of a substance use disorder. Utilize clinical judgment	O'Connor et al. (2018)
Anxiety	All adults aged 64 years and younger, including pregnant and postpartum persons (grade B).	No specific guidelines for screening intervals; use clinical judgment and assessment of individual patient risk factors	O'Connor et al. (2023a)
Depression	All adults aged 19+, including pregnant and postpartum persons (grade B).	No specific guidelines for screening intervals; use clinical judgment and assessment of individual patient risk factors	O'Connor et al. (2023b)

(continued)

Table 4.3 (continued)

Condition	Screening recommendation	Special considerations	References
Unhealthy drug use[a]	All adults aged 18+ including pregnant and postpartum persons (grade B)	No specific guidelines for screening intervals. Screening should only occur if accurate diagnosis, treatment, and appropriate care can be offered or referred. Utilize clinical judgment	Patnode et al. (2020)
Intimate partner violence (IPV)	All women of reproductive age (including adolescents and women in their 40 s; grade B). Insufficient evidence to suggest screening with older or vulnerable adults (grade I)	No specific guidelines for screening intervals; use clinical judgment and assessment of individual patient risk factors	Curry et al. (2018)
Suicide risk	Insufficient evidence to suggest separate screening for suicide risk with adults, including pregnant and postpartum persons and older adults (grade I)	Many depression screeners include items that assess suicidality, which still yield useful information; always consider individual patient risk factors and clinical judgment when determining whether to screen for suicidal risk	O'Connor et al. (2023b)
Tobacco use	All adults aged 18+ including pregnant and postpartum persons (grade A)	No specific guidelines for screening intervals. Do not avoid screening with adolescents if there are current or suspected diagnoses of a substance use disorder. Utilize clinical judgment	Patnode et al. (2021)

[a] The AAFP differs from the USPSTF regarding screening recommendations for drug use. The AAFP declared that the evidence is insufficient to suggest screening adolescents and adults for unhealthy drug use, except for suspected opioid use. The AAFP recommends that clinicians selectively screen adults 18+ for opioid abuse if effective treatment and psychosocial supports can be offered (Grade C; American Academy of Family Physicians, n.d.)

American College of Obstetricians and Gynecologists (ACOG) As with the USPSTF and the AAFP, ACOG has specific recommendations for various screening practices, including BH screening for perinatal individuals and those receiving well-woman services (many of which are aligned with USPSTF recommendations). Recommendations are based off the strength and quality of existing evidence for each respective diagnosis. ACOG provides recommendations either strongly for or against specific practices as well as conditional recommendations that are based on individual patient characteristics. ACOG also provides a rating for the quality of evidence (high, moderate, low, very low). ACOG notes "good practice points" when given a recommendation based off limited or non-existent evidence. Aside from recommended screening practices, ACOG has published committee opinions regarding the screening of tobacco, drug, and alcohol use as well as sexual assault history. Screening recommendations for ACOG are listed in Table 4.4. See the ACOG Practice Guideline Number 4 for more specific details about behavioral health screening (American College of Obstetricians and Gynecologists, 2023).

Table 4.4 ACOG screening guidelines

Condition	Screening recommendation	Special considerations	References
Alcohol use	All individuals seeking obstetric-gynecologic care should be screened at least yearly and within the first trimester of pregnancy	Screening for alcohol use at the initial prenatal visit is recommended; continued screening should be based on clinical judgment	American College of Obstetricians and Gynecologists (2011)
Anxiety	All individuals receiving well-woman, pre-pregnancy, prenatal, and postpartum care (strong recommendation)	Screening for perinatal anxiety should occur at the initial prenatal visit, near or in the third trimester, and at postpartum visits	American College of Obstetricians and Gynecologists (2023)
Depression	All individuals receiving well-woman, pre-pregnancy, prenatal, and postpartum care (strong recommendation)	Screening for perinatal depression should occur at the initial prenatal visit, near or in the third trimester, and at postpartum visits	American College of Obstetricians and Gynecologists (2023)
Drug use	Universal screening is recommended regardless of if there is an absence, or presence, of certain risk factors (e.g., adherence to prenatal care, race, age, co-occurring conditions)	Screening for substance use should occur at the initial prenatal visit. Providers should consider ethical and legal considerations when screening for substances	American College of Obstetricians and Gynecologists (2012)
Perinatal bipolar disorder	All individuals receiving prenatal and postpartum care (conditional recommendation, depending on patient risk factors)	Screening for bipolar disorder should happen in tandem with other screening measures at least at the initial prenatal visit. Individuals should be screened for bipolar disorder before initiating pharmacotherapy for anxiety and/or depression	American College of Obstetricians and Gynecologists (2023)

(continued)

Table 4.4 (continued)

Condition	Screening recommendation	Special considerations	References
Perinatal suicide risk	All individuals who affirmatively endorse a self-harm or suicide risk question (either by screener or discussion) should complete a full suicide risk assessment (strong recommendation)	No specific guidelines for screening intervals, though questions regarding suicide risk are typically included in depression screeners	American College of Obstetricians and Gynecologists (2023)
Postpartum psychosis	Universal screening is not recommended due to the rarity of the diagnosis; however, providers should be aware of patient risk factors and should use clinical judgment	Clinicians should provide immediate medical attention for postpartum psychosis (strong recommendation)	American College of Obstetricians and Gynecologists (2023)
Sexual assault	All individuals seeking obstetric-gynecologic care should be screened for sexual assault history	Additional screening for symptoms of PTSD and substance use should also be considered with an affirmative history	American College of Obstetricians and Gynecologists (2019)
Tobacco use	Universal screening is recommended for women during the pre-pregnancy, pregnancy, and postpartum periods	Screening for tobacco use at the initial prenatal visit is recommended; continued screening should be based on clinical judgment	American College of Obstetricians and Gynecologists (2020)

American Academy of Pediatrics (AAP) The AAP along with Bright Futures published the *Bright Futures Guidelines, Fourth Edition* for providers regarding overall best practices with the pediatric population, including recommendations for comprehensive screening practices for children and adolescents ranging from birth to age 21 (Hagan Jr. et al., 2017). For detailed descriptions and recommendations, please see Hagan Jr. et al. (2017). Notably, the guidelines include Grade A and Grade B recommendations made by the USPSTF, recommendations endorsed by the Centers for Disease Control and Prevention (CDC) Community Guide, and other services endorsed by the AAP. For the purposes of this chapter, specific neurodevelopmental and BH recommendations made by the AAP, along with other commonly presenting concerns, are included in Table 4.5.

Table 4.5 AAP screening guidelines

Condition	Screening Recommendation	Special Considerations	Reference
Alcohol use	No formal recommendation to specifically screen for alcohol use with children due to insufficient evidence. Universal screening is recommended from age 11 through 21 at each well-child visit or unless otherwise indicated. AAP suggests increased screening efforts (i.e., SBIRT) with adolescents	Providers should use clinical judgment and individual patient risk factors when deciding whether or not to screen for alcohol use	Committee on Substance Use and Prevention (2016), Hagan Jr. et al. (2017)
Anxiety	Universal screening for anxiety for children ages 8–18. At each well-child visit or unless otherwise indicated	Screening should consider including social determinants of health, racism, poverty, and relationships, which may be contributing to anxiety	O'Connor et al. (2023a)
Attention-deficit/ hyperactivity disorder (ADHD)	From age 4 to age 18, children presenting with academic or behavioral problems and symptoms of inattention, hyperactivity, or impulsivity should be screened for ADHD	Providers should concurrently screen for other comorbid conditions (e.g., anxiety, depression, oppositional defiant disorder, language disorders, autism spectrum disorder, sleep apnea) to help with diagnostic certainty	Wolraich et al. (2019)
Autism Spectrum disorder (ASD)	Universal screening for ASD at the child's 18-month and 2-year well-child visit	ASD screening should be administered in conjunction with other regular developmental and social/emotional/ behavioral screeners	Council on Children With Disabilities, Section on Developmental Behavioral Pediatrics, Bright Futures Steering Committee,, and Medical Home Initiatives for Children With Special Needs Project Advisory Committee (2006)

(continued)

Table 4.5 (continued)

Condition	Screening Recommendation	Special Considerations	Reference
Depression	Universal screening for children aged 12+ at each well-child visit or unless otherwise indicated	It is also recommended that maternal depression screening be completed from 1-month of age up to 6-months of age	United States Preventative Services Task Force (2016)
Unhealthy drug use	No formal recommendation to specifically screen for drug use with children due to insufficient evidence. Universal screening is recommended from age 11 through 21 at each well-child visit or unless otherwise indicated. AAP suggests increased screening efforts (i.e., SBIRT) with adolescents	Providers should use clinical judgment and individual patient risk factors when deciding whether to screen for drug use	Committee on Substance Use and Prevention (2016), Hagan Jr. et al. (2017)
Social determinants of health (SDoH)	Social determinants of health should be screened with every patient encounter	Clinicians should consider how SDoH are documented in the patient's chart so that patients are protected from unnecessary involvement of outside agencies (e.g., child protective services)	Council on Children With Disabilities, Section on Developmental Behavioral Pediatrics, Bright Futures Steering Committee,, and Medical Home Initiatives for Children With Special Needs Project Advisory Committee (2006)
Specific learning disorders	No formal recommendation to specifically screen for learning disorders; however, broadband universal screening of developmental trajectory should occur at well-child visits	If a patient presents with academic underachievement concerns, providers are encouraged to complete a medical exam consisting of history (grades, school supports, risk factors), physical exam (dermatologic, neurologic, dysmorphology, growth parameters, handwriting, sensorium). Refer for psychosocial evaluation as needed	Curtin et al. (2019)

(continued)

Table 4.5 (continued)

Condition	Screening Recommendation	Special Considerations	Reference
Speech and language	No formal recommendation to specifically screen for speech and language concerns due to insufficient evidence; however, broadband universal screening should occur at 9-month, 18-month, and 2.5-year well-child visits, or as otherwise indicated	Regular screening at well-child visits should help to identify speech and language concerns early so that appropriate referrals for intervention can be made	Council on Children With Disabilities, Section on Developmental Behavioral Pediatrics, Bright Futures Steering Committee,, and Medical Home Initiatives for Children With Special Needs Project Advisory Committee (2006)
Suicide risk	Universal screening for all children aged 12+ at well-child visits unless otherwise indicated	Screening interval is up to clinical judgment, though typically no more than once a month and at least 1 year	American Academy of Pediatrics (n.d.)
Tobacco use	Providers should focus efforts to prevent tobacco use initiation and provide anticipatory guidance by the age of 5. Universal screening is recommended from age 11 through 21 at each well-child visit or unless otherwise indicated. AAP suggests increased screening efforts (i.e., SBIRT) with adolescents	As part of broadband screening, exposure to secondhand smoke should also be assessed	Committee on Substance Use and Prevention (2016), Hagan Jr. et al. (2017)

Key Points

- BH screening is a crucial step in early symptom identification and management but cannot be used alone. Screening in conjunction with a collaborative plan with the patient is the goal.
- BH screening is an important factor in overall patient health improvement and patient satisfaction.
- There are multiple time-saving ways to implement BH screening within the primary care clinic, if done thoughtfully and with consideration to clinic flow, patient characteristics, and screeners chosen.

- PCPs should ensure that screeners used are psychometrically valid and reliable.
- When in doubt, refer to your specific medical organization (e.g., AAP, AAFP, ACOG) for screening guidelines.

References

Aggarwal, S., Taljard, L., Wilson, Z., & Berk, M. (2017). Evaluation of modified patient health Questionnaire-9 teen in South African adolescents. *Indian Journal of Psychological Medicine, 39*(2), 143–145. https://doi.org/10.4103/0253-7176.203124

American Academy of Family Physicians. (n.d.). *Opioid use disorder screening*. https://www.aafp.org/family-physician/patient-care/clinical-recommendations/all-clinical-recommendations/oud.html

American Academy of Pediatrics. (n.d.). *Suicide: Blueprint for youth suicide prevention*. https://www.aap.org/en/patient-care/blueprint-for-youth-suicide-prevention/

American College of Obstetricians and Gynecologists. (2011). Committee opinion no. 496: At-risk drinking and alcohol dependence: Obstetric and gynecologic implications. *Obstetrics & Gynecology, 118*(2), 383. https://doi.org/10.1097/AOG.0b013e31822c9906

American College of Obstetricians and Gynecologists. (2012). Committee Opinion No. 524: Opioid abuse, dependence, and addiction in pregnancy. *Obstetrics & Gynecology, 119*(5), 1070. https://doi.org/10.1097/AOG.0b013e318256496e

American College of Obstetricians and Gynecologists. (2019). ACOG Committee opinion no. 777: Sexual assault. *Obstetrics & Gynecology, 133*(4), e296. https://doi.org/10.1097/AOG.0000000000003178

American College of Obstetricians and Gynecologists. (2020). Tobacco and nicotine cessation during pregnancy: ACOG committee opinion, number 807. *Obstetrics & Gynecology, 135*(5), e221–e229. https://doi.org/10.1097/AOG.0000000000003822

American College of Obstetricians and Gynecologists. (2023). Screening and diagnosis of mental health conditions during pregnancy and postpartum: ACOG clinical practice guideline no. 4. *Obstetrics & Gynecology, 141*(6), 1232. https://doi.org/10.1097/AOG.0000000000005200

Ashman, J. J., Rui, P., & Okeyode, T. (2019). Characteristics of office-based physician visits, 2016. https://stacks.cdc.gov/view/cdc/62369

Bastien, C. H., Vallières, A., & Morin, C. M. (2001). Validation of the insomnia severity index as an outcome measure for insomnia research. *Sleep Medicine, 2*(4), 297–307. https://doi.org/10.1016/S1389-9457(00)00065-4

Biel, M. G., Tang, M. H., & Zuckerman, B. (2020). Pediatric mental health care must be family mental health care. *JAMA Pediatrics, 174*(6), 519–520. https://doi.org/10.1001/jamapediatrics.2020.0065

Birmaher, B., Brent, D. A., Chiappetta, L., Bridge, J., Monga, S., & Baugher, M. (1999). Psychometric properties of the screen for child anxiety related emotional disorders (SCARED): A replication study. *Journal of the American Academy of Child & Adolescent Psychiatry, 38*(10), 1230–1236. https://doi.org/10.1097/00004583-199910000-00011

Birmaher, B., Khetarpal, S., Brent, D., Cully, M., Balach, L., Kaufman, J., & Neer, S. M. (1997). The screen for child anxiety related emotional disorders (SCARED): Scale construction and psychometric characteristics. *Journal of the American Academy of Child & Adolescent Psychiatry, 36*(4), 545–553. https://doi.org/10.1097/00004583-199704000-00018

Committee on Substance Use and Prevention. (2016). Substance use screening, brief intervention, and referral to treatment. *Pediatrics, 138*(1), e20161210. https://doi.org/10.1542/peds.2016-1210

Council on Children With Disabilities, Section on Developmental Behavioral Pediatrics, Bright Futures Steering Committee, & Medical Home Initiatives for Children With Special Needs Project Advisory Committee. (2006). Identifying infants and young children with developmental disorders in the medical home: An algorithm for developmental surveillance and screening. *Pediatrics, 118*(1), 405–420. https://doi.org/10.1542/peds.2006-1231

Cox, J. L., Holden, J. M., & Sagovsky, R. (1987). Detection of postnatal depression: Development of the 10-item Edinburgh postnatal depression scale. *The British Journal of Psychiatry, 150*(6), 782–786. https://doi.org/10.1192/bjp.150.6.782

Curry, S. J., Krist, A. H., Owens, D. K., Barry, M. J., Caughey, A. B., Davidson, K. W., Doubeni, C. A., Epling, J. W., Jr., Kemper, A. R., Kubik, M., Kurth, A., Landefeld, S., Mangione, C. M., Silverstein, M., Simon, M. A., Tseng, C.-W., & Wong, J. B. (2018). Screening for intimate partner violence, elder abuse, and abuse of vulnerable adults: US preventive services task force final recommendation statement. *JAMA, 320*(16), 1678–1687. https://doi.org/10.1001/jama.2018.14741

Curtin, M. J., Willis, D. R., & Enneking, B. (2019). Specific learning disabilities: The family physician's role. *American Family Physician, 100*(10), 628–635.

Drake, E., & Valenstein, M. (2021). *Behavioral health integration into primary care.* https://edhub.ama-assn.org/steps-forward/module/2782794

Faulstich, M. E., Carey, M. P., Ruggiero, L., Enyart, P., & Gresham, F. (1986). Assessment of depression in childhood and adolescence: An evaluation of the Center for Epidemiological Studies Depression Scale for children (CES-DC). *American Journal of Psychiatry, 143*(8), 1024–1027. https://doi.org/10.1176/ajp.143.8.1024

Gardner, W., Murphy, M., Childs, G., Kelleher, K., Pagano, M., Jellinek, M., McInerny, T., Wasserman, R., Nutting, P., & Chiappetta, L. (1999). The PSC-17: A brief pediatric symptom checklist with psychosocial problem subscales. *Ambulatory Child Health, 5*(3), 225–236.

Garg, A., Toy, S., Tripodis, Y., Silverstein, M., & Freeman, E. (2015). Addressing social determinants of health at well child care visits: A cluster RCT. *Pediatrics, 135*(2), e296–e304. https://doi.org/10.1542/peds.2014-2888

Hagan, J. F., Jr., Shaw, J. S., Duncan, P. M., & American Academy of Pediatrics. (2017). *Bright futures guidelines for health supervision of infants, children, and adolescents* (4th ed.). American Academy of Pediatrics. https://publications.aap.org/aapbooks/monograph/478/Bright-Futures-Guidelines-for-Health-Supervision

Harrison, P. A., & Sidebottom, A. C. (2008). Systematic prenatal screening for psychosocial risks. *Journal of Health Care for the Poor and Underserved, 19*(1), 258–276.

Hine, C. E., Howell, H. B., & Yonkers, K. A. (2008). Integration of medical and psychological treatment within the primary health care setting. *Social Work in Health Care, 47*(2), 122–134. https://doi.org/10.1080/00981380801970244

Hirschfeld, R. M. A. (2002). The mood disorder questionnaire: A simple, patient-rated screening instrument for bipolar disorder. *The Primary Care Companion for CNS Disorders, 4*(1), 25565. https://doi.org/10.4088/PCC.v04n0104

Horowitz, L. M., Snyder, D. J., Boudreaux, E. D., He, J.-P., Harrington, C. J., Cai, J., Claassen, C. A., Salhany, J. E., Dao, T., Chaves, J. F., Jobes, D. A., Merikangas, K. R., Bridge, J. A., & Pao, M. (2020). *Validation of the ask suicide-screening questions for adult medical inpatients: A brief tool for all ages.* ClinicalKey. https://www.clinicalkey.com/#!/content/playContent/1-s2.0-S0033318220301201?returnurl=https:%2F%2Flinkinghub.elsevier.com%2Fretrieve%2Fpii%2FS0033318220301201%3Fshowall%3Dtrue&referrer=

Humeniuk, R., Holmwood, C., Beshara, M., & Kambala, A. (2016). ASSIST-Y V1.0: First-stage development of the WHO alcohol, smoking and substance involvement screening test (ASSIST) and linked brief intervention for young people. *Journal of Child & Adolescent Substance Abuse, 25*(4), 384–390. https://doi.org/10.1080/1067828X.2015.1049395

Humeniuk, R. E., Henry-Edwards, S., Ali, R. L., Poznyak, V., & Monteiro, M. (2010). *The alcohol, smoking and substance involvement screening test (ASSIST).* https://www.who.int/publications/i/item/978924159938-2

Iverson, K. M., King, M. W., Gerber, M. R., Resick, P. A., Kimerling, R., Street, A. E., & Vogt, D. (2015). Accuracy of an intimate partner violence screening tool for female VHA patients: A replication and extension. *Journal of Traumatic Stress, 28*(1), 79–82. https://doi.org/10.1002/jts.21985

Juhnke, G. A. (1996). The adapted-sad persons: A suicide assessment scale designed for use with children. *Elementary School Guidance and Counseling, 30*(4), 252–258.

Kazak, A. E., Nash, J. M., Hiroto, K., & Kaslow, N. J. (2017). Psychologists in patient-centered medical homes (PCMHs): Roles, evidence, opportunities, and challenges. *American Psychologist, 72*(1), 1–12. https://doi.org/10.1037/a0040382

Kessler, R. (2012). Mental health care treatment initiation when mental health services are incorporated into primary care practice. *The Journal of the American Board of Family Medicine, 25*(2), 255–259. https://doi.org/10.3122/jabfm.2012.02.100125

Knight, J. R., Shrier, L. A., Bravender, T. D., Farrell, M., Vander Bilt, J., & Shaffer, H. J. (1999). A new brief screen for adolescent substance abuse. *Archives of Pediatrics & Adolescent Medicine, 153*(6), 591–596. https://doi.org/10.1001/archpedi.153.6.591

Kraepelien, M., Blom, K., Forsell, E., Hentati Isacsson, N., Bjurner, P., Morin, C. M., Jernelöv, S., & Kaldo, V. (2021). A very brief self-report scale for measuring insomnia severity using two items from the insomnia severity index—Development and validation in a clinical population. *Sleep Medicine, 81*, 365–374. https://doi.org/10.1016/j.sleep.2021.03.003

Kroenke, K., Spitzer, R. L., & Williams, J. B. W. (1999). *Patient health questionnaire-9*. APA PsycTests. https://doi.org/10.1037/t06165-000

Kroenke, K., Spitzer, R. L., Williams, J. B. W., Monahan, P. O., & Löwe, B. (2007). Anxiety disorders in primary care: Prevalence, impairment, comorbidity, and detection. *Annals of Internal Medicine, 146*(5), 317–325. https://doi.org/10.7326/0003-4819-146-5-200703060-00004

McNeely, J., Wu, L.-T., Subramaniam, G., Sharma, G., Cathers, L. A., Svikis, D., Sleiter, L., Russell, L., Nordeck, C., Sharma, A., O'Grady, K. E., Bouk, L. B., Cushing, C., King, J., Wahle, A., & Schwartz, R. P. (2016). Performance of the tobacco, alcohol, prescription medication, and other substance use (TAPS) tool for substance use screening in primary care patients. *Annals of Internal Medicine, 165*(10), 690–699. https://doi.org/10.7326/M16-0317

Mueller, A. E., Segal, D. L., Gavett, B., Marty, M. A., Yochim, B., June, A., & Coolidge, F. L. (2015). Geriatric anxiety scale: Item response theory analysis, differential item functioning, and creation of a ten-item short form (GAS-10). *International Psychogeriatrics, 27*(7), 1099–1111. https://doi.org/10.1017/S1041610214000210

Mulvaney-Day, N., Marshall, T., Downey Piscopo, K., Korsen, N., Lynch, S., Karnell, L. H., Moran, G. E., Daniels, A. S., & Ghose, S. S. (2018). Screening for behavioral health conditions in primary care settings: A systematic review of the literature. *Journal of General Internal Medicine, 33*(3), 335–346. https://doi.org/10.1007/s11606-017-4181-0

National Alliance on Mental Illness. (2023). *Mental health by the numbers. NAMI*. https://www.nami.org/about-mental-illness/mental-health-by-the-numbers/.

National Association of Community Health Centers. (2016). Protocol for responding to and assessing patients' assets, risks, and experiences (PRAPARE). https://prapare.org/wp-content/uploads/2024/04/PRAPARE-English.pdf

National Institute on Alcohol Abuse and Alcoholism (NIAAA). (n.d.). *Alcohol screening and brief intervention for youth: A practitioner's guide*. Retrieved October 14, 2024, from https://www.niaaa.nih.gov/alcohols-effects-health/professional-education-materials/alcohol-screening-and-brief-intervention-youth-practitioners-guide

National Institute on Drug Abuse (NIDA). (n.d.). *NIDA quick screen V1.0F*. Retrieved September 18, 2024, from https://nida.nih.gov/sites/default/files/pdf/nmassist.pdf

O'Connor, E., Henninger, M., Perdue, L. A., Coppola, E. L., Thomas, R., & Gaynes, B. N. (2023b). *Screening for depression, anxiety, and suicide risk in adults: A systematic evidence review for the U.S. Preventive Services Task Force*. Agency for Healthcare Research and Quality (US). http://www.ncbi.nlm.nih.gov/books/NBK592805/

O'Connor, E. A., Henninger, M. L., Perdue, L. A., Coppola, E. L., Thomas, R. G., & Gaynes, B. N. (2023a). Anxiety screening: Evidence report and systematic review for the US preventive services task force. *JAMA, 329*(24), 2171–2184. https://doi.org/10.1001/jama.2023.6369

O'Connor, E. A., Perdue, L. A., Senger, C. A., Rushkin, M., Patnode, C. D., Bean, S. I., & Jonas, D. E. (2018). Screening and behavioral counseling interventions to reduce unhealthy alcohol use in adolescents and adults: Updated evidence report and systematic review for the US preventive services task force. *JAMA, 320*(18), 1910–1928. https://doi.org/10.1001/jama.2018.12086

Ogundele, M. O., & Morton, M. (2022). Classification, prevalence and integrated care for neurodevelopmental and child mental health disorders: A brief overview for paediatricians. *World Journal of Clinical Pediatrics, 11*(2), 120–135. https://doi.org/10.5409/wjcp.v11.i2.120

Owens, J. A., & Dalzell, V. (2005). Use of the 'BEARS' sleep screening tool in a pediatric residents' continuity clinic: A pilot study. *Sleep Medicine, 6*(1), 63–69. https://doi.org/10.1016/j.sleep.2004.07.015

Patnode, C. D., Henderson, J. T., Melnikow, J., Coppola, E. L., Durbin, S., & Thomas, R. (2021). *Interventions for tobacco cessation in adults, including pregnant women: An evidence update for the U.S. Preventive Services Task Force.* Agency for Healthcare Research and Quality (US). http://www.ncbi.nlm.nih.gov/books/NBK567066/

Patnode, C. D., Perdue, L. A., Rushkin, M., & O'Connor, E. A. (2020). *Screening for unhealthy drug use in primary care in adolescents and adults, including pregnant persons: Updated systematic review for the U.S. Preventive Services Task Force.* Agency for Healthcare Research and Quality (US). http://www.ncbi.nlm.nih.gov/books/NBK558174/

Patterson, W. M., Dohn, H. H., Bird, J., & Patterson, G. A. (1983). Evaluation of suicidal patients: The SAD PERSONS scale. *Psychosomatics, 24*(4), 343–349. https://doi.org/10.1016/S0033-3182(83)73213-5

Petterson, S., Miller, B. F., Payne-Murphy, J. C., & Phillips, R. L., Jr. (2014). Mental health treatment in the primary care setting: Patterns and pathways. *Families, Systems & Health, 32*(2), 157–166. https://doi.org/10.1037/fsh0000036

Posner, K., Brown, G. K., Stanley, B., Brent, D. A., Yershova, K. V., Oquendo, M. A., Currier, G. W., Melvin, G. A., Greenhill, L., Shen, S., & Mann, J. J. (2011). The Columbia–Suicide Severity Rating Scale: Initial validity and internal consistency findings from three multisite studies with adolescents and adults. *American Journal of Psychiatry, 168*(12), 1266–1277. https://doi.org/10.1176/appi.ajp.2011.10111704

Prins, A., Bovin, M. J., Smolenski, D. J., Marx, B. P., Kimerling, R., Jenkins-Guarnieri, M. A., Kaloupek, D. G., Schnurr, P. P., Kaiser, A. P., Leyva, Y. E., & Tiet, Q. Q. (2016). The primary care PTSD screen for DSM-5 (PC-PTSD-5): Development and evaluation within a veteran primary care sample. *Journal of General Internal Medicine, 31*(10), 1206–1211. https://doi.org/10.1007/s11606-016-3703-5

Radloff, L. S. (1977). The CES-D scale: A self-report depression scale for research in the general population. *Applied Psychological Measurement, 1*(3), 385–401. https://doi.org/10.1177/014662167700100306

Reppeto, H., Tuning, C., Olsen, D. H., Mullane, A., & Smith, C. (2021). Triple aim: Benefits of behavioral health providers in primary care. *Journal of Health Psychology, 26*(2), 205–213. https://doi.org/10.1177/1359105318802949

Robins, D. L., Barton, M., & Fein, D. (2018). *Modified checklist for autism in toddlers, revised with follow-up.* https://southcountypediatrics.wustl.edu/files/2024/09/M-CHAT-R_F_Rev_Aug2018.pdf

Rogers, R., Hartigan, S. E., & Sanders, C. E. (2021). Identifying mental disorders in primary care: Diagnostic accuracy of the connected mind fast check (CMFC) electronic screen. *Journal of Clinical Psychology in Medical Settings, 28*(4), 882–896. https://doi.org/10.1007/s10880-021-09820-1

Russell, M. (1994). New assessment tools for risk drinking during pregnancy: T-ACE, TWEAK, and others. *Alcohol Health and Research World, 18*(1), 55–61.

Sachser, C., Berliner, L., Holt, T., Jensen, T. K., Jungbluth, N., Risch, E., Rosner, R., & Goldbeck, L. (2017). International development and psychometric properties of the child and adolescent trauma screen (CATS). *Journal of Affective Disorders, 210*, 189–195. https://doi.org/10.1016/j.jad.2016.12.040

Salinas, A., Crenshaw, J. T., Gilder, R. E., & Gray, G. (2023). Implementing the evidence: Routine screening for depression and anxiety in primary care. *Journal of American College Health, 72*(8), 2893–2898. https://doi.org/10.1080/07448481.2022.2138406

Saunders, J. B., Aasland, O. G., Babor, T. F., De La Fuente, J. R., & Grant, M. (1993). Development of the alcohol use disorders identification test (AUDIT): WHO collaborative project on early detection of persons with harmful alcohol consumption-ii. *Addiction, 88*(6), 791–804. https://doi.org/10.1111/j.1360-0443.1993.tb02093.x

Sayre, M., Lapham, G. T., Lee, A. K., Oliver, M., Bobb, J. F., Caldeiro, R. M., & Bradley, K. A. (2020). Routine assessment of symptoms of substance use disorders in primary care: prevalence and severity of reported symptoms. *Journal of General Internal Medicine, 35*(4), 1111–1119. https://doi.org/10.1007/s11606-020-05650-3

Segal, D. L., June, A., Payne, M., Coolidge, F. L., & Yochim, B. (2010). Development and initial validation of a self-report assessment tool for anxiety among older adults: The geriatric anxiety scale. *Journal of Anxiety Disorders, 24*(7), 709–714. https://doi.org/10.1016/j.janxdis.2010.05.002

Sheikh, J. I., & Yesavage, J. A. (1986). 9/geriatric depression scale (GDS): Recent evidence and development of a shorter version. *Clinical Gerontologist, 5*(1–2), 165–173. https://doi.org/10.1300/J018v05n01_09

Smith, C. J., Pollard, E., Stein, A. J., Ober-Reynolds, S., Kirwan, J., Malligo, A., Matthews, N. L., Openden, D., & Melmed, R. D. (2015). A method for universal screening of elementary school students: Development of the social challenges screening questionnaire. *Journal of Applied School Psychology, 31*(2), 115–140. https://doi.org/10.1080/15377903.2014.995391

Sohal, H., Eldridge, S., & Feder, G. (2007). The sensitivity and specificity of four questions (HARK) to identify intimate partner violence: A diagnostic accuracy study in general practice. *BMC Family Practice, 8*(1), 49. https://doi.org/10.1186/1471-2296-8-49

Spitzer, R. L., Kroenke, K., Williams, J. B. W., & Löwe, B. (2006). *Generalized anxiety disorder 7*. APA PsycTests. https://doi.org/10.1037/t02591-000

Sun, J., McPhillips, M. V., Chen, K.-C., Zang, Y., Li, J., Oehlke, J., Brewster, G. S., & Gooneratne, N. S. (2021). Primary care provider evaluation and management of insomnia. *Journal of Clinical Sleep Medicine, 17*(5), 1083–1091. https://doi.org/10.5664/jcsm.9154

Thielke, S., Vannoy, S., & Unützer, J. (2007). Integrating mental health and primary care. *Primary Care; Clinics in Office Practice, 34*(3), 571–592. https://doi.org/10.1016/j.pop.2007.05.007

United States Preventative Services Task Force. (2016). Screening for depression in children and adolescents: U.S. preventive services task force recommendation statement. *Annals of Internal Medicine, 164*(5), 360. https://www.acpjournals.org/doi/full/10.7326/M15-2957?journalCode=aim

United States Preventive Services Task Force. (2018). *Grade definitions | United States preventive services taskforce*. https://www.uspreventiveservicestaskforce.org/uspstf/about-uspstf/methods-and-processes/grade-definitions.

United States Preventive Services Task Force. (n.d.). *Task Force at a glance | United States Preventive Services Taskforce*. https://www.uspreventiveservicestaskforce.org/uspstf/about-uspstf/task-force-at-a-glance

Wolraich, M. L., Hagan, J. F., Jr., Allan, C., Chan, E., Davison, D., Earls, M., Evans, S. W., Flinn, S. K., Froehlich, T., Frost, J., Holbrook, J. R., Lehmann, C. U., Lessin, H. R., Okechukwu, K., Pierce, K. L., Winner, J. D., & Zurhellen, W. (2019). Clinical practice guideline for the diagnosis, evaluation, and treatment of attention-deficit/hyperactivity disorder in children and adolescents. *Pediatrics, 144*(4), e20192528. https://doi.org/10.1542/peds.2019-2528

Wolraich, M. L., Lambert, W., Doffing, M. A., Bickman, L., Simmons, T., & Worley, K. (2003). Psychometric properties of the Vanderbilt ADHD diagnostic parent rating scale in a referred population. *Journal of Pediatric Psychology, 28*(8), 559–568. https://doi.org/10.1093/jpepsy/jsg046

Chapter 5
Risk Assessment for the Primary Care Provider

Kaylee Jackson PhD, Mariah Montgomery PhD, Brandon Williamson MD, FAAFP, and Katelin Dias PhD

Primary care offices are one of the primary points of contact for patients with suicidal ideation (SI), homicidal ideation (HI), nonsuicidal self-injury (NSSI), and abuse or neglect (Ahmedani et al., 2014; Olfson et al., 2014). These appointments with patients are frequently unexpected, unplanned, and, at times, disruptive to the PCP's schedule. Appointments just before lunch or before the clinic closes are common and add time pressure. The availability of support staff (behavioral health (BH), nursing) and additional outpatient resources are often limited. The convergence of potential patient acuity and practice constraints necessitates a protocolized approach to assessing and managing these patients in the office (Brodsky et al., 2018; Spottswood et al., 2022). Education on risk management, developing clear protocols for staff involved, and utilization of BH integration when available can help PCPs better manage at-risk patients under their care (Spottswood et al., 2022).

Prevalence of Self-Directed Violence

Suicide is one of the leading causes of death in the United States. The 2022 National Survey on Drug Use and Health found that among US adults, 5.2% (13.2 million people) had serious thoughts of suicide, and 0.6% (1.6 million people) attempted suicide (Substance Abuse and Mental Health Services Administration, 2022). For youth aged 12–17, 13.4% (3.4 million people) reported serious thoughts of suicide, and 3.7% (1.7 million people) attempted suicide (Centers for Disease Control and

K. Jackson PhD (✉) · B. Williamson MD, FAAFP · K. Dias PhD
Naresh K. Vashisht College of Medicine, Department of Primary Care and Rural Medicine, Texas A&M University, Bryan, TX, USA
e-mail: kayleejanae@tamu.edu

M. Montgomery PhD
Dell Medical School, University of Texas at Austin, Austin, TX, USA

M. L. C. Williamson and D. L. Terry (eds.), *Essentials for Treating Behavioral Health in Primary Care*, https://doi.org/10.1007/978-3-032-09558-9_5

Prevention, 2024a; Substance Abuse and Mental Health Services Administration, 2022).

For individuals who die by suicide, contact with primary care is common, with 44% seeking care in the month prior to death (Stene-Larsen & Reneflot, 2019). Older adults and women may be even more likely to seek out care from a PCP prior to suicidal behavior (Luoma et al., 2002; Stene-Larsen & Reneflot, 2019). PCPs are well poised to intervene with suicidal patients and should be prepared with the knowledge and skills to do so.

Risk Assessment Language

PCPs should become familiar with the numerous terms related to suicide and risk assessment (see Table 5.1).

Screening Recommendations

The risk of suicide and other harmful behaviors is present in primary care (Stene-Larsen & Reneflot, 2019). However, there is not a clear consensus from regulating bodies on routine suicide screening and which screening tools should be utilized (see Table 5.2). While the Joint Commission recommends assessing suicide risk in all patients, the US Preventative Services Task Force (USPSTF) has not found sufficient evidence to make this recommendation (U.S. Preventive Services Task Force, 2023). Rather, the USPSTF, along with the American Academy of Family Physicians, recommends routine screening for depression in all patients ages 12 and up (LeFevre, 2014; U.S. Preventive Services Task Force, 2023). The American Academy of Pediatrics recommends universal screening of suicide risk in youth over the age of 12 and screening when clinically indicated for youth aged eight to 12 (American Academy of Pediatrics, 2023).

PCPs should work with their organizations to develop protocols to identify individuals who are at risk for suicide (Spottswood et al., 2022). Considerations when developing protocols can include recommendations by governing bodies, the overall patient population typically served, and the availability of additional staff to assist in risk assessment (Spottswood et al., 2022).

Conducting Risk Assessments

Risk assessments consist of four primary components: (1) identification of risk factors, (2) identification of protective factors, (3) inquiry about ideation, intent, and plans, and (4) judgment of risk level and determination of interventions (Montana

Table 5.1 Suicide and risk assessment terminology (Harmer et al., 2024; Minnesota Department of Health, 2019; Williamson et al., 2019; Yip et al., 2012)

Suicidal ideation (SI)/homicidal ideation (HI)	Thoughts about engaging in behaviors resulting in the death of oneself or others
Intent	The intent of an individual to engage in behaviors to harm self or others and an awareness that this act will be completed in the near future
Plan	How the injurious behavior will be completed, including means and timeline
Means	What is used to carry out the injurious behavior (e.g., weapon, vehicle, medication)
Suicidal self-directed injurious behavior (SIB)	Deliberate behavior that results in injury or death by suicide or the potential for death by suicide
Nonsuicidal self-injurious behavior (NSSI)	Deliberate behavior that results in injury to the body without the intent to complete suicide
Safety plan	Written list of warning signs, coping strategies, and means reduction to reduce the likelihood of engagement in behavior that could result in the death of oneself or others
Means reduction	Strategies to reduce availability or ease of access to lethal means for engaging in behaviors that could result in the death of oneself or others
Passive ideation	Desire to die or hurt someone else without a plan to engage in injurious behavior (e.g., "I don't want to wake up tomorrow")
Active ideation	Current, specific thoughts (e.g., "I want to kill myself") about the death of oneself or others
Low risk	Ideation with no intent or plan
Moderate risk	Ideation with some level of intent but can maintain safety
High risk	Ideation, intent, and plan are all present, and the patient is unable to maintain safety
Acute risk	Risk factors that are currently present
Chronic risk	Risk factors that have been present for a substantial length of time over the course of a person's life
Warning signs	Thoughts, feelings, or behaviors a patient portrays that may indicate they are thinking about harming themselves or others (e.g., feeling hopeless, recent suicide attempt, withdrawing from social connections)

(continued)

Table 5.1 (continued)

Protective factors	Factors that reduce risk (e.g., social support, reasons for living, coping skills)
Risk factors	Factors that contribute to risk (e.g., depression, substance abuse, social isolation)
Frequency	How often and the last time a patient experiences ideation, plan, or intent
Intensity	The magnitude of the ideations
Duration	How long do ideations persist before subsiding
Type of means/lethality of means	Objects a patient would likely use to engage in injurious behavior (weapon, medication, vehicle) and how likely the means are to be lethal
Access of means	A patient's access to the objects they would plan to use to engage in injurious behavior
Preparatory behaviors	Acts of preparation prior to engaging in injurious behavior often before active harm has begun (e.g., selling valuables, giving away pets)

Table 5.2 Screening recommendations

Recommendation	Source
Conduct a risk assessment when a patient screens positive for suicidality	Joint commission, APA, WICHE MHP & SPRC, USPSTF, VA/DoD
Address immediate safety needs and appropriate treatment setting	Joint commission
Review personal and medical history for suicide risk factors	Joint commission
Screen all patients for suicidal ideation	Joint commission
Screen for depression in adult populations, including pregnant and postpartum persons	USPSTF, APA
Complete a safety plan after a positive screen for suicide	SPRC, VA/DoD, WICHE MHP & SPRC

American Psychiatric Association (APA) (2010), U.S. Preventive Services Task Force (2023), Department of Veterans Affairs and Department of Defense (2019), Western Interstate Commission for Higher Education Mental Health Program and Suicide Prevention Resource Center (2017), National Action Alliance for Suicide Prevention (2018), The Joint Commission (2016)

Department of Public Health and Human Services, n.d.; Western Interstate Commission for Higher Education Mental Health Program and Suicide Prevention Resource Center, 2017). PCPs should rely on multiple data points, such as results from screening tools and clinical interviews, to make decisions about risk levels and interventions (Department of Veterans Affairs and Department of Defense, 2019).

Confidentiality and Privacy Considerations Providers should be familiar with the ethical and legal guidelines regarding patient and provider confidentiality and be prepared to discuss these issues explicitly with their patients. While some laws are universal across the country, others vary by state, such as the duty to report warn another party if a patient threatens to harm them (Johnson et al., 2014). PCPs should familiarize themselves with their own jurisdiction's laws and guidelines regarding the duty to warn and the reporting of abuse.

> Practice this statement: "Just as a reminder, your health information is private unless you tell me you are going to hurt yourself or someone else and cannot stay safe, or if you share any instances of real or suspected abuse of a child, older adult, or adult with disabilities."

In many practices, patients sign informed consent documents at the onset of the patient/provider relationship. They may not be aware of the specific circumstances that allow their provider to breach confidentiality to maintain their safety or abide by reporting laws. PCPs may consider reminding patients when conducting risk assessments that they are obligated to keep health information private unless the patient poses an imminent risk to themselves or someone else or discloses actual or suspected abuse of a child, adult with disabilities, or older adult (see below for practice). This conversation can help to build trust and rapport between the patient and provider. When patients clearly understand what may happen when they disclose sensitive information, such as suicidal thoughts, they may be more willing to disclose (Richards et al., 2019). Discussing limits to confidentiality early also reduces the risk of rupturing the patient-provider relationship when confidentiality must be broken (Richards et al., 2019). For further discussion on communication, please refer to Chap. 2.

Risk and Protective Factors There is no typical at-risk patient, and numerous factors can increase or decrease a patient's risk for suicide (See Table 5.3). These can include precipitating events, such as job loss or financial hardship, or static factors, such as age, gender, sexuality, or ethnicity (Suicide Prevention Resource Center, n.d.; Berman, 2018; Centers for Disease Control and Prevention, 2024b; Raue et al., 2014). For example, the 2023 National Survey on the Mental Health of LGBTQ Young People reported that 41% of LGBTQ+ youth surveyed had seriously considered suicide in the last year; nearly half of transgender and non-binary youth surveyed reported seriously considering suicide (The Trevor Project, 2023). Understanding these risk factors can aid providers in the screening and assessment process.

When conducting risk assessments, PCPs should be aware of warning signs such as isolation, increased substance use, feeling trapped, or feeling like a burden that may put patients at greater risk for suicide (Centers for Disease Control and Prevention, 2024b).

Table 5.3 Risk and protective factors (Suicide Prevention Resource Center, n.d.; Berman, 2018; Centers for Disease Control and Prevention, 2024b; Department of Veterans Affairs and Department of Defense, 2019; Prins, 2014; Raue et al., 2014)

Risk factors for suicidal behaviors	Protective factors for suicidal behaviors
– Prior suicidal behaviors	– Effective behavioral health care
– Substance abuse	– Social support
– Depression/mental illness	– Positive coping skills
– Access to lethal means	– Life satisfaction
– Family death by suicide	– Reasons for living
– Social isolation/loss of relationship(s)	– Strong sense of cultural identity
– Chronic disease and disability	– Social connection
– Lack of access to behavioral health care	– Reduced access to lethal means
– Financial hardship	– Cultural, religious, or moral objections to injurious behaviors
– Discrimination/victimization	
– History of trauma	
– Recent psychiatric hospitalization	
– Male gender	
– American Indian/Alaskan native; non-Hispanic white race	
– Veteran or active-duty military	
– Domestic violence	
– LGBTQIA+ individuals	
– Involvement in the justice system	

Inquiry About Ideation, Intent, and Plans PCPs should use direct language when inquiring about risk (Department of Veterans Affairs and Department of Defense, 2019). Practicing asking questions can help providers feel more comfortable discussing sensitive topics (Department of Veterans Affairs and Department of Defense, 2019). Physicians should inquire about ideation, intent, and plans during a risk assessment (Montana Department of Public Health and Human Services, n.d.; Western Interstate Commission for Higher Education Mental Health Program and Suicide Prevention Resource Center, 2017). They should also inquire about any history of injurious behaviors and identify relevant risk and protective factors that may increase or decrease the likelihood of current or future behaviors that would harm themselves or others (Montana Department of Public Health and Human Services, n.d.; Department of Veterans Affairs and Department of Defense, 2019; Western Interstate Commission for Higher Education Mental Health Program and Suicide Prevention Resource Center, 2017). When assessing for ideation, PCPs should inquire about the nature of the thoughts (i.e., whether they are active or passive) and their frequency, intensity, and duration (Department of Veterans Affairs and Department of Defense, 2019; Western Interstate Commission for Higher Education Mental Health

Current and past ideation, intent, and plans

Ideation

It is not uncommon for people going through similar situations to have thoughts of hurting or killing themselves (someone else).
Have you had thoughts like this?
Can you describe the thoughts you have been having? (Nature)
When did the thoughts begin? (Duration)
How often do they occur? (Frequency and Intensity)

Intent

Do you have any intention of acting on these thoughts?
How likely are you to act on the thoughts of killing yourself (someone else)?

Plans

Have you thought of a plan of how you would kill yourself (someone else)?
Can you describe the plans you have made?
Do you have a timeline to carry out this plan?
Have you gathered the things you need to carry out this plan?
Do you have access to firearms or other items you might use to harm yourself (someone else) in your home?

Previous attempts or behaviors, including self-aborted attempts because the patient changed their mind, intervention, or the method failed.

Have you done anything before to try to hurt or kill yourself (someone else)?
If yes: Can you describe what happened? How long ago did it happen? What stopped you?

Protective and risk factors that are relevant to the patient.

Is there anything that helps or worsens these thoughts or urges?
What things would stop you from acting on these thoughts or plans?

Fig. 5.1 Risk assessment questions (Department of Veterans Affairs and Department of Defense, 2019; Western Interstate Commission for Higher Education Mental Health Program and Suicide Prevention Resource Center, 2017)

Program and Suicide Prevention Resource Center, 2017). Direct questions, such as the ones below (see Fig. 5.1), can guide the risk assessment and gather the necessary information.

Suicide Risk Assessment Tools

PC offices may utilize screening tools to aid in the risk assessment process. These tools can be used in a variety of ways. They can be administered to every patient, and then a clinical interview can be conducted if patients screen positive, or they can be used as a supplement to routine risk assessment questions.

Columbia Suicide Severity Rating Scale (C-SSRS) The C-SSRS is a universal screening tool for suicide risk. It is free and widely available in two versions: a "screen" and the full three-page assessment (Posner et al., 2011). This assessment is written to aid providers in quickly assessing the severity of suicidal ideation and behaviors. The C-SSRS has strong validity data supporting its use in adolescent (Gipson et al., 2015) and adult (Posner et al., 2011) populations. Further, it has been translated into many languages and is available for provider access online. Further, research has demonstrated the C-SSRS to predict short-term suicidal behavior in high-risk adolescent populations (Conway et al., 2017). However, some have noted unclear navigation instructions, making adherence to the full administration protocol difficult (Giddens et al., 2014).

Suicide Assessment Five-Step Evaluation and Triage (SAFE-T) The SAFE-T was developed in alignment with the American Psychiatric Association Practice Guidelines for the Assessment and Treatment of Patients with Suicidal Behaviors (Suicide Prevention Resource Center, 2009). It is available in a "pocket card" format and a mobile application called "Suicide Safe," increasing ease of access. Clinically, the SAFE-T is frequently used with both adolescents and adults and has strong clinical foundations. However, there are currently no published studies evaluating its validity or effectiveness.

Ask Suicide Screening Questions Toolkit (ASQ) The ASQ toolkit includes a brief suicide safety assessment (BSSA), which is designed for time-limited settings and can be completed in 15 min or less (National Institute of Mental Health (NIMH), n.d.). It is available for free in 24 languages and in both adult and youth versions. The BSSA guides the provider through assessing the patient's frequency of SI, plan, and past behavior. In addition, it aids in determining related risk factors (e.g., impulsivity, substance misuse) and protective factors (e.g., social support, reasons for living). The BSSA also provides examples of how to ask risk-related questions to youth and aids the provider in determining the next steps (e.g., emergency psychiatric evaluation, non-urgent mental health follow-up). Studies have demonstrated the ASQ to be a valid measure for assessing suicide risk in adults (Horowitz et al., 2020) and youth (Aguinaldo et al., 2021).

The Patient Health Questionnaire (PHQ): Item 9 Item 9 of the PHQ evaluates if the patient has had passive suicidal thoughts in the last 2 weeks (Kroenke et al., 1999). The PHQ is frequently used to screen for depression in PC settings, with positive endorsement item 9 being used as an indicator that further risk assessment is needed. This method is supported by studies demonstrating endorsement of item 9 as a strong predictor of a suicide attempt (Simon et al., 2013). However, in subsequent studies, PHQ item 9 has been found insufficient as a risk screening tool when used alone, with frequent false positives (Na et al., 2018). Taken together, these findings suggest that while the PHQ item 9 is an indicator of potential suicide risk, further clinical assessment is needed when a patient is positive. When the patient endorses suicidal thoughts on the PHQ then a full risk assessment should be conducted (ideation, intent, plan, means).

Precautions on the Use of Screeners

Screening tools can be useful for identifying patients needing a more substantial risk assessment. They should complement a clinical interview and not be used as a standalone tool to make decisions about a patient's level of risk (Department of Veterans Affairs and Department of Defense, 2019). An exception may be the C-SSRS, which shows high sensitivity and specificity in identifying self-injurious behaviors (Posner et al., 2011). Additionally, if using screening tools, PCPs should ensure that policies are in place when patients screen positive for risk and that positive screens are not overlooked or left untreated (Western Interstate Commission for Higher Education Mental Health Program and Suicide Prevention Resource Center, 2017).

Assessing for Other Types of Risk

Although suicidal risk is most often discussed, other types of risk may present in primary care and need to be screened for.

Homicidal Ideation While less common, PCPs should not overlook homicidal risk in patients (Paulson & Hidaka, 2022). Assessing for homicidal risk is similar to assessing for suicidal risk, and physicians should ask about ideation, intent, plans, and previous behaviors that may indicate harm toward others (Sher & Rice, 2015). PCPs should also be aware of cultural colloquialisms that patients may use when assessing for homicidal risk (e.g., "I'm so mad I could kill him").

Nonsuicidal Self-Injury (NSSI) Not all self-injurious behaviors have suicidal intent but still require the PCPs attention (National Institute for Health and Care Excellence, 2022). When assessing suicidal ideations, PCPs should also ask whether patients have ever thought about or tried to harm themselves without the intent to die and inquire about the frequency and means of the behavior (National Institute for Health and Care Excellence, 2022). Using neutral, compassionate language can be helpful when approaching these conversations. Common NSSI behaviors include cutting, burning, or picking. If not seen acutely, an observant clinician frequently will find evidence of NSSI during an exam for another reason. While considered a distinct entity from SI, NSSI conveys significant risk for future suicide attempts (Asarnow et al., 2011; Cox et al., 2012; Selby et al., 2015). PCPs should consider the potential lethality of self-harm behaviors even if suicidal intent is not present (e.g., need for stitches, cutting too deep) and discuss these risks with their patients during the visit.

Abuse and Neglect Abuse of older persons, also called elder abuse, can include physical, emotional, sexual abuse, financial abuse, and neglect (Patel et al., 2021). Individuals in long-term care facilities are at higher risk for abuse. Additional risk factors include female gender, social isolation, physical disability, and dementia. Despite an estimated rate of 10% of adults over 65 experiencing abuse, it is often missed in primary care, and many PCPs report not feeling equipped to detect elder abuse (Jones et al., 1997).

Strategies that can aid providers in the assessment of abuse include paying close attention to medical history, including frequent injuries, missed follow-up appointments, and delays in the treatment of illness and injury (Jandu et al., 2024). While these factors could be explained by other variables (e.g., medical conditions impacting cognitive abilities or lack of transportation), they may alert providers to a need for screening for elder abuse and community resources. When screening for elder abuse, PCPs should try to ask their patient questions about their safety and well-being in a private space, if possible. Studies show that patients are less likely to disclose abuse with others in the room (Lachs & Pillemer, 2015). Several screeners have been designed to support providers in assessing elder abuse, including the Elder Abuse Suspicion Index (EASI), the Elder Assessment Instrument (EAI), and the Older Adult Psychological Abuse Measure (OAPAM) (Gallione et al., 2017).

PCPs also play a vital role in assessing child abuse and neglect (CAN). Currently, an estimated 1 in 7 children in the US experience maltreatment (Centers for Disease Control and Prevention, 2024c). CAN impacts children from all racial and ethnic backgrounds and socioeconomic statuses. Notably, providers have been shown to report potential CAN disproportionately, with more reports being made regarding children from minoritized racial and ethnic groups (US Preventive Services Task Force, 2024); further, some studies have demonstrated missed CAN in white families (Viswanathan et al., 2024). Therefore, PCPs must assess for child abuse regularly and know common signs while maintaining awareness of potential biases. PCPs should stay up to date with ethical and legal guidelines as well as recommendations for best practice. In most states, providers are exempt from civil and criminal liability when a report of possible CAN is made in good faith; failure to report CAN can result in legal consequences and harm to the patient. Steps providers can take to aid them in assessment for CAN include reviewing all available medical records, conducting a thorough examination, asking relevant questions to the patient and their caregiver, and consulting with experienced colleagues (St. Claire, 2009). When communicating concerns with caregivers, approach the topic with compassion and clarity, emphasizing the goal of ensuring the child's safety and well-being. Providing families with information on support services and resources is vital to help mitigate stress and assist in addressing underlying issues contributing to abuse and neglect. Collaboration with multidisciplinary teams and ongoing education in recognizing signs of potential abuse and neglect further enhances PCPs' ability to protect vulnerable children.

Special Populations

PCPs should be particularly aware when assessing risk with vulnerable populations, such as minors, older adults, pregnant individuals, and patients with disabilities.

Minors When assessing risk in pediatric populations, it is important to first discuss limits of confidentiality with both the minor and their parent/guardian using clear language and providing an opportunity to ask questions. Parent/guardians may feel concerned about asking their child about suicide risk due to myths that asking about suicide will cause suicidal thoughts. Myths such as this one are common, and having psychoeducation available to guardians may be important. Research investigating the efficacy of depression screening tools in evaluating suicide risk among pediatric populations highlights that depression screeners alone missed nearly one-third of at-risk children (Horowitz et al., 2021). Given these findings, PCPs may wish to ask pediatric patients directly about their suicide risk or use a suicide-specific screening tool.

Fatal suicides among children under the age of eight are infrequent. Nevertheless, studies reveal discrepancies in suicide rates, indicating that Black children between the ages of five and 12 are twice as likely to experience death by suicide compared to their White counterparts (Bridge et al., 2018).

Warning signs of suicide risk in youth under age 12 include (but are not limited to) (American Academy of Pediatrics, 2023):

- Talking about wanting to die
- Dramatizations of death such as acting out, choking, hanging, or using a firearm to end their life
- Self-harming behaviors
- Giving away treasured toys or possessions

When assessing suicide risk, as well as other forms of risk such as abuse and neglect, minors may feel more comfortable disclosing this information without their guardian in the room (American Academy of Pediatrics, 2023). Questions can be straightforward (e.g., "Has an adult ever made you feel unsafe?").

Older Adults For older adults, it is crucial to consider socio-environmental factors like social isolation, financial stability, and physical health to assess suicide risk accurately (De Mendonça Lima et al., 2021). Older adults are also at heightened risk for suicide early in treatment for serious medical illness (e.g., dementia, end-stage renal disease) (Beghi et al., 2021). Moreover, research indicates that many older adults who report suicidal ideation in primary care settings do not meet the criteria for a depressive disorder (Raue et al., 2010, 2014), continuing to highlight the importance of suicide-specific screening.

Pregnant Individuals When working with pregnant individuals, the American College of Gynecologists (ACOG) recommends screening for depression, anxiety, and psychosis, which may increase the risk of suicide or infanticide (American College of Obstetricians and Gynecologists, 2023a, 2023b). PCPs should consider risk factors that may increase the likelihood of self-harm or SI, including known mental health disorders, substance misuse, younger age, being unmarried, complications during pregnancy or birth, and a history of fetal or infant loss (American

College of Obstetricians and Gynecologists, 2023a). PCPs should also counsel pregnant patients on the benefits and risks of psychopharmacotherapy during pregnancy and initiate medications or behavioral health interventions when necessary (American College of Obstetricians and Gynecologists, 2023a); abrupt discontinuation of psychotropic drugs during pregnancy may increase the risk of mental health-related deaths (American College of Obstetricians and Gynecologists, 2023a).

Managing Barriers to Risk Assessment and Provider Reactions

Discussing suicide with patients can elicit many emotions within PCPs. However, nonjudgmental listening and empathy are paramount during these conversations. They may help patients be more likely to report ideation and risk to their PCP (Richards et al., 2019). PCPs may want to practice having these conversations beforehand to help them be more comfortable with their patients' emotions. Overreacting to patients reporting risk or reading off a checklist may be counterproductive (Richards et al., 2019).

Consider these barriers and potential solutions when conducting risk assessments:

Barrier to risk assessment	Potential intervention
The patient shuts down when asking questions and refuses to continue with the risk assessment	• Use motivational interviewing and empathy to try and re-engage the patient • Warmly and clearly remind the patient of your mandated role as their healthcare provider and the next steps if they refuse or are unable to participate in the risk assessment process (e.g., a higher level of care for psychiatric evaluation)[a]
The patient consistently reports high risk at follow-up appointments	• Emphasize protective factors and use the decision tree to choose the appropriate level of care • Involve BH providers in the area or on your team
The patient becomes very emotional when discussing risk	• Stay calm, nonjudgmental, and empathic • Balance the use of active listening, validation, and redirection to the risk assessment process
Communication barriers due to disability status	• Psychoeducation and safety planning with caregivers (e.g., warning signs and means restriction) • If your patient is unable to communicate their risk status but has displayed warning signs or suicidal behaviors, referral to a higher level of care may be necessary for a full evaluation

[a] The next steps will vary based on your state and the indications you have for the patient's risk level (e.g., wounds from SIB, indications of a suicide attempt, statements made by the patient, etc.).

The goal is to provide clear expectations so the patient can make an informed choice regarding participation in the risk assessment process

What Not to Do

Panic

PCPs should aim to stay calm and empathetic when working with at-risk patients (Richards et al., 2019).

Contract for Safety

Safety contracts—verbal or written contracts requiring patients to guarantee that they will not commit suicide—are not evidence-based (Hoffman, 2013). PCPs may become less vigilant in assessing risk when using contracts, and they are counterproductive to empowering patients to keep themselves safe (Hoffman, 2013).

Forcing the Issue

When a patient expresses imminent risk of harm to themselves or others, PCPs face both legal and ethical obligations to respond appropriately; however, these obligations are nuanced, and legal requirements vary from state to state. It is imperative for PCPs to think critically about the balance of their ethical and legal obligations to patient safety as well as their ethical obligation to respect their patients' right to autonomy. While safety is paramount, it is critical that PCPs strive to respect patient autonomy as much as possible when navigating these conversations. For example, if a patient is unwilling to engage fully in safety planning but can demonstrate future-oriented thinking and describe actionable steps toward maintaining safety, PCPs may not need to force the patient to continue in the intervention.

Ask Leading Questions

Framing questions in ways that make patients less likely to answer them honestly (e.g., "You're not thinking about committing suicide, *are you*?") is unhelpful. Leading questions often result in patients feeling that they cannot be honest with their PCP, which provides an inaccurate assessment of the patient's risk (Western Interstate Commission for Higher Education Mental Health Program and Suicide Prevention Resource Center, 2017).

Guilt Tripping

PCPs may be inclined to evoke guilt to help patients recognize reasons for living. For example, saying, "What about how sad your family will feel?" or "Can you imagine how your mom would feel finding you like that?" may lead to the patient shutting down or feeling as if the PCP does not understand what they are experiencing (Richards et al., 2019). These statements can also have a similar effect to leading questions. Instead, the PCP can utilize curiosity to understand the patient, such as, "You mentioned your family earlier; are they an important reason to keep living (Western Interstate Commission for Higher Education Mental Health Program and Suicide Prevention Resource Center, 2017)?" This allows the patient's experience to be centered in the conversation rather than others (e.g., the family).

Next Steps

After gathering information from multiple sources (screening measures, chart review, clinical interview), PCPs will utilize their clinical judgment to determine the patient's level of risk and assist in selecting an appropriate intervention. The decision tree below (see Fig. 5.2) can be a helpful tool to aid in selecting the appropriate level of risk and corresponding intervention.

Interventions for Risk

After conducting the risk assessment and determining the level of risk the patient presents with, PCPs can use that information to select an appropriate intervention. In clinics with an integrated BH team (IBH), this may be the time when clinic staff may contact BH for support, or it may be earlier in the process, depending on their own clinic's processes. For PCPs working in a setting without an (IBH), the focus should be on managing the risk and balancing the disruption of clinic flow. Workflow may vary depending on individual clinic policy and may include nursing or other support staff.

Managing Clinic Flow In an established IBH setting, the PCP may take a more limited history and initiate a visit with a BH provider for further risk stratification and safety planning. In the more common setting without BH support, it is recommended a protocol be put in place that provides a high standard of care while minimally disrupting clinic flow (Spottswood et al., 2022). Any specific protocol will be highly dependent on the model of BH the clinic utilizes (see Chap. 12).

For instance, upon identifying SI in a patient, the PCP may have an in-room readily available checklist that reviews risk factors and safety factors, assists with determining severity, and lists the next steps. A safety plan can be available in each

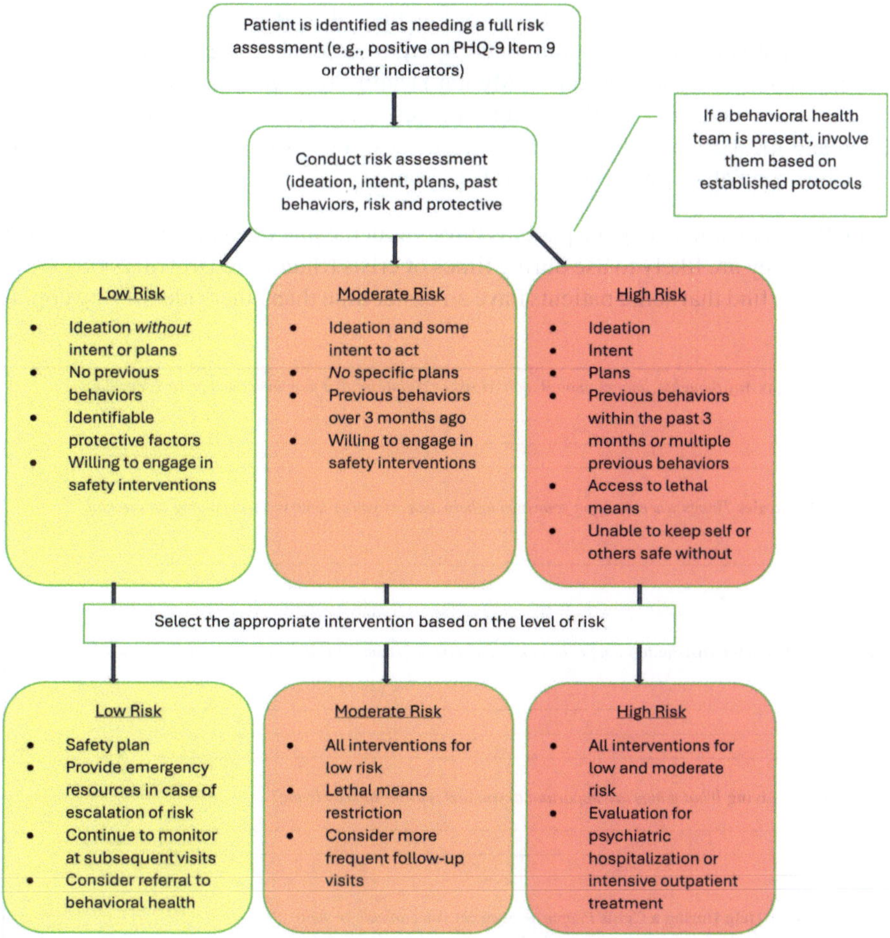

Fig. 5.2 Risk assessment decision tree (Montana Department of Public Health and Human Services, n.d.; Western Interstate Commission for Higher Education Mental Health Program and Suicide Prevention Resource Center, 2017)

exam room, similar to other resources, to be completed without leaving the room. A smart phrase can also be developed and easily entered into the electronic health record with the required fields to be completed. The PCP or ancillary staff can schedule a short-term follow-up with permission for overbooking established as part of the protocol.

Safety Plans Safety plans are written lists of coping skills and resources that patients can use during a crisis (Stanley & Brown, 2008). They should be brief, use the patient's own words, and be easy to read (Stanley & Brown, 2008). Safety plans have been shown to decrease suicidal behaviors in patients with suicidal ideation (Stanley et al., 2018). PCPs can use premade safety plan templates (like the one below in Fig. 5.3) or design their own, but they should be easily accessible and used with patients during appointments (Spottswood et al., 2022; Western Interstate Commission for Higher Education Mental Health Program and Suicide Prevention Resource Center, 2017). PCPs can tailor the resources and crisis lines for their population and local community to fit their needs best. For example, The Trevor Project crisis line specializes in serving LGBTQ+ youth.

PCPs should aim to engage patients throughout the process and help them identify strategies they are likely to use during times of crisis (Stanley & Brown, 2008). PCPs are likely to find that some patients have an easier time than others identifying coping

Warning Signs *Any thoughts, images, moods, behaviors, or situations that may indicate a crisis is developing.*

1. ______________________________
2. ______________________________
3. ______________________________

Coping Strategies *Things you can do on your own to help distract you or keep you from acting on suicidal thoughts.*

1. ______________________________
2. ______________________________
3. ______________________________

People or Places for Distraction *People or places that can help distract you from suicidal thoughts and help keep you safe.*

1. ______________________________
2. ______________________________
3. ______________________________

Reasons for Living *What things are important to you and reasons to keep living?*

1. ______________________________
2. ______________________________
3. ______________________________

Resources for Help During a Crisis *People or agencies you can call for help.*

Mental Health Professional: ____________ Phone #: ________________

Closest Emergency Room: ____________ Phone #: __________ Address: ____________

Local Mental Health Authority Crisis Number: ________________

Name: ____________ Phone #: ______________

Name: ____________ Phone #: ______________

Name: ____________ Phone #: ______________

National Suicide Hotline #: 988 (Call or Text; Veterans can press 1)

The Trevor Project (LGBTQ+ Hotline): (866) 488-7386

Making the Environment Safe *What steps can you take to make your environment safer during a crisis, like limiting access to dangerous items you might use to harm yourself?*

1. ______________________________
2. ______________________________
3. ______________________________

Fig. 5.3 Blank safety plan (Suicide Prevention Resource Center, n.d.; Western Interstate Commission for Higher Education Mental Health Program and Suicide Prevention Resource Center, 2017)

skills, reasons for living, and people that they can contact for help. When encountering patients who have difficulty completing the safety plan, PCPs can rely on Motivational Interviewing strategies to help engage them (Miller & Rollnick, 2013). Patients should also be encouraged to identify as many strategies in each category as possible—whether only one or several (Western Interstate Commission for Higher Education Mental Health Program and Suicide Prevention Resource Center, 2017). Consider the completed example below (see Fig. 5.4) and how one might efficiently help patients complete their safety plans.

After completing the safety plan, patients should be given a copy and encouraged to keep it where they will routinely see it (such as on a mirror or a picture on their phone) to access it during a crisis quickly (Western Interstate Commission for Higher Education Mental Health Program and Suicide Prevention Resource Center, 2017). PCPs may also recommend cell phone applications for patients, such as the Suicide

Warning Signs *Any thoughts, images, moods, behaviors, or situations that may indicate a crisis is developing.*
1. _*Being alone in my room at night and feeling anxious*_______________
2. _*Getting into a fight with my partner*_______________
3. ___*Thinking that I will never be good enough*_______________

Coping Strategies *Things you can do on your own to help distract you or keep you from acting on suicidal thoughts.*
1. _*Listening to my favorite podcast*_______________
2. _*Taking a deep breath and reminding myself of all the people who care about me*_______
3. ___*Watching TV*_______________

People or Places for Distraction *People or places that can help distract you from suicidal thoughts and help keep you safe.*
1. _*Go for a walk around my neighborhood*_______________
2. _*Calling my cousin Bobby*_______________
3. ___*Playing with my pets*_______________

Reasons for Living *What things are important to you and reasons to keep living?*
1. _*My family*_______________
2. _*My pets*_______________
3. _*Seeing my life improve for the better*_______________

Resources for Help During a Crisis *People or agencies you can call for help.*
Mental Health Professional: ___*Dr. Jones*__ Phone #: _*(888) 123-4567*________
Closest Emergency Room: _*Southlake ER 123 W 2nd St., Yourtown, NY Phone #: (888) 234-2345*_
Local Mental Health Authority Crisis Number: _*(888) 345-5678*_______________
Name: __Bobby____________ Phone #: _______________
Name: __Shelly____________ Phone #: _______________
Name: _______________ Phone #: _______________
National Suicide Hotline #: 988 (Call or Text; Veterans can press 1)
The Trevor Project (LGBTQ+ Hotline): (866) 488-7386
Making the Environment Safe *What steps can you take to make your environment safer during a crisis, like limiting access to dangerous items you might use to harm yourself?*
1. _*Give my partner the key to the gun safe*_______________
2. _*Talk to my partner about distributing my medications*_______________
3.______________________________

Fig. 5.4 Completed example safety plan

Safety Plan phone application or the VA Safety Plan (Inquiry Health LLC, 2020; US Department of Veterans Affairs (VA), 2023).

Lethal Means Restriction

During the safety planning process, all patients may benefit from a brief conversation about keeping their environment safe from lethal means that they could harm themselves with, such as firearms, sharps, or medications (Department of Veterans Affairs and Department of Defense, 2019; Spottswood et al., 2022; Western Interstate Commission for Higher Education Mental Health Program and Suicide Prevention Resource Center, 2017). For patients who are at moderate or high risk of suicide, lethal means restriction is an evidence-based intervention that can reduce their risk of suicide (Montana Department of Public Health and Human Services, n.d.). Lethal means restriction involves discussing the means a patient has access to and collaboratively developing a plan to reduce the access to the means (even temporarily). Plans could include obtaining gun locks, having a trusted family member dispense medications, or reducing the supply of medications while the patient is in crisis.

Firearms Restriction

Firearms are used in almost half of all completed suicides in the United States (Ehlman et al., 2022). PCPs should be aware of the cultural attitudes around firearms among the population that they serve to help guide conversations (Simonetti et al., 2021). PCPs working with rural, veteran, or military patients, who may be more likely to own firearms, should consider regularly discussing firearm safety (Anestis & Capron, 2016; Parker et al., 2017). PCPs should also discuss firearm safety with parents who own firearms, as adolescents who die by suicide with a firearm are most likely to use a gun owned by their parents (Johnson et al., 2010) While some patients who own firearms may have value-based reasons for owning firearms that may serve as a barrier to means restriction, emphasizing that the changes are voluntary and temporary may help when having these conversations with them (Knapp, 2023; Simonetti et al., 2021).

Escalating Care for High-Risk Patients If a patient has been identified as high-risk, their care should be escalated (Paulson & Hidaka, 2022; Western Interstate Commission for Higher Education Mental Health Program and Suicide Prevention Resource Center, 2017). This may involve transporting them to the nearest emergency department or calling the local mental health authority for an evaluation. Providers should work with their organizations to develop clear protocols for escalating care for high-risk individuals so that they know what to do when a situation arises. PCPs can refer patients for an involuntary psychiatric evaluation if they pose an immediate risk (Johnson & Stern, 2014).

PCPs to be mindful when escalating care for patients of color, who may be more vulnerable when interacting with law enforcement (Vitiello & Moseley, 2021). When recommending crisis or emergency lines, PCPs should be mindful of recommending 911 as a resource during a BH emergency for patients of color and consider alternative resources in the area that may be safer for them to utilize or they may be more likely to engage with (Drustrup et al., 2023).

Interventions for Homicidal Ideation

Safety planning and lethal means restriction (especially firearms) are effective interventions for homicidal risk (Sher & Rice, 2015). Providers should also be aware of legislation and regulations governing the duty to warn in their state or province. In the US, at least 20 states mandate that physicians warn others if their patient poses a threat to others (Johnson et al., 2014). If a patient discloses intent to harm another person, PCPs should be aware of whether they are mandated to disclose this information or are protected from liability if they choose to disclose it.

NSSI Interventions

NSSI can be conceptualized as a maladaptive coping skill (Kilburn & Whitlock, 2009). When working with patients engaging in NSSI, physicians can help patients identify alternative, more adaptive coping skills to replace the self-harming behaviors (National Institute for Health and Care Excellence, 2022). These coping skills can be included in safety plans (PCPs can utilize the same templates that are used for SI), and restriction of lethal means can be used to remove objects that the patient is using to harm themselves (National Institute for Health and Care Excellence, 2022). Alternative coping skills should be tailored to the individual and can be distracting (e.g., listening to music, going for a walk), sensory (e.g., squeezing ice, eating flavorful food), comforting (talking to close others, taking a hot bath), or other things the patient needs during an urge to self-harm (Kilburn & Whitlock, 2009).

Documentation and Follow-Up Care

PC staff should thoroughly document the risk assessment, plan, interventions, and any consultations or care transitions during the visit (Western Interstate Commission for Higher Education Mental Health Program and Suicide Prevention Resource Center,

2017). Storing copies of screening measures and safety plans is good practice and can help with follow-up care (Western Interstate Commission for Higher Education Mental Health Program and Suicide Prevention Resource Center, 2017).

PCPs may initiate pharmacotherapy, refer to BH, or utilize IBH teams (Department of Veterans Affairs and Department of Defense, 2019; Western Interstate Commission for Higher Education Mental Health Program and Suicide Prevention Resource Center, 2017). In addition, they should closely follow up with patients in their clinic to monitor their risk and intervene, as necessary. Follow-up and check-ins can be facilitated through the help of support staff in addition to provider utilization (see Chap. 13). Developing protocols within medical charts to flag high-risk patients and enlisting the help of patients' loved ones to engage them in care can be valuable tools to promote follow-up care (Western Interstate Commission for Higher Education Mental Health Program and Suicide Prevention Resource Center, 2017).

Key Points

- PCPs should develop clear protocols for assessing and managing risk in their clinic.
- PCPs should familiarize themselves with risk screening tools and clinical interviewing questions.
- Safety planning is the primary effective intervention for risk—safety contracts are *ineffective.*
- PCPs should aim to stay calm, lead with curiosity, and utilize support staff when available.

References

Aguinaldo, L. D., Sullivant, S., Lanzillo, E. C., Ross, A., He, J.-P., Bradley-Ewing, A., Bridge, J. A., Horowitz, L. M., & Wharff, E. A. (2021). Validation of the ask suicide-screening questions (ASQ) with youth in outpatient specialty and primary care clinics. *General Hospital Psychiatry, 68*, 52–58. https://doi.org/10.1016/j.genhosppsych.2020.11.006

Ahmedani, B. K., Simon, G. E., Stewart, C., Beck, A., Waitzfelder, B. E., Rossom, R., Lynch, F., Owen-Smith, A., Hunkeler, E. M., Whiteside, U., Operskalski, B. H., Coffey, M. J., & Solberg, L. I. (2014). Health care contacts in the year before suicide death. *Journal of General Internal Medicine, 29*(6), 870–877. https://doi.org/10.1007/s11606-014-2767-3

American Academy of Pediatrics. (2023). *Screening for suicide risk in clinical practice.* https://www.aap.org/en/patient-care/blueprint-for-youth-suicide-prevention/strategies-for-clinical-settings-for-youth-suicide-prevention/screening-for-suicide-risk-in-clinical-practice/

American College of Obstetricians and Gynecologists. (2023a). Screening and diagnosis of mental health conditions during pregnancy and postpartum: ACOG clinical practice guideline no. 4. *Obstetrics and Gynecology, 141*(6), 1232–1261. https://doi.org/10.1097/AOG.0000000000005200

American College of Obstetricians and Gynecologists. (2023b). Treatment and management of mental health conditions during pregnancy and postpartum: ACOG clinical practice guideline no. 5. *Obstetrics and Gynecology, 141*(6), 1262–1288. https://doi.org/10.1097/AOG.0000000000005202

American Psychiatric Association (APA). (2010). *Practice guideline for the assessment and treatment of patients with suicidal behaviors*. https://psychiatryonline.org/pb/assets/raw/sitewide/practice_guidelines/guidelines/suicide.pdf
Anestis, M., & Capron, D. W. (2016). The associations between state veteran population rates, handgun legislation, and statewide suicide rates. *Journal of Psychiatric Research, 74*, 30–34. https://doi.org/10.1016/j.jpsychires.2015.12.014
Asarnow, J. R., Porta, G., Spirito, A., Emslie, G., Clarke, G., Wagner, K. D., Vitiello, B., Keller, M., Birmaher, B., McCracken, J., Mayes, T., Berk, M., & Brent, D. A. (2011). Suicide attempts and nonsuicidal self-injury in the treatment of resistant depression in adolescents: Findings from the TORDIA study. *Journal of the American Academy of Child & Adolescent Psychiatry, 50*(8), 772–781. https://doi.org/10.1016/j.jaac.2011.04.003
Beghi, M., Butera, E., Cerri, C. G., Cornaggia, C. M., Febbo, F., Mollica, A., Berardino, G., Piscitelli, D., Resta, E., Logroscino, G., Daniele, A., Altamura, M., Bellomo, A., Panza, F., & Lozupone, M. (2021). Suicidal behaviour in older age: A systematic review of risk factors associated to suicide attempts and completed suicides. *Neuroscience & Biobehavioral Reviews, 127*, 193–211. https://doi.org/10.1016/j.neubiorev.2021.04.011
Berman, A. L. (2018). Risk factors proximate to suicide and suicide risk assessment in the context of denied suicide ideation. *Suicide and Life-threatening Behavior, 48*(3), 340–352. https://doi.org/10.1111/sltb.12351
Bridge, J. A., Horowitz, L. M., Fontanella, C. A., Sheftall, A. H., Greenhouse, J., Kelleher, K. J., & Campo, J. V. (2018). Age-related racial disparity in suicide rates among US youths from 2001 through 2015. *JAMA Pediatrics, 172*(7), 697–699. https://doi.org/10.1001/jamapediatrics.2018.0399
Brodsky, B. S., Spruch-Feiner, A., & Stanley, B. (2018). The zero suicide model: Applying evidence-based suicide prevention practices to clinical care. *Frontiers in Psychiatry, 9*. https://doi.org/10.3389/fpsyt.2018.00033
Centers for Disease Control and Prevention. (2024a). *About child abuse and neglect*. Child Abuse and Neglect Prevention. https://www.cdc.gov/child-abuse-neglect/about/index.html.
Centers for Disease Control and Prevention. (2024b). *Preventing child abuse and neglect*. Child Abuse and Neglect Prevention. https://www.cdc.gov/child-abuse-neglect/prevention/index.html.
Centers for Disease Control and Prevention. (2024c). *Risk and protective factors for suicide*. Suicide Prevention. https://www.cdc.gov/suicide/risk-factors/index.html.
Conway, P. M., Erlangsen, A., Teasdale, T. W., Jakobsen, I. S., & Larsen, K. J. (2017). Predictive validity of the Columbia-suicide severity rating scale for short-term suicidal behavior: A Danish study of adolescents at a high risk of suicide. *Archives of Suicide Research, 21*(3), 455–469. https://doi.org/10.1080/13811118.2016.1222318
Cox, L. J., Stanley, B. H., Melhem, N. M., Oquendo, M. A., Birmaher, B., Burke, A., Kolko, D. J. J., Zelazny, J. M., Mann, J. J., Porta, G., & Brent, D. A. (2012). A longitudinal study of nonsuicidal self-injury in offspring at high risk for mood disorder. *The Journal of Clinical Psychiatry, 73*(6), 10597. https://doi.org/10.4088/JCP.11m07250
De Mendonça Lima, C. A., De Leo, D., Ivbijaro, G., & Svab, I. (2021). Suicide prevention in older adults. *Asia-Pacific Psychiatry, 13*(3), e12473. https://doi.org/10.1111/appy.12473
Department of Veterans Affairs & Department of Defense. (2019). *VA/DoD clinical practice guideline for the assessment and management of patients at risk for suicide*. https://www.healthquality.va.gov/guidelines/MH/srb/VADoDSuicideRiskFullCPGFinal5088212019.pdf
Drustrup, D., Kivlighan, D. M., & Ali, S. R. (2023). Decentering the use of police: An abolitionist approach to safety planning in psychotherapy. *Psychotherapy, 60*(1), 51–62. https://doi.org/10.1037/pst0000422
Ehlman, D. C., Yard, E., Stone, D. M., Jones, C. M., & Mack. (2022). Changes in suicide rates—United States, 2019 and 2020. *MMWR. Morbidity and Mortality Weekly Report, 71*. https://doi.org/10.15585/mmwr.mm7108a5

Gallione, C., Dal Molin, A., Cristina, F. V. B., Ferns, H., Mattioli, M., & Suardi, B. (2017). Screening tools for identification of elder abuse: A systematic review. *Journal of Clinical Nursing, 26*(15–16), 2154–2176. https://doi.org/10.1111/jocn.13721

Giddens, J. M., Sheehan, K. H., & Sheehan, D. V. (2014). The Columbia-suicide severity rating scale (C-SSRS): Has the "gold standard" become a liability? *Innovations in Clinical Neuroscience, 11*(9–10), 66–80.

Gipson, P. Y., Agarwala, P., Opperman, K. J., Horwitz, A., & King, C. A. (2015). Columbia-suicide severity rating scale: Predictive validity with adolescent psychiatric emergency patients. *Pediatric Emergency Care, 31*(2), 88. https://doi.org/10.1097/PEC.0000000000000225

Harmer, B., Lee, S., Rizvi, A., & Saadabadi, A. (2024). Suicidal ideation. In *StatPearls*. StatPearls Publishing. http://www.ncbi.nlm.nih.gov/books/NBK565877/

Hoffman, R. M. (2013). *Contracting for safety: A misused tool.* Pennsylvania Patient Safety Authority. https://patientsafety.pa.gov:443/ADVISORIES/Pages/201306_82.aspx

Horowitz, L. M., Mournet, A. M., Lanzillo, E., He, J.-P., Powell, D. S., Ross, A. M., Wharff, E. A., Bridge, J. A., & Pao, M. (2021). Screening pediatric medical patients for suicide risk: Is depression screening enough? *Journal of Adolescent Health, 68*(6), 1183–1188. https://doi.org/10.1016/j.jadohealth.2021.01.028

Horowitz, L. M., Snyder, D. J., Boudreaux, E. D., He, J.-P., Harrington, C. J., Cai, J., Claassen, C. A., Salhany, J. E., Dao, T., Chaves, J. F., Jobes, D. A., Merikangas, K. R., Bridge, J. A., & Pao, M. (2020). *Validation of the Ask Suicide-Screening Questions for adult medical inpatients: A brief tool for all ages*. https://www.clinicalkey.com/#!/content/playContent/1-s2.0-S0033318220301201?returnurlhttps://www.linkinghub.elsevier.com2/retrieve2/pii2/S00333182203012013/showall=true&referrer=

Inquiry Health LLC. (2020). *MoodTools* (version 1.6.7) [Mobile app]. App store. https://apps.apple.com/us/app/moodtools-depression-aid/id1012822112

Jandu, J. S., Mohanaselvan, A., Johnson, M. J., & Fertel, H. (2024). Elder abuse. In *StatPearls*. StatPearls Publishing. https://www.ncbi.nlm.nih.gov/sites/books/NBK560883/

Johnson, J. M., & Stern, T. A. (2014). Involuntary hospitalization of primary care patients. *The Primary Care Companion for CNS Disorders, 16*(3), PCC.13f01613. https://doi.org/10.4088/PCC.13f01613

Johnson, R., Persad, G., & Sisti, D. (2014). The Tarasoff rule: The implications of interstate variation and gaps in professional training. *The Journal of the American Academy of Psychiatry and the Law, 42*(4), 469–477.

Johnson, R. M., Barber, C., Azrael, D., Clark, D. E., & Hemenway, D. (2010). Who are the owners of firearms used in adolescent suicides? *Suicide & Life-Threatening Behavior, 40*(6), 609. https://doi.org/10.1521/suli.2010.40.6.609

Jones, J. S., Veenstra, T. R., Seamon, J. P., & Krohmer, J. (1997). Elder mistreatment: National survey of emergency physicians. *Annals of Emergency Medicine, 30*(4), 473–479. https://doi.org/10.1016/S0196-0644(97)70007-6

Kilburn, E., & Whitlock, J. (2009). *Distraction techniques and alternative coping strategies*. Cornell University. https://www.selfinjury.bctr.cornell.edu/documents/distraction-tech-and-alts.pdf

Knapp, S. (2023). Lethal means counseling for suicidal firearm owners. *Journal of Contemporary Psychotherapy, 53*(4), 279–287. https://doi.org/10.1007/s10879-023-09588-5

Kroenke, K., Spitzer, R. L., & Williams, J. B. W. (1999). Patient health questionnaire-9. https://doi.org/10.1037/t06165-000

Lachs, M. S., & Pillemer, K. A. (2015). Elder abuse. *New England Journal of Medicine, 373*(20), 1947–1956. https://doi.org/10.1056/NEJMra1404688

LeFevre, M. L. (2014). Screening for suicide risk in adolescents, adults, and older adults in primary care: U.S. preventive services task force recommendation statement. *Annals of Internal Medicine, 160*(10), 719–726. https://doi.org/10.7326/M14-0589

Luoma, J. B., Martin, C. E., & Pearson, J. L. (2002). Contact with mental health and primary care providers before suicide: A review of the evidence. *American Journal of Psychiatry, 159*(6), 909–916. https://doi.org/10.1176/appi.ajp.159.6.909

Miller, W. R., & Rollnick, S. (2013). *Motivational interviewing: Helping people change* (3rd ed., p. 482). Guilford Press.

Minnesota Department of Health. (2019). *Suicidal ideation risk assessment*. https://www.health.state.mn.us/people/syringe/suicide.pdf

Montana Department of Public Health & Human Services. (n.d.). *Suicide prevention in primary care settings*. https://dphhs.mt.gov/suicideprevention/toolkit/primarycare

Na, P. J., Yaramala, S. R., Kim, J. A., Kim, H., Goes, F. S., Zandi, P. P., Vande Voort, J. L., Sutor, B., Croarkin, P., & Bobo, W. V. (2018). The PHQ-9 item 9 based screening for suicide risk: A validation study of the patient Health questionnaire (PHQ)−9 item 9 with the Columbia suicide severity rating scale (C-SSRS). *Journal of Affective Disorders, 232*, 34–40. https://doi.org/10.1016/j.jad.2018.02.045

National Action Alliance for Suicide Prevention. (2018). *Recommended standard care for people with suicide risk: Making health care suicide safe*. https://theactionalliance.org/sites/default/files/action_alliance_recommended_standard_care_final.pdf

National Institute for Health and Care Excellence. (2022). *Self-harm: Assessment, management and preventing recurrence*. https://www.nice.org.uk/guidance/ng225/evidence/p-skills-required-by-staff-in-specialist-settings-pdf-403069580827

National Institute of Mental Health (NIMH). (n.d.). *Ask suicide-screening questions (ASQ) toolkit*. Retrieved November 11, 2024, from https://www.nimh.nih.gov/research/research-conducted-at-nimh/asq-toolkit-materials

Olfson, M., Kroenke, K., Wang, S., & Blanco, C. (2014). Trends in office-based mental health care provided by psychiatrists and primary care physicians. *The Journal of Clinical Psychiatry, 75*(3), 21732. https://doi.org/10.4088/JCP.13m08834

Parker, K., Horowitz, J., Igielnik, R., Oliphant, B., & Brown, A. (2017). *America's complex relationship with guns: An in-depth look at the attitudes and experiences of U.S. adults*. Pew Research Center. https://assets.pewresearch.org/wp-content/uploads/sites/3/2017/06/06151541/Guns-Report-FOR-WEBSITE-PDF-6-21.pdf

Patel, K., Bunachita, S., Chiu, H., Suresh, P., Patel, U. K., Patel, K., Bunachita, S., Chiu, H., Suresh, P., & Patel, U. K. (2021). Elder abuse: A comprehensive overview and physician-associated challenges. *Cureus, 13*. https://doi.org/10.7759/cureus.14375

Paulson, D., & Hidaka, B. (2022). Improving family medicine residents' confidence to assess and manage psychiatric crises in an outpatient clinic. *Journal of Primary Care & Community Health, 13*, 21501319221119943. https://doi.org/10.1177/21501319221119943

Posner, K., Brown, G. K., Stanley, B., Brent, D. A., Yershova, K. V., Oquendo, M. A., Currier, G. W., Melvin, G. A., Greenhill, L., Shen, S., & Mann, J. J. (2011). The Columbia–suicide severity rating scale: Initial validity and internal consistency findings from three multisite studies with adolescents and adults. *American Journal of Psychiatry, 168*(12), 1266–1277. https://doi.org/10.1176/appi.ajp.2011.10111704

Prins, S. J. (2014). Prevalence of mental illnesses in U.S. state prisons: A systematic review. *Psychiatric Services, 65*(7), 862–872. https://doi.org/10.1176/appi.ps.201300166

Raue, P. J., Ghesquiere, A. R., & Bruce, M. L. (2014). Suicide risk in primary care: Identification and management in older adults. *Current Psychiatry Reports, 16*(9), 466. https://doi.org/10.1007/s11920-014-0466-8

Raue, P. J., Morales, K. H., Post, E. P., Bogner, H. R., Have, T. T., & Bruce, M. L. (2010). The wish to die and 5-year mortality in elderly primary care patients. *The American Journal of Geriatric Psychiatry, 18*(4), 341–350. https://doi.org/10.1097/JGP.0b013e3181c37cfe

Richards, J. E., Whiteside, U., Ludman, E. J., Pabiniak, C., Kirlin, B., Hidalgo, R., & Simon, G. (2019). Understanding why patients may not report suicidal ideation at a health care visit prior to a suicide attempt: A qualitative study. *Psychiatric Services, 70*(1), 40–45. https://doi.org/10.1176/appi.ps.201800342

Selby, E. A., Kranzler, A., Fehling, K. B., & Panza, E. (2015). Nonsuicidal self-injury disorder: The path to diagnostic validity and final obstacles. *Clinical Psychology Review, 38*, 79–91. https://doi.org/10.1016/j.cpr.2015.03.003

Sher, L., & Rice, T. (2015). Prevention of homicidal behaviour in men with psychiatric disorders. *The World Journal of Biological Psychiatry, 16*(4), 212–229. https://doi.org/10.3109/15622975.2015.1028998

Simon, G. E., Rutter, C. M., Peterson, D., Oliver, M., Whiteside, U., Operskalski, B., & Ludman, E. J. (2013). Does response on the PHQ-9 depression questionnaire predict subsequent suicide attempt or suicide death? *Psychiatric Services, 64*(12), 1195–1202. https://doi.org/10.1176/appi.ps.201200587

Simonetti, J. A., Wortzel, H. S., & Matarazzo, B. B. (2021). Therapeutic risk management and firearm-related lethal means safety. *Journal of Psychiatric Practice, 27*(6), 456. https://doi.org/10.1097/PRA.0000000000000586

Spottswood, M., Lim, C. T., Davydow, D., & Huang, H. (2022). Improving suicide prevention in primary care for differing levels of behavioral health integration: A review. *Frontiers in Medicine, 9*. https://doi.org/10.3389/fmed.2022.892205

St. Claire, K. (2009). What to do when it might be child abuse. *AMA Journal of Ethics, 11*(2), 111–116. https://doi.org/10.1001/virtualmentor.2009.11.2.ccas2-0902

Stanley, B., & Brown, G. K. (2008). *Safety planning guide: A quick guide for clinicians*. https://sprc.org/wp-content/uploads/2023/01/SafetyPlanningGuide-Quick-Guide-for-Clinicians.pdf

Stanley, B., Brown, G. K., Brenner, L. A., Galfalvy, H. C., Currier, G. W., Knox, K. L., Chaudhury, S. R., Bush, A. L., & Green, K. L. (2018). Comparison of the safety planning intervention with follow-up vs usual care of suicidal patients treated in the emergency department. *JAMA Psychiatry, 75*(9), 894–900. https://doi.org/10.1001/jamapsychiatry.2018.1776

Stene-Larsen, K., & Reneflot, A. (2019). Contact with primary and mental health care prior to suicide: A systematic review of the literature from 2000 to 2017. *Scandinavian Journal of Public Health, 47*(1), 9–17. https://doi.org/10.1177/1403494817746274

Substance Abuse and Mental Health Services Administration. (2022). *Highlights for the 2022 national survey on drug use and health*. https://www.samhsa.gov/data/sites/default/files/reports/rpt42731/2022-nsduh-main-highlights.pdf

Suicide Prevention Resource Center. (2009). *Suicide assessment five-step evaluation and triage SAFE-T pocket card*. Suicide Prevention Resource Center. https://sprc.org/online-library/suicide-assessment-five-step-evaluation-and-triage-safe-t-pocket-card/

Suicide Prevention Resource Center. (n.d.). *Risk and protective factors*. Suicide Prevention Resource Center. https://sprc.org/risk-and-protective-factors/

The Joint Commission. (2016). *Detecting and treating suicide ideation in all settings*. Detecting and Treating Suicide Ideation in All Settings. 56. https://psnet.ahrq.gov/issue/detecting-and-treating-suicide-ideation-all-settings

The Trevor Project. (2023). *2023 U.S. national survey on the mental health of LGBTQ young people*. The Trevor Project. https://www.thetrevorproject.org/

U.S. Preventive Services Task Force. (2023). *Depression and suicide risk in adults: Screening*. https://www.uspreventiveservicestaskforce.org/uspstf/recommendation/screening-depression-suicide-risk-adults#fullrecommendationstart

US Department of Veterans Affairs (VA). (2023). *Safety plan* [Mobile app]. App Store. https://apps.apple.com/us/app/safety-plan/id1663044514

US Preventive Services Task Force. (2024). Primary care interventions to prevent child maltreatment: US preventive services task force recommendation statement. *JAMA, 331*(11), 951–958. https://doi.org/10.1001/jama.2024.1869

Viswanathan, M., Rains, C., Hart, L. C., Doran, E., Sathe, N., Hudson, K., Ali, R., Jonas, D. E., Chou, R., & Zolotor, A. J. (2024). Primary care interventions to prevent child maltreatment: Evidence report and systematic review for the US preventive services task force. *JAMA, 331*(11), 959–971. https://doi.org/10.1001/jama.2024.0276

Vitiello, E., & Moseley, D. D. (2021). Navigating care from afar: Ethical considerations for police welfare checks. *Psychiatric Services, 72*(11), 1345–1347. https://doi.org/10.1176/appi.ps.202000732

Western Interstate Commission for Higher Education Mental Health Program & Suicide Prevention Resource Center. (2017). *Suicide prevention toolkit for primary care practices. A guide for primary care providers and medical practice managers.* https://www.wiche.edu/wp-content/uploads/2018/10/Suicide_Prevention_Toolkit_US_April_2018.pdf

Williamson, M. L. C., Hogue, G., Cotter, J., Roberman, S., Neal, G., & Williamson, B. (2019). Suicide screening: How to recognize and treat at-risk adults. *The Journal of Family Practice, 68*(9), 505–510.

Yip, P. S., Caine, E., Yousuf, S., Chang, S.-S., Wu, K. C.-C., & Chen, Y.-Y. (2012). Means restriction for suicide prevention. *The Lancet, 379*(9834), 2393–2399. https://doi.org/10.1016/S0140-6736(12)60521-2

Chapter 6
Mental Status and Cognition Considerations for Older Adults

Max Zubatsky PhD, Jamil Neme MD, and Danielle L. Terry PhD, ABPP

Older Adults and Healthcare

With 22% of the United States (U.S.) population expected to be over the age of 65 by 2060, the readiness of the healthcare workforce to treat older adult patients in primary care and other outpatient settings has never been more important (Wismann et al., 2024). The scarcity of geriatricians in the United States will be a continuing workforce epidemic, given that older adults are living longer with more chronic illnesses. PCPs make most initial dementia diagnoses, are central to post-diagnostic care, and have a growing role in the dementia care workforce. Alzheimer's and dementia-related disorders (ADRD) have become some of the fastest growing presenting issues that PCPs are assessing and treating in practice.

As a result of this workforce shortage, PCPs will face the precarious task of treating a high number of older adult patients. This trend will require PCPs and other specialists to find effective strategies to detect and prevent further health problems in this population (Lester et al., 2020). This shortage is especially concerning in rural and underserved areas. In these areas there are fewer on-site providers and support staff will force physicians to take on greater responsibilities for each patient, often missing important assessment and diagnostic information at early appointments.

Identifying the signs and symptoms of memory loss in older adult patients can be challenging for PCPs. Currently, in the primary care setting, as many as two-thirds of people with dementia may be misdiagnosed (i.e., the neurocognitive syndrome and neurologic etiology are misidentified), and there is often a significant delay between symptom onset and diagnosis. As a result, early mild cognitive impairment

M. Zubatsky PhD · J. Neme MD
Saint Louis University School of Medicine, St. Louis, MO, USA
e-mail: max.zubatsky@health.slu.edu

D. L. Terry PhD, ABPP (✉)
Guthrie Medical Group, Sayre, PA, USA
e-mail: danielle.terry@guthrie.org

M. L. C. Williamson and D. L. Terry (eds.), *Essentials for Treating Behavioral Health in Primary Care*, https://doi.org/10.1007/978-3-032-09558-9_6

(MCI) may be missed due to a lack of formalized testing available. As a result of decreased access to assessment, behavioral health (BH) and other specialties may not be included (Bradford et al., 2009; Shinagawa et al., 2016). Given that a large percentage of PCPs do not get formalized training in geriatric diagnosis and symptoms (Dai & Peterson, 2020), this presents a troubling trend for healthcare.

Older, underserved patients face access to care and insurance barriers when having to afford the costs associated with dementia-related symptoms. With the rising costs for medication and advanced treatment options, there are greater disparities in populations trying to slow the progression of memory loss issues (Kim et al., 2023). PCPs will continue to face the challenges of taking on a growing number of older adult patients onto their panels, treating more complex conditions in this age group. This chapter will focus on practical considerations, including assessment of initial concerns related to cognition and mental status, management of concerns, and ways to facilitate family and community involvement.

The Initial Presentation

Patients who have cognitive concerns may present in both emergent and non-emergent ways. Concerns may arise based upon observations by the PCP, observations or concerns raised by family members or friends, and, less likely, the patients themselves. Making a timely diagnosis and communication to the patient and family helps alleviate any ambiguity around memory complications and confusions. The PCP is often responsible for the continuity of care after the initial months of a diagnosis. Responsibilities may include arranging specific referrals, medication recommendations, and coordination with caregivers to attend to specific complications and symptoms (Moore et al., 2018).

While it is important to attend to more pressing medical needs, it can be useful to consider what the cognitive status was of the individual that led them to their current predicament. For example, someone presenting with an acute concern related to dangerously high or low glucose readings may stem from an inability to remember or manage medications properly. Neglecting assessment of the "why" or context (See Chap. 2) within which an older adult presents with current concerns may result in missing an essential component of safe and responsible treatment.

Co-occurring Health Issues with Memory Loss

Cognitive impairment in older adults has a variety of possible causes, including medication side effects; metabolic and/or endocrine dysfunction; delirium due to illness (such as a urinary tract or COVID-19 infection); depression; and dementia, including Alzheimer's disease, vascular dementia, Lewy body dementia, and frontotemporal disorders. Those on dementia medications are usually taking a higher rate of other medications for existing health-related complications, often causing counteracting side effects (Mueller et al., 2018). Although taking multiple dementia medications may be necessary for the management of memory loss, higher polypharmacy utilization can lead to greater drug interaction problems and larger risk for adverse drug reactions (Ruangritchankul et al., 2020).

Psychosocial complications often exist for those with memory loss and neurodegenerative disorders. Behavioral and psychological symptoms such as delusions, hallucinations, and agitation are common in persons with dementia. These conditions often contribute to significant distress in patients as well as familial and professional caregivers (Rao et al., 2020). Depression and chronic stress have been cited as modifiable risk factors for different types of dementia. Low mood has been seen as not only a complication for those with memory problems but can advance the risk of cognitive decline for older adults who are often homebound or isolated(Luo et al., 2023; Singh-Manoux et al., 2017).

Persons with dementia can also present with increased health and lifestyle risks. Those with diagnosed forms of dementia have elevated rates of premature mortality and increased risk of suicide (See Chap. 5), especially among patients with both dementia and psychiatric comorbidities. Those with more advanced forms of dementia can also suffer from onset of severe chronic conditions such as cardiovascular disease, chronic kidney disease, dental problems, diabetes, and other neurological conditions (Snowden et al., 2017).

For those that are presenting for more routine care, comprehensive geriatric assessments are important for PCPs to determine the medical, psychological, and functional capabilities of an older adult patient. These assessments are vital in detecting underlying issues of individuals, reducing future hospitalizations, and increasing the life span in older adults (Ellis et al., 2011). For PCPs, the comprehensive assessment should be proficient because, as society ages, older adults will constitute a high percentage of patients in outpatient settings. The Medicare Annual Wellness Visit (MAWV) is one medical encounter that includes the key elements of geriatric assessment performed by PCPs. The MAWV and other routine assessments help inform care teams not only about specific health concerns, but form preventative care plans to help older adults thrive (Tatum III et al., 2018).

During the initial assessment, the mental status examination (MSE) is an essential tool to help inform PCPs to make important health, psychiatric, and cognitive interpretations of the patient. The MSE includes a historic report from the patient and observational data gathered by the physician throughout the patient encounter. The PCP should ensure that the patient is in a comfortable and non-judgmental environment to get the best reports from an initial assessment of the patient's capacity (Snyderman & Rovner, 2009; Wiley et al., 2024). The interview may include some brief observations during the encounter to assess the non-verbal and motor skills of the patient. The PCP may also use specific standardized tools to assess certain cognitive or health indicators for certain memory, cognitive, and spatial awareness testing (see Table 6.1). Brief assessments such as the Mini Mental Status Examination, Saint Louis University Mental Status Examination, and the Montreal Cognitive Assessment offer key indicators for memory loss at initial appointments.

Table 6.1 Cognitive assessments for older adult patients in primary care

Assessment	Number of items/scoring	Targeted areas	Length of time to complete
Mini status mental examination (MMSE)	30 point assessment. A score of 25 or higher indicates a normal range of cognition	Assesses cognitive impairment, specifically in orientation, attention, short-term memory, language skills, visual and spatial relationships, and follow instructions	7–8 min
Montreal cognitive assessment (MOCA)	30 item test that assesses a range of items. Score of 25 or less may indicate some form of cognitive impairment	Explores short-term memory, visuospatial abilities, executive functions, attention, concentration, language, and orientation to time and place	10–12 min
Mini-cog	5 point scale with two questions	Looks at spatial recognition and recall of items, to be administered as a quick screener	3–5 min
AD8 test	8 items on a 3-point rating scale, with 0–1 indicating normal range for cognition	Items that assess for forgetfulness, recall, interests, and daily functioning	4–5 min
General practitioner assessment of cognition (GPCOG)	9 items, with a score of 9 indicates cognitively intact	Investigates reasoning perception and other cognitive abilities to detect mild cognitive impairment	Less than 4 min
Saint Louis university mental status exam (SLUMS)	30-point assessment. 27 points or higher indicates normal cognitive functioning	Assesses for a range of cognitive, memory, recall, and spatial recognition abilities	10–12 min
Rapid geriatric assessment: Rapid cognitive screen (RCS)	4 questions, with a 10-point scale. 8 or higher indicates normal range	A brief screening for memory, executive functioning, recall and spatial orientation	2–3 min

Components of the Mental Status Exam

There are ten components of the MSE to help inform the PCPs of specific motor, cognitive, and functional areas of the older adult: appearance, behavior, speech, mood, affect, thoughts, perception, cognition, patient insights and judgment, and clinical judgment. The PCP needs to take time in conducting a thorough assessment, not just writing verbatim the patient's words and reports, but also tracking non-verbal feedback from the patient's facial and body expressions. Additionally, elements such as age, culture, gender, cognitive functioning, and language of the patient needs to be considered in the MSE report (Finney et al., 2016; Norris et al., 2016). Cognitive functioning and memory are two important areas of the MSE for PCPs to consider when working with older adults. Screening for these issues is a useful strategy when conditions are common and treatable even if not curable. This may allow for enhanced treatment planning at the early or asymptomatic asymptomatic stage (Siddiqui et al., 2023). Even in the absence of dementia, age-related cognitive decline impacts specific types of memories and brain structures in humans (Crimmins, 2015). However, many older adults who present with these symptoms in usual care often never receive a diagnosis, let alone a comprehensive evaluation to determine any risk factors of complications in the patient's life (Kotagal et al., 2015).

Assessment Around Cognitive Issues

- Conducting a comprehensive biopsychosocial-spiritual assessment: PCPs would benefit in taking a holistic and systemic approach in any cognitive assessment in primary care. Often, PCPs miss the underlying mental, cognitive, and social mechanisms that increase complications for those with memory concerns. Considering spirituality in aging adults is often crucial to understanding the context related to treatment and end of life decisions (See Chap. 2).
- Building therapeutic rapport: Given the stigma and shame associated with memory loss, physicians need to be attentive to therapeutic skills such as joining, humor, curiosity, and empathy to make older adults more comfortable at these appointments. Families with individuals diagnosed with dementia need PCPs who are supportive and transparent about the continued risks and symptoms that should be anticipated.
- Safety considerations for home and in public: Individuals with diagnosed memory issues are often at greater risk for falls and unexpected accidents. Allied health professionals and community health workers are important providers for PCPs to consider for families who are navigating in-home and external healthcare services. Medical teams should also provide education to patients and care partners about safety precautions in public, including the risks of driving with increasing memory loss concerns.

  PCPs are positioned to detect certain changes in thinking and behavior that might indicate dementia, as reported by the individual or by family members. After the diagnosis, PCPs must find ways to help offer strategies and information to the family at several phases of the disease. With the rise in older adult patients with cognitive challenges in our healthcare system, PCPs will be tasked with increasing requests for medical care along with caregiving and familial support among this population (Bernstein Sideman et al., 2023).

Some of the practice skills with patients at any stage and severity of dementia-related disorders should include:

- Responsibility for educating patients and family members about the progression of symptoms and ways to prevent complications in the home.
- Navigating referrals to help find the best specialists to help detect further diagnostic or behavioral issues.
- Developing trusting relationships with caregivers and other care partners of the patient, where open communication and trust is developed over time.
- Initiating conversations with patients' families to focus on a shared understanding of values, wishes and other preferences of those living with dementia.
- Evaluating the strains on caregivers and facilitating multiple services to decrease burden, improve quality of life, and enable caregivers to provide at-home care.

The Role of Family and Friends

Caregivers and family members also play key roles in helping to report signs and symptoms of their loved ones with memory loss or cognitive challenges. Although they can relay additional information to the medical team, their attendance at initial appointments can be inconsistent due to scheduling conflicts, work, or other commitments. Dementia caregivers also experience high levels of caring stress, anxiety, depression, and other emotional strains (Shin & Kim, 2022). This leaves the patient's self-report as one of the only factors for PCPs to determine any potential diagnosis of memory loss or form of dementia-related disorders. There are also cultural and community factors that often make it challenging for patients to disclose personal struggles with memory recall and other types of cognitive processes (Kim et al., 2023).

PCPs should be mindful of the types of referrals given to newly diagnosed patients with dementia or some type of memory loss. Often, caregivers and care partners need time to process how their lifestyle and daily management will look different because of their loved one's new diagnosis. Patients also need time to process what the context of the diagnosis will mean in their life and how proactive they want to be in effectively managing these new symptoms. If possible, working around caregiver schedules to ensure they are involved in primary care visits, and using the electronic medical record as a tool for communication with the caregiver (especially if the patient is combative or defensive) may be helpful.

The Geriatric 4Ms

One key role of providers is to cover what is called the "GERIATRIC 4Ms," which includes Mentation, Mobility, Medications, and What Matters Most (Lester et al., 2020; Molnar & Frank, 2019; see Fig. 6.1). These anchor measures help plan out an older adult's management of care, which is largely connected to the cognitive capabilities of the patient. Healthcare facilities have been charged with moving toward

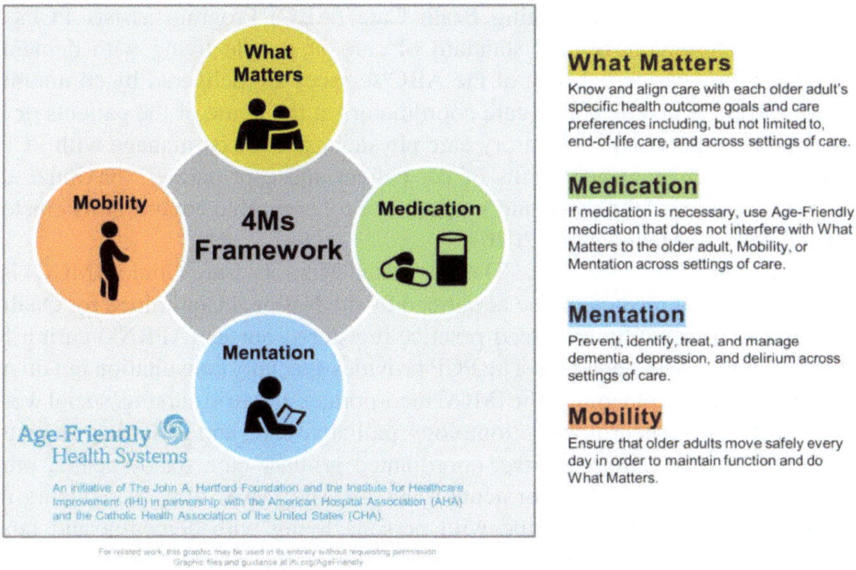

Fig. 6.1 4Ms framework of an age-friendly health system (Institute for Healthcare Improvement, 2024)

Age Friendly Health Centers, with the goal of creating a system that could better prevent avoidable harms, better patient care, and stronger support for caregivers and families (Fulmer et al., 2018). PCPs are now being asked to cover many of these metrics in usual care encounters for older adults. With PCPs often overwhelmed with the demanding tasks and caseloads in practices, covering these essential health indicators for older adults can be challenging in ambulatory visits (Boustani et al., 2007).

Interventions to Work with Memory Loss

- Primary care has evolved in the way that care can be provided by integrated teams. Unfortunately, most psychosocial and community models of dementia care and intervention focus only on specific dementia diagnoses such as Alzheimer's disease (Morhardt et al., 2015). These models are multi-dimensional in how they address the core components of dementia, and how a person might access and travel through such services (Lewis et al., 2023). Collaboration and continuity of services can help the PCP organize effective treatment plans and utilize the expertise of community providers to address specific memory loss complications.

- The ABC program: The Aging Brain Care (ABC) Program assists PCPs in achieving the recommended standard of care of people living with dementia and their care partners. Much of the ABC services are delivered by community health workers and dementia care coordinators at the home of the patients or by telephone, supervised by memory care physicians. They co-manage with PCPs, enhance self-management skills of the patient and care partner, maximize the coping behavior of the dyad, and support care for comorbid conditions (Feinstein et al., 2017; LaMantia et al., 2016).
- Integrated memory care clinic: The Integrated Memory Care Clinic (IMCC) is a patient-centered medical home as defined by the National Committee for Quality Assurance directed by advanced practice registered nurses (APRNs) caring for persons living with dementia. The PCP provides specialty consultation but do not direct care or care planning. The IMCC incorporates geriatric nursing, social work, and APRNs from neurology, gerontology, palliative care, and geriatric psychiatry. APRNs provide comprehensive, coordinated primary care for dementia, other chronic conditions, and minor acute illnesses. The IMCC aims at reducing the dementia burden by partnering with persons living with dementia and families through a palliative-oriented, dementia-informed medical home approach (Clevenger et al., 2018).
- MIND at home: The Maximizing Independence (MIND) at home dementia care coordination program is a coordinated protocol to address cognitive and memory symptoms (Samus et al., 2014). The program can be designed to address individual needs by addressing how medications are organized, fall and other safety risks, available community resources and caregiver support. Patients and caregivers work with a memory care coordinator, who is a nonclinical community health worker, as well as a team that includes a geriatric psychiatrist, registered nurse, and an occupational therapist. The team, which often is led by the direction of the PCP, conducts an in-home assessment followed by implementation of care plans based on six strategies: resource referrals, attention to environmental safety, dementia care education, behavior management skills training, informal counseling and problem-solving.

Pharmacological Treatments

Medications have been seen as the first line of treatment for early stages of memory loss and cognitive decline in primary care. Managing the changes associated with dementia requires a thoughtful approach from the medical team, weighing the risks of medications based on the stage of diagnosis and other co-occurring issues associated with memory problems. Patients and caregivers should always be aware that polypharmacy options are not a cure for dementia and do not alter the underlying disease process. In view of their modest efficacy, potential side effects and high cost, a thorough discussion with the patient and family is recommended.

Four of the most common medications (under the group called Cholinesterase Inhibitors) are indicated for several forms of dementia, including Alzheimer's disease: donepezil, rivastigmine, galantamine, and memantine. While these medications will not reverse the course of cognitive decline, they may stall the progression for those between mild to moderate stages of dementia. Adjustments to these medications should be dependent on risks of side effects, ineffective benefits, or other co-occurring issues for patients. In recent years, newly approved medications for dementia-related disorders have been available to the public with mixed reviews (Huang et al., 2023). Aducanumab and Lecanemab have received FDA approval. With all medications it is important to consider patient selection, surveillance for adverse events, and clinician preparedness for use of these medications for older adult patients (Cummings et al., 2022).

Non-pharmacological Treatments Provided by Behavioral Health Providers

Non-pharmacological interventions and treatments for memory loss, as well as those with brain damage and neurodegenerative disorders, have gained much attention in recent years. There is momentum for referrals to these interventions due to limited efficacy in drug therapies and lack of other medical treatments that slow the progression of memory and cognition (Cotelli et al., 2012). Behavioral and psychological symptoms of dementia (BPSDs) are among the most distressing sequelae of Alzheimer's disease and related dementias. While behavioral and educational approaches might help address some of the underlying mood and emotional areas of dementia, these approaches often lack effectiveness to treat the memory issues of patients. PCPs are not required to handle dementia care independently, but are encouraged to use their network of referrals and other community resources for the underlying psychosocial and behavioral aspects of the disease. While little is offered on-site regarding non-medication interventions, PCPs are encouraged to familiarize themselves with BH and educational resources to help their patients improve memory, mood, reminiscence, and other socialization skills (Moore et al., 2018).

Cognitive Stimulation Therapy Cognitive Stimulation Therapy (CST) is a psychosocial group intervention for individuals with mild to moderate dementia. CST is based upon cognitive stimulation, reality orientation, reminiscence therapy, and validation therapy (Spector et al., 2003). It incorporates aspects of holistic therapies and includes a guided curriculum. Usually, it is delivered twice a week for 45 min over 7 weeks. The 14-themed sessions are outlined in the manual *Making a Difference: An Evidenced-Based Group Program to Offer Cognitive Stimulation Therapy for People with Dementia* (Spector et al., 2020). Each session follows a structured protocol that uses themes of reminiscence and validation therapy to help participants develop new memory links based on past stories and memories. Improvements in cognition, mood, and quality of life factors were improved for long-term CST maintenance groups (Aguirre et al., 2010; Streater et al., 2012).

Reminiscence Therapy Reminiscence therapy involves eliciting recall of past events, activities, and memories via photographs, familiar items from the past, music and/or movies. Typically, recalling recent memories will be more difficult for individuals with neurocognitive disorders, while longer term memories of personal importance may be more accessible and available to the patient. This therapy encourages individuals to talk about previous experiences. This decreases the cognitive demand while encouraging those preserved abilities. Reminiscence has been identified as an effective means of improving mood in persons with dementia, but results are mixed regarding a definite cognitive benefit. PCPs can make referrals to BH providers to help facilitate this intervention in either individual or group settings. These encounters are typically once per week focusing on free recall of memories within the context of a focused life review (Woods et al., 2018). One strategy for the PCP to assist the patient with reminiscence is to inquire about positive memories from a patient's life and ask the patient, patient's family, and/or the caregiver(s) to bring a picture to the PCP visit to discuss briefly with your patient to increase positive memory recall.

Social Prescribing Social prescribing, also known as community referrals, requires health professionals to refer individuals to non-clinical services. This is a holistic approach to address health needs. These are prescribed to promote creativity and improve quality of life (Gallacher & Burns, 2021). The aim is to use a person-centered approach to connect people with unmet non-medical needs to community assets (public or private). These community assets are the available resources in the physical environment, in hopes of increasing social connections and thus improving long-term health outcomes (Percival et al., 2022).

The implementation and utilization of social prescribing from PCPs has been seen globally around memory and cognition. In Asia, healthcare facilities have partnered with care teams and social care networks to help find meaningful activities in the community to help stimulate cognition (Wang & Yu, 2023). Clinicians in Canada tailored social events and interventions based on the number of chronic conditions associated with older adult health and cognitive functioning. Participants not only found individual and community benefits but reported better rapport and coordination with their healthcare team (Ghogomu et al., 2024). In the UK, support services are now offered at community centers for older adults who do not have other sources of support provided from their healthcare team.

Other Considerations

- Age-friendly health systems: PCPs who work routinely with older adults may want to find ways to market or label their site as senior friendly. The development of an Age-Friendly Health System (Institute for Healthcare Improvement, 2024) status allows providers and clinics to market their practice to quality older adult care for a range of issues, including memory loss.

- Find and connect with dementia care specialist: Nurse Practitioners can receive advanced training to work with the biopsychosocial issues of older adults with memory complications. PCPs can often utilize these specialists to help manage co-occurring conditions and other areas of the patient at follow-up encounters.
- Integrating behavioral health services: Although PCPs and other medical professionals can adequately assess and treat ADRD, the incorporation of BH services to address co-occurring psychosocial and community needs is essential. For PCPs who have integrated behavioral health services on-site (See Chap. 12), including these providers into conversations with caregivers and families about the continued complications and management of the disease will be paramount.
- Educating caregivers early in the treatment process: One of the more frequent complaints from caregivers (family and professionals alike) is the lack of communication and upfront information from their medical team during initial appointments around memory loss. Caregivers should be intentionally and strategically incorporated into treatment plans for medical management, social engagement, resource decision-making, and connections to behavioral health and other specialists.
- In-home strategies that involve family and other care partners: Caregivers are tasked with managing many daily living activities for loved ones with memory and cognitive issues. Multidisciplinary care teams (social work, behavioral health, community healthcare workers, nursing) offer vital information for families to keep the home environment safe and accessible for patients. Additional services often provided in the home include physical therapy, occupational therapy, and other home healthcare options.
- Awareness of loneliness and social isolation: During the COVID-19 pandemic, healthcare providers saw the profound effects of being isolated from society for those patients with memory loss. As caregivers and care partners continue to struggle to find meaningful activities for their loved ones with memory and cognitive challenges, PCPs would benefit from assessing for loneliness and isolation more in this population. Providers would benefit from including a loneliness/ social isolation question into their yearly evaluations and wellness visits with older adult patients and engaging in social prescribing to connect these individuals to community resources (Lahlou & Daaleman, 2021).

Conclusions

Due to the increasing rates of cognitive impairment and other co-occurring issues related to memory loss, PCPs will be at the forefront of managing older adult neurological issues for years to come. Given the high volume of patients seen in primary care and other larger healthcare settings, PCPs need to be equipped with conducting brief screening approaches, and interventions to help detect cognitive functioning and other neurological areas in older adults (Lang & Bland, 2019). If the geriatrics workforce does not increase, provider-patient ratio will remain 1:3000 in usual care for older adult patients in the memory and cognitive issues in older adults would help address the growing demand for additional services in primary care settings. Given that PCPs will continue to be the lead medical provider to effectively screen, assess and treat memory loss issues, attending to the biopsychosocial and systemic dimensions of care will be important in the coming years.

Key Points

- PCPs should be knowledgeable in how to conduct a mental status examination and other brief observations in routine care.
- Family members and primary caregivers are key individuals to help inform the PCP about specific memory impairment and cognitive declines in their loved ones.
- Integrated teams with multiple providers involved in the older adult's care can help coordinate services and treatment plans efficiently.
- Even though medications help to slow the progression of memory decline in older adult patients, there are still few psychosocial interventions to help stimulate memory and mood in this population.

References

Aguirre, E., Spector, A., Hoe, J., Russell, I. T., Knapp, M., Woods, R. T., & Orrell, M. (2010). Maintenance cognitive stimulation therapy (CST) for dementia: A single-blind, multi-Centre, randomized controlled trial of maintenance CST vs CST for dementia. *Trials, 11*(1), 46. https://doi.org/10.1186/1745-6215-11-46

Bernstein Sideman, A., Gilissen, J., Harrison, K. L., Garrett, S. B., Terranova, M. J., Ritchie, C. S., & Geschwind, M. D. (2023). Caregiver experiences navigating the diagnostic journey in a rapidly progressing dementia. *Journal of Geriatric Psychiatry and Neurology, 36*(4), 282–294. https://doi.org/10.1177/08919887221135552

Boustani, M., Sachs, G., & Callahan, C. M. (2007). Can primary care meet the biopsychosocial needs of older adults with dementia? *Journal of General Internal Medicine, 22*(11), 1625–1627. https://doi.org/10.1007/s11606-007-0386-y

Bradford, A., Kunik, M. E., Schulz, P., Williams, S. P., & Singh, H. (2009). Missed and delayed diagnosis of dementia in primary care: Prevalence and contributing factors. *Alzheimer Disease & Associated Disorders, 23*(4), 306. https://doi.org/10.1097/WAD.0b013e3181a6bebc

Clevenger, C. K., Cellar, J., Kovaleva, M., Medders, L., & Hepburn, K. (2018). Integrated memory care clinic: Design, implementation, and initial results. *Journal of the American Geriatrics Society, 66*(12), 2401–2407. https://doi.org/10.1111/jgs.15528

Cotelli, M., Manenti, R., Zanetti, O., & Miniussi, C. (2012). Non-pharmacological intervention for memory decline. *Frontiers in Human Neuroscience, 6*. https://doi.org/10.3389/fnhum.2012.00046

Crimmins, E. M. (2015). Lifespan and healthspan: Past, present, and promise. *The Gerontologist, 55*(6), 901–911. https://doi.org/10.1093/geront/gnv130

Cummings, J., Rabinovici, G. D., Atri, A., Aisen, P., Apostolova, L. G., Hendrix, S., Sabbagh, M., Selkoe, D., Weiner, M., Salloway, S., & Alzheimer's Disease and Related Disorders Therapeutics

Working Group. (2022). Aducanumab: Appropriate use recommendations update. *The Journal of Prevention of Alzheimer's Disease, 9*(2), 221–230. https://doi.org/10.14283/jpad.2022.34

Dai, M., & Peterson, L. E. (2020). Characteristics of family medicine residency graduates, 1994-2017: An update. *The Annals of Family Medicine, 18*(4), 370–373. https://doi.org/10.1370/afm.2535

Ellis, G., Whitehead, M. A., Robinson, D., O'Neill, D., & Langhorne, P. (2011). Comprehensive geriatric assessment for older adults admitted to hospital: Meta-analysis of randomised controlled trials. *BMJ, 343*, d6553. https://doi.org/10.1136/bmj.d6553

Feinstein, D. R., Connelly, D. J., & Feinstein, M. (2017). *Integrating behavioral health and primary care.* Oxford University Press.

Finney, G. R., Minagar, A., & Heilman, K. M. (2016). Assessment of mental status. *Neurologic Clinics, 34*(1), 1–16. https://doi.org/10.1016/j.ncl.2015.08.001

Fulmer, T., Mate, K. S., & Berman, A. (2018). The age-friendly health system imperative. *Journal of the American Geriatrics Society, 66*(1), 22–24. https://doi.org/10.1111/jgs.15076

Gallacher, J., & Burns, A. (2021). Social prescribing for dementia. *The Lancet Neurology, 20*(9), 707–708. https://doi.org/10.1016/S1474-4422(21)00208-8

Ghogomu, E. T., Welch, V., Yaqubi, M., Dewidar, O., Barbeau, V. I., Biswas, S., Card, K., Hsiung, S., Muhl, C., Nelson, M., Salzwedel, D. M., Saragosa, M., Yu, C., Mulligan, K., & Hébert, P. (2024). PROTOCOL: Effects of social prescribing for older adults: An evidence and gap map. *Campbell Systematic Reviews, 20*(2), e1382. https://doi.org/10.1002/cl2.1382

Huang, L.-K., Kuan, Y.-C., Lin, H.-W., & Hu, C.-J. (2023). Clinical trials of new drugs for Alzheimer disease: A 2020–2023 update. *Journal of Biomedical Science, 30*(1), 83. https://doi.org/10.1186/s12929-023-00976-6

Institute for Healthcare Improvement. (2024). *Age-friendly health systems.* https://www.ihi.org/networks/initiatives/age-friendly-health-systems

Kim, S., Yoon, H., & Jang, Y. (2023). Access to primary healthcare and discussion of memory loss with a healthcare provider in adults with subjective cognitive decline: Does race/ethnicity matter? *Behavioral Sciences, 13*(11), 955. https://doi.org/10.3390/bs13110955

Kotagal, V., Langa, K. M., Plassman, B. L., Fisher, G. G., Giordani, B. J., Wallace, R. B., Burke, J. R., Steffens, D. C., Kabeto, M., Albin, R. L., & Foster, N. L. (2015). Factors associated with cognitive evaluations in the United States. *Neurology, 84*(1), 64–71. https://doi.org/10.1212/WNL.0000000000001096

Lahlou, R. M., & Daaleman, T. P. (2021). Addressing loneliness and social isolation in older adults. *American Family Physician, 104*(1), 85–87.

LaMantia, M. A., Perkins, A. J., Gao, S., Austrom, M. G., Alder, C. A., French, D. D., Litzelman, D. K., Cottingham, A. H., & Boustani, M. A. (2016). Response to depression treatment in the aging brain care medical home model. *Clinical Interventions in Aging, 11*, 1551–1558. https://doi.org/10.2147/CIA.S109114

Lang, C. E., & Bland, M. D. (2019). Impaired motor control and neurologic rehabilitation in older adults. In *Guccione's geriatric physical therapy*. Elsevier Health Sciences.

Lester, P. E., Dharmarajan, T. S., & Weinstein, E. (2020). The looming geriatrician shortage: Ramifications and solutions. *Journal of Aging and Health, 32*(9), 1052–1062. https://doi.org/10.1177/0898264319879325

Lewis, S., Triandafilidis, Z., Curryer, C., Jeong, S. Y.-S., Goodwin, N., Carr, S., & Davis, D. (2023). Models of care for people with dementia approaching end of life: A rapid review. *Palliative Medicine, 37*(7), 915–930. https://doi.org/10.1177/02692163231171181

Luo, J., Beam, C. R., & Gatz, M. (2023). Is stress an overlooked risk factor for dementia? A systematic review from a lifespan developmental perspective. *Prevention Science, 24*(5), 936–949. https://doi.org/10.1007/s11121-022-01385-1

Molnar, F., & Frank, C. C. (2019). Optimizing geriatric care with the GERIATRIC 5Ms. *Canadian Family Physician, 65*(1), 39–39.

Moore, A., Frank, C., & Chambers, L. W. (2018). Role of the family physician in dementia care. *Canadian Family Physician, 64*(10), 717–719.

Morhardt, D., Weintraub, S., Khayum, B., Robinson, J., Medina, J., O'Hara, M., Mesulam, M., & Rogalski, E. J. (2015). The CARE pathway model for dementia: Psychosocial and rehabilitative strategies for care in young-onset dementias. *The Psychiatric Clinics of North America, 38*(2), 333–352. https://doi.org/10.1016/j.psc.2015.01.005

Mueller, C., Molokhia, M., Perera, G., Veronese, N., Stubbs, B., Shetty, H., Codling, D., Huntley, J., & Stewart, R. (2018). Polypharmacy in people with dementia: Associations with adverse health outcomes. *Experimental Gerontology, 106*, 240–245. https://doi.org/10.1016/j.exger.2018.02.011

Norris, D. R., Clark, M. S., & Shipley, S. (2016). The mental status examination. *American Family Physician, 94*(8), 635–641.

Percival, A., Newton, C., Mulligan, K., Petrella, R. J., & Ashe, M. C. (2022). Systematic review of social prescribing and older adults: Where to from here? *Family Medicine and Community Health, 10*(Suppl 1), e001829. https://doi.org/10.1136/fmch-2022-001829

Rao, G. P., Sivakumar, P. T., Srivastava, S., & Sidana, R. C. (2020). Cognitive therapy and family intervention for patients with dementia and psychosis. *Indian Journal of Psychiatry, 62*(Suppl 2), S183. https://doi.org/10.4103/psychiatry.IndianJPsychiatry_769_19

Ruangritchankul, S., Peel, N. M., Hanjani, L. S., & Gray, L. C. (2020). Drug related problems in older adults living with dementia. *PLoS One, 15*(7), e0236830. https://doi.org/10.1371/journal.pone.0236830

Samus, Q. M., Johnston, D., Black, B. S., Hess, E., Lyman, C., Vavilikolanu, A., Pollutra, J., Leoutsakos, J.-M., Gitlin, L. N., Rabins, P. V., & Lyketsos, C. G. (2014). A multidimensional home-based care coordination intervention for elders with memory disorders: The maximizing independence at home (MIND) pilot randomized trial. *The American Journal of Geriatric Psychiatry, 22*(4), 398–414. https://doi.org/10.1016/j.jagp.2013.12.175

Shin, J. H., & Kim, J. H. (2022). Family caregivers of people with dementia associate with poor health-related quality of life: A nationwide population-based study. *International Journal of Environmental Research and Public Health, 19*(23), 16252. https://doi.org/10.3390/ijerph192316252

Shinagawa, S., Catindig, J. A., Block, N. R., Miller, B. L., & Rankin, K. P. (2016). When a little knowledge can be dangerous: False-positive diagnosis of behavioral variant frontotemporal dementia among community clinicians. *Dementia and Geriatric Cognitive Disorders, 41*(1-2), 99–108. https://doi.org/10.1159/000438454

Siddiqui, M., Nyahoda, T., Traber, C., Elliott, S., Wang, V., Toledo-Franco, L., & Rodin, M. B. (2023). Screening for cognitive impairment in primary care: Rationale and tools. *Missouri Medicine, 120*(6), 431–439.

Singh-Manoux, A., Dugravot, A., Fournier, A., Abell, J., Ebmeier, K., Kivimäki, M., & Sabia, S. (2017). Trajectories of depressive symptoms before diagnosis of dementia: A 28-year follow-up study. *JAMA Psychiatry, 74*(7), 712–718. https://doi.org/10.1001/jamapsychiatry.2017.0660

Snowden, M. B., Steinman, L. E., Bryant, L. L., Cherrier, M. M., Greenlund, K. J., Leith, K. H., Levy, C., Logsdon, R. G., Copeland, C., Vogel, M., Anderson, L. A., Atkins, D. C., Bell, J. F., & Fitzpatrick, A. L. (2017). Dementia and co-occurring chronic conditions: A systematic literature review to identify what is known and where are the gaps in the evidence? *International Journal of Geriatric Psychiatry, 32*(4), 357–371. https://doi.org/10.1002/gps.4652

Snyderman, D., & Rovner, B. W. (2009). Mental status examination in primary care: A review. *American Family Physician, 80*(8), 809–814.

Spector, A., Thorgrimsen, L., Woods, B., Royan, L., Davies, S., Butterworth, M., & Orrell, M. (2003). Efficacy of an evidence-based cognitive stimulation therapy programme for people with dementia: Randomised controlled trial. *The British Journal of Psychiatry, 183*(3), 248–254. https://doi.org/10.1192/bjp.183.3.248

Spector, A., Woods, B., Stoner, R. C., & Orrell, M. (2020). *Making a difference 1: An evidence based group program to offer cognitive stimulation therapy (CST) to people with dementia* (2nd ed.). https://www.ucl.ac.uk/international-cognitive-stimulation-therapy/publications/cst-manuals

Streater, A., Spector, A., Aguirre, E., Hoe, J., Hoare, Z., Woods, R., Russell, I., & Orrell, M. (2012). Maintenance cognitive stimulation therapy (CST) in practice: Study protocol for a randomized controlled trial. *Trials, 13*(1), 91. https://doi.org/10.1186/1745-6215-13-91

Tatum, P. E., III, Talebreza, S., & Ross, J. S. (2018). Geriatric assessment: An office-based approach. *American Family Physician, 97*(12), 776–784.

Wang, H., & Yu, X. (2023). Strengthening implementation research on social prescribing in mental healthcare for older adults in Western Pacific region. *The Lancet Regional Health, 35*, 100721. https://doi.org/10.1016/j.lanwpc.2023.100721

Wiley, A. T., Dreher, J. W., & London, J. D. (2024). Mental status examination in primary care. *American Family Physician, 109*(1), 51–60.

Wismann, A., Kleszynski, K., Jelinek, D., Hand, R., Lich, B., Wickersham, E., & Jennings, L. A. (2024). An age-friendly approach to primary care in an academic health system. *Journal of the American Geriatrics Society, 72*(S3), S23–S35. https://doi.org/10.1111/jgs.18848

Woods, B., O'Philbin, L., Farrell, E. M., Spector, A. E., & Orrell, M. (2018). Reminiscence therapy for dementia. *Cochrane Database of Systematic Reviews, 3*. https://doi.org/10.1002/14651858.CD001120.pub3

[illegible]

Chapter 7
Psychopharmacology for the Primary Care Provider

Ryan Laschober MD, FAAFP, Lance Kelley PhD, and Zach Sartor MD, FAAFP

General Prescribing Principles

The Role of Psychopharmacology in Treatment Psychopharmacology is a crucial element of the primary care management of behavioral health (BH) conditions (Hughes et al., 2024). Evidence-based psychopharmacological interventions have been shown to significantly enhance the quality of life for patients with BH conditions. However, the primary care provider (PCP) needs an understanding of the principles of prescribing such medication to be as effective as possible. This section provides clinicians with the standard approach to choosing a pharmacological treatment option for any BH condition. Importantly, these are general rules and may not apply to all patients or all situations, but they will be helpful in most cases. They will provide a launching point for PCPs who prescribe medications for treating BH conditions.

Collaborative Prescribing Collaborative prescribing occurs when the PCP works with the patient to identify the goals for treatment alongside the patient as opposed to a more conventional or "paternalistic" approach. A collaborative approach can improve adherence and lead to better therapeutic effects.

Risk-Benefit Assessment A thorough risk-benefit assessment is fundamental before prescribing psychotropic medication. A risk-benefit assessment is a systematic and ongoing evaluation of a medication's efficacy and safety. This process primarily

R. Laschober MD, FAAFP · L. Kelley PhD (✉) · Z. Sartor MD, FAAFP
The Waco Guide to Psychopharmacology®, Waco Family Medicine, Waco, TX, USA
e-mail: Lance.Kelley@wacofamilymedicine.org

R. Laschober MD, FAAFP
e-mail: ryan.laschober@wacofamilymedicine.org

Z. Sartor MD, FAAFP
e-mail: Zach.Sartor@wacofamilymedicine.org

M. L. C. Williamson and D. L. Terry (eds.), *Essentials for Treating Behavioral Health in Primary Care*, https://doi.org/10.1007/978-3-032-09558-9_7

involves weighing two key aspects: the benefits, which encompass both the therapeutic effectiveness and the enhancement of quality of life, and the risks, which include the safety profile of the medication and the likelihood of unintended adverse events that are predicted based on the drug's mechanism of action (Curtin & Schulz, 2011). This assessment may also include cost.

Getting in Front of "The Guinea Pig" Phenomenon

BH conditions vary widely in how they respond to psychopharmacological interventions. This reality inevitably leads to a natural trial-and-error process in prescribing, where patients may need to try multiple medications or dosages before finding the one that effectively manages their symptoms without intolerable side effects. This is commonly referred to as the "guinea pig" phenomenon, as patients often report feeling like experimental subjects during the process of finding the right medication and dosage. When PCPs anticipate this concern, they can discuss it openly and establish specific, measurable objectives for treatment. Moreover, openly discussing clinical decision support tools with a patient may also be beneficial as they offer reassurance that an evidence-based treatment plan is in place.

Treatment Targets Establishing clear, individualized treatment targets is critical for guiding therapeutic decisions and measuring progress. Determining the desired outcome informs whether a treatment is successful, unsuccessful, or partially successful. Is the goal remission or significantly reducing a particular symptom or constellation? Although, understandably, a patient may desire to eliminate a set of symptoms, this is often an unrealistic expectation. For example, in the context of clinical trials for obsessive-compulsive disorder (OCD), a "full response" to treatment is often defined as achieving a 35% reduction in the severity of symptoms (Tolin et al., 2015).

Shared Decision-Making Shared decision-making (SDM), where the PCP and patient collaborate to make decisions about the next treatment steps, is foundational to patient-centered care. Two experts contribute to effective SDM: Patients as experts in their own lives and perceived needs (Coulter & Collins, 2011) and PCPs as experts on evidence-based treatment options. SDM is linked to improved adherence to medical decisions, decreased medical errors, reduced stigma, and greater patient engagement (Slade, 2017). To realize the benefits of SDM, prescribing clinicians should share the latest evidence-based treatment options, potential benefits, and risks and elicit from patients their preferences, concerns, and values. This process may involve including BH providers, family members, and peer support into integrated care teams with primary care. By embedding shared decision-making into the fabric of primary care, clinicians honor a patient's right to self-determination and promote transparency about treatment options.

Psychopharmacology in Action

Navigating the complexities of psychopharmacologic medications requires an appropriate understanding of their initiation, titration, continuation, and the management of common side effects, as well as their discontinuation. Fortunately, a wealth of resources stands ready to guide healthcare professionals through these critical decisions. This section aims to serve as an essential tool in this journey, offering evidence-based insights and practical guidance for optimizing patient care in psychopharmacology within primary care settings.

Medication Initiation and Titration

Starting Medication When commencing treatment with psychopharmaceuticals, the guiding principle should be to begin at the lowest dose approved by the FDA for the specific condition being treated. The commonly adopted mantra in this context is to "start low and go slow," emphasizing a cautious and gradual approach to dosage increases.

The titration of psychopharmaceuticals is a nuanced process that must be tailored to each patient's response to treatment. While some individuals may exhibit improvement within the first 2 weeks of pharmacotherapy, others might show significant progress in the 6–8 weeks. The essence of adequate titration lies in starting with the lowest FDA-approved dose for a given condition and increasing steadily as clinically indicated and tolerable. This approach involves adjusting the medication dose every 1–4 weeks until one of three potential outcomes results: achieving an adequate therapeutic response, reaching the maximum dose approved by the FDA without a meaningful response, or encountering intolerable side effects. Insufficient dose titration is a common error seen in primary care psychopharmacology, underscoring the importance of carefully evaluating previous medication trials, including the doses used.

Side effects might emerge as doses are adjusted upward, often resolving within a few weeks. Managing these side effects can involve maintaining the current dose, reducing the dose, or discontinuing the medication through a gradual tapering process over several weeks in the case of intolerable side effects.

At the beginning of the treatment process, clinicians must communicate with patients that adjusting medication doses is a standard and expected part of managing their therapy. By setting this expectation, clinicians can foster a sense of preparedness and partnership. This approach helps to build a solid therapeutic alliance between the patient and clinician, laying the groundwork for a collaborative and transparent treatment journey.

Adherence Concerns about adherence to treatment regimens are common and can arise from various factors. One significant contributor to incomplete adherence is the need for sufficient follow-up intervals. Research by Posternak and

Zimmerman (2007) has demonstrated that more frequent follow-up visits can significantly improve adherence rates to antidepressant therapies. This finding highlights the importance of regular monitoring and support from healthcare clinicians to assist patients in reaching their goals.

Moreover, the onset of side effects during the initial weeks of treatment can deter patients from continuing pharmacotherapy. Providing appropriate anticipatory guidance, strategies for symptom management, and setting realistic expectations can be pivotal in helping patients navigate these early challenges. Ensuring patients understand the transient nature of many side effects and the potential for symptom improvement can foster greater adherence.

Lastly, the stigma and misconceptions surrounding behavioral health conditions can also hinder adherence. These societal perceptions can lead to premature discontinuation of antidepressants, as individuals may feel discouraged by the negative views associated with their treatment.

Evaluating Treatment Response

Trial Response Assessing the effectiveness of psychopharmacological treatments involves a multifaceted approach, incorporating patient self-reporting, clinician evaluations, observations of functional improvements, and standardized psychometric tools. Measurement-based care (MBC) is a systematic approach to tracking a patient's progress through standardized instruments, such as the Patient Health Questionnaire-9 (PHQ-9) for depression or the Generalized Anxiety Disorder Scale (GAD-7) for anxiety (Kroenke et al., 1999; Spitzer et al., 2006). These tools are critical in clinical settings for guiding treatment decisions, enhancing patient outcomes, and tailoring care to individual needs. By establishing a baseline at the outset of treatment and comparing subsequent scores, healthcare teams can accurately gauge treatment response, adjust interventions as needed, and actively involve patients in their treatment plans.

Findings from significant studies like the Star*D trial (Rush et al., 2004) underscore the importance of MBC. The trial demonstrated that using standardized measures and protocols in treatment can lead to equally positive outcomes in primary care and psychiatric settings. This highlights the effectiveness of MBC in leveling the playing field across different care environments and communities.

An exemplary MBC tool is the PHQ-9, a validated instrument renowned for its sensitivity (88%) and specificity (85%) in screening for major depression. Appropriate for individuals aged 12 and above, it serves as a screening tool and a method for assessing treatment response. The PHQ-9 quantifies response as follows: a reduction of symptoms by more than 50% indicates a successful response, a 25–49% improvement suggests a partial response and less than 25% improvement is considered an inadequate response. Such metrics enable clinicians to monitor the efficacy of medications and make collaborative and impactful treatment decisions (Table 7.1). Integrating MBC tools like the PHQ-9 into routine care is crucial for optimizing treatment strategies and ensuring patients receive the most effective interventions for their needs. See Chap. 4 for additional information on screening measures.

Adequate Trial Length Determining the appropriate duration for medication trials is crucial in psychopharmacology. The length of these trials can vary significantly, depending on the medication class used and the specific condition it's intended to treat. For instance, in the treatment of major depressive disorder (MDD), the standard duration for a trial of SSRIs (Selective Serotonin Reuptake Inhibitors) is typically 6 to 8 weeks at the maximum tolerable and indicated dose before considering the treatment unsuccessful. On the other hand, treating OCD with SSRIs usually requires a longer commitment, with trials extending from 8 to 12 weeks at the maximum tolerable and advised dose to assess effectiveness accurately. For regularly updated disorder-specific trial lengths, reference The Waco Guide to Psychopharmacology® (Laschober et al., n.d.).

Especially in managing major depressive disorder, one of the most frequently encountered conditions in behavioral health, it's established that a minimum trial period of 6–8 weeks at the highest tolerable dose is necessary. This recommendation is supported by evidence indicating that up to one-third of patients who do not show a response at the 2-week mark may begin to respond by the sixth week. This underscores the importance of patience and persistence in the treatment of MDD, ensuring that decisions regarding the efficacy of a medication are made based on an adequate trial length.

Switching Medications In behavioral health treatment, it becomes necessary to transition a patient from one medication to another (Table 7.2, Table 7.3).

Switching medications depends on several factors, including the characteristics of the medicines involved, their effects on metabolic enzymes, and their pharmacological classes. For some medications, a direct switch, where the new medication is started the day after discontinuing the old one, is possible and safe. This approach is often referred to as dose-equivalent switching. However, in other cases, a more gradual process known as cross-tapering is required. Cross-tapering involves slowly

Table 7.1 Trial length for tolerable psychopharmacology doses (Laschober et al., n.d.)

Behavioral health condition	Typical minimum pharmacotherapy trial length at maximum clinically indicated and tolerable dose	Potential MBC tool(s)
Major depressive disorder	6–8 weeks	PHQ-9 (>12), CES-D (</=12), postpartum (Edinburgh)
Generalized anxiety disorder	6–8 weeks	GAD-7
Posttraumatic stress disorder	6–8 weeks	PCL-5
ADHD	1–2 weeks (stimulants), 6 weeks (nonstimulants)	Vanderbilt (pediatrics), ASRS (adults)

Table 7.2 Titration guide

From ↓ / To →	Sertraline Citalopram Escitalopram	Fluoxetine	Paroxetine Fluvoxamine	Duloxetine Venlafaxine Desvenlafaxine	Bupropion	Mirtazapine	Vortioxetine Vilazodone	Tricyclic Antidepressants
Sertraline Citalopram Escitalopram	Start new medication 1 day after stopping old medication Consider a quick cross-taper for high doses of medication before starting new medication Example: -Sertraline 200 mg taper to 100 mg for 2-3 days while starting new medication	Start new medication 1 day after stopping old medication Consider a quick cross-taper for high doses of medication before starting new medication Example: -Sertraline 200 mg taper to 100 mg for 2-3 days while starting new medication	Start new medication 1 day after stopping old medication Consider a quick cross-taper for high doses of medication before starting new medication Example: -Sertraline 200 mg taper to 100 mg for 2-3 days while starting new medication	Cross taper medications over 1-2 weeks	Start new medication 1 day after stopping old medication Consider a quick cross-taper for high doses of medication before starting new medication Example: -Sertraline 200 mg taper to 100 mg for 2-3 days while starting new medication	Start new medication 1 day after stopping old medication Consider a quick cross-taper for high doses of medication before starting new medication Example: -Sertraline 200 mg taper to 100 mg for 2-3 days while starting new medication	Start new medication 1 day after stopping old medication Consider a quick cross-taper for high doses of medication before starting new medication Example: -Sertraline 200 mg taper to 100 mg for 2-3 days while starting new medication	Start new medication 1 day after stopping old medication Consider a quick taper for high doses of medication before starting new medication Example: -Sertraline 200 mg taper to 100 mg for 2-3 days before starting new medication
Fluoxetine	Stop old medication and start new medication at least 1 week later	-	Stop old medication and start new medication at least 1 week later	Stop old medication and start new medication at least 1 week later	Start new medication 1 day after stopping old medication	Stop old medication and start new medication at least 1 week later	Stop old medication and start new medication at least 1 week later	Stop old medication and start new medication at least 1 week later
Paroxetine Fluvoxamine	Cross taper medications over 2 weeks	Cross taper medications over 2 weeks	Cross taper medications over 2 weeks	Cross taper medications over 2 weeks	Add new medication then taper old medication slowly over 2 weeks	Add new medication then taper old medication slowly over 2 weeks	Cross taper medications over 2 weeks	Slowly taper old medication over 2 weeks Start new medication 1 day after stopping old medication
Duloxetine Venlafaxine Desvenlafaxine	Cross taper medications over 1-2 weeks	Cross taper medications over 2 weeks	Cross taper medications over 1-2 weeks	Cross taper medications over 1-2 weeks	Add new medication then taper old medication slowly over 1-2 weeks	Add new medication then taper old medication slowly over 1-2 weeks	Cross taper medications over 1-2 weeks	Slowly taper old medication over 1-2 weeks Start new medication 1 day after stopping old medication
Bupropion	Start new medication 1 day after stopping old medication	Start new medication 1 day after stopping old medication	Add new medication then taper old medication slowly over 1-2 weeks Example: start new medication and taper bupropion by 150 mg every 1-2 weeks	Add new medication then taper old medication slowly over 1-2 weeks Example: start new medication and taper bupropion by 150 mg every 1-2 weeks	-	Add new medication then taper old medication slowly over 1-2 weeks Example: start new medication and taper bupropion by 150 mg every 1-2 weeks	Add new medication then taper old medication slowly over 1-2 weeks Example: start new medication and taper bupropion by 150 mg every 1-2 weeks	Add new medication then taper old medication slowly over 1-2 weeks Example: start new medication and taper bupropion by 150 mg every 1-2 weeks
Mirtazapine	Start new medication 1 day after stopping old medication	Start new medication 1 day after stopping old medication	Start new medication 1 day after stopping old medication	Start new medication 1 day after stopping old medication	Start new medication 1 day after stopping old medication	-	Start new medication 1 day after stopping old medication	Slowly taper old medication over 1-2 weeks Start new medication 1 day after stopping old medication
Vortioxetine Vilazodone	Start new medication 1 day after stopping old medication (taper high doses)	Start new medication 1 day after stopping old medication	Start new medication 1 day after stopping old medication	Start new medication 1 day after stopping old medication	Start new medication 1 day after stopping old medication	Start new medication 1 day after stopping old medication	-	Slowly taper old medication over 1-2 weeks Start new medication 1 day after stopping old medication
Tricyclic Antidepressants	Slowly taper old medication over 1-2 weeks Doses less than 50 mg do not need to be tapered Start new medication 1 day after stopping old medication	Slowly taper old medication over 1-2 weeks Doses less than 50 mg do not need to be tapered Start new medication 1 day after stopping old medication	Slowly taper old medication over 1-2 weeks Doses less than 50 mg do not need to be tapered Start new medication 1 day after stopping old medication	Slowly taper old medication over 1-2 weeks Doses less than 50 mg do not need to be tapered Start new medication 1 day after stopping old medication	Cross taper medications over 1-2 weeks Doses less than 50 mg do not need to be tapered	Slowly taper old medication over 1-2 weeks Doses less than 50 mg do not need to be tapered Start new medication 1 day after stopping old medication	Slowly taper old medication over 1-2 weeks Doses less than 50 mg do not need to be tapered Start new medication 1 day after stopping old medication	Cross taper medications over 1-2 weeks Doses less than 50 mg do not need to be tapered

Table 7.3 Titration guide continued

From ↓ / To →	Antipsychotics	Lithium	Valproic Carbamazepine Lamotrigine
Antipsychotics	Cross taper agents over 2 weeks Monitor for emerging side effects and need for additional titration Consider a longer cross tapers may be needed for higher doses of antipsychotics	Start and titrate new medication to an effective dose then taper antipsychotic over a course of 2 weeks Monitor for emerging side effects and need for additional titration Consider a longer cross tapers may be needed for higher doses of antipsychotics	Start and titrate new medication to effective dose then taper antipsychotic over a course of 2 weeks Monitor for emerging side effects and need for additional titration Consider a longer cross tapers may be needed for higher doses of antipsychotics
Lithium	Start and titrate antipsychotic to an effective dose then taper lithium over a course of 2 weeks	-	Start and titrate new medication to an effective dose then taper lithium over a course of 2 weeks
Valproic Acid Carbamazepine Lamotrigine	Start antipsychotic and taper mood stabilizer over a course of 2 weeks	Start and titrate new medication to an effective dose then taper old medication over a course of 2 weeks	Taper old medication completely over 2 weeks prior to starting new medication

decreasing the dose of the initial medication while gradually increasing the dose of the new medicines. This method helps to minimize withdrawal effects from the first medication. It reduces the risk of adverse reactions from the new medication, ensuring a smoother and safer transition for the patient.

Tapering and/or Discontinuing Medications The approach to discontinuing a medication is tailored to the particular drug, considering factors such as its half-life and how long the patient has taken it. It is generally recommended to gradually reduce the pharmacotherapy dosage over several weeks. This methodical process helps mitigate withdrawal symptoms and allows for adjustment to the decreasing levels of medication.

Leveraging Resources to Elevate Practice

In the intricate realm of BH medication management, the necessity for evidence-based psychopharmacology resources cannot be overstated. While reviewing guidelines and scholarly articles is foundational to a clinician's comprehension of psychopharmacological treatments, access to a reliable point-of-care resource is unparalleled. Clinical decision support tools (CDSTs) are designed to seamlessly integrate evidence-based guidelines, literature reviews, and expert consensus into daily patient care. Committee on Quality of Health Care in America (2001) highlights the significance of such tools in its report "Crossing the Quality Chasm," advocating for clinical tools that systematically apply current knowledge to the decision-making process in healthcare. Furthermore, the Chronic Care Model (CCM), championed by E.H. Wagner, emphasizes the importance of embedding evidence-based clinical guidelines into everyday practice, democratizing access to specialized knowledge (Coleman et al., 2009).

Drawing inspiration from these principles, *The Waco Guide to Psychopharmacology in Primary Care®* was created to address the routine and complex aspects of BH care in primary care (Laschober et al., n.d.). These tools are indispensable for PCPs, offering them the latest evidence to inform their treatment strategies. *The Waco Guide to Psychopharmacology in Primary Care®* was developed by Waco Family Medicine Residency faculty in consultation with faculty in the Department of Psychiatry within the Division of Professional and Public Education at Massachusetts General Hospital. It aims to synthesize the highest-quality evidence with expert opinions to support PCPs in their busy practices. To develop the tools, we used a modified consensus-building process. A dependable resource becomes essential given the complexities of tracking treatment durations, failed medication trials, and other specifics. This compendium, featuring over 100 clinical decision support tools, aims to enhance evidence-based prescribing practices for BH conditions within the primary care setting. *The Waco Guide to Psychopharmacology in Primary Care®* is recognized by the American Medical Association's Behavioral Health Integration Collaborative and the American College of Physicians. Notably, it is a freely available resource, developed without industry funding, and accessible across various platforms, including its website, iOS, and Android apps.

The Waco Guide to Psychopharmacology in Primary Care Guide® comprehensively covers a broad spectrum of topics pertinent to psychopharmacology in primary care—from indications for pharmacotherapy and initial dosing strategies to titration methods, management of side effects, determination of treatment durations, guidelines for medication switching, and considerations for next steps following unsuccessful trials. This guide is an indispensable national resource, facilitating the application of evidence-based practices in managing BH conditions in primary care settings. Moreover, the Waco Guide was studied and proven effective as an instrument for medical education. Researchers from the University of Texas Medical Branch at Galveston used *The Waco Guide to Psychopharmacology in Primary Care®* as the curricular resource to develop training for obstetrical residents and other medical learners, showing the guide's utility in significantly improving clinicians' ability to manage BH conditions (Mallya et al., 2024).

Practical Prescribing Considerations

This section aims to equip clinicians with practical prescribing considerations, offering additional guidance in making informed psychopharmacological decisions beyond the standard practices described in previous sections. These topics greatly influence treatment decisions and will serve as guiding principles throughout all psychopharmacological practice. By bridging the gap between theory and practice, this section will support PCPs in their mission to provide holistic and patient-centered BH care, ensuring that the principles of efficacy, safety, and patient preference guide every prescribing decision.

Cost The economic aspect of prescribing psychopharmacological treatments is essential, as the financial burden significantly impacts patient adherence. Generic medications, which can reduce costs by up to 85% compared to branded counterparts, often present a viable, cost-effective solution (U.S. Food and Drug Administration, 2021). Fortunately, many medications from standard pharmaceutical classes—SSRIs, mood stabilizers, hypnotics—have wide availability as generic formulations, ensuring that clinicians have the option of using effective yet affordable psychopharmacological treatments. A common concern among clinicians and patients may be that brand-name medications work better than generic ones; however, research has contradicted this (Kesselheim et al., 2008; Tian et al., 2020). New medications, which are under patent and unavailable as generics, tend to offer hope for newer, more effective treatment options. However, rarely do newer medications offer benefits for effectiveness; instead, they offer tolerability or other non-effectiveness advantages. Therefore, novel medications necessary for treatment will occasionally be available as brand names.

For example, a novel dextromethorphan-bupropion combination antidepressant is only available under the brand name Auvelity®. The clinical effectiveness data show separation from placebo: a −15.9 point reduction on the Montgomery-Åsberg Depression Rating Scale, or MADRS, for the medication group in a clinical trial; however, the effect of sertraline (generic for Zoloft®) in similar studies is nearly identical (−15.7 point reduction on the MADRS; Friedli et al., 2017; Iosifescu et al., 2022). However, clinical data show that Auvelity® works quickly, with benefits shown in up to 2 weeks.

If clinicians and patients decide on a treatment plan that requires a brand-name medication, insurance coverage may provide the necessary benefits for coverage. However, suppose the patient's insurance plan does not. In that case, many pharmaceutical manufacturers offer patient assistance programs or coupon programs to make newer medications that are not available as generic to patients without insurance coverage or when insurance plans do not otherwise cover the medication.

The use of generics, patient assistance, consumer-facing resources (e.g., GoodRx®), and adhering to insurance formularies allow PCPs to mitigate financial barriers for patients, ensuring that cost does not impede access to necessary treatment.

Balancing Effectiveness and Tolerability The core of psychopharmacological treatment lies in the balance between therapeutic effectiveness and side effect tolerability. Evidence suggests several first-line agents offer comparable efficacy for most BH conditions but differ in side-effect profiles. For example, most antidepressants have similar effectiveness (Cipriani et al., 2009). However, tolerability varies widely. Tricyclic antidepressants and selective serotonin reuptake inhibitors have numbers needed to treat of four and six, respectively, yet the numbers needed to harm are 5–11 and 24–94 (Arroll et al., 2005).

Additionally, clinicians can leverage the differences in tolerability and side-effect profiles between medications to address clinical symptoms individually. For example, mirtazapine is an option to treat depression, but it is often sedating and leads to weight gain. Therefore, a patient who is underweight or with poor appetite related to depression or with significant sleep issues as co-occurring symptoms may greatly benefit from this choice of medication. To optimize patient outcomes, clinicians must tailor medication choices to individual patient needs, considering the potential benefits and the side-effect burden.

Ease of Administration The likelihood of patient adherence increases with the ease of medication administration. Oral medications with once-daily dosing are preferred for their convenience and simplicity, which can significantly enhance treatment adherence (Medic et al., 2013). However, alternative delivery systems such as transdermal patches or long-acting injectables may offer substantial benefits for conditions or patients where adherence is challenging. While potentially more costly upfront, these alternatives can improve long-term adherence and patient outcomes. Additionally, clinicians should consider the half-life of medications when recommending treatment, especially when adherence is a concern (Andrade, 2022). For example, venlafaxine may be a poor choice for a patient who misses frequent doses of medicines in a week due to the high association of discontinuation syndrome. In this case, fluoxetine, with its long half-life, might be the best option.

Anticipatory Counseling

Effective treatment begins with anticipatory counseling, where clinicians set realistic expectations about the treatment, including potential side effects and the typical timeline for therapeutic effects to become noticeable. This counseling is crucial for BH treatments, where therapeutic effects may take weeks to manifest. Clear, upfront communication can preemptively address concerns, improve adherence and satisfaction, and may assist the clinician in developing a stronger therapeutic alliance.

Polypharmacy and Deprescribing

In primary care, polypharmacy is typically the rule, not the exception. The concurrent use of multiple medications increases the risk of adverse drug interactions and side effects. A systematic review approach to deprescribing—evaluating each medication's current value against its risks—can help minimize these risks and simplify treatment regimens. Regular medication reviews can identify opportunities to reduce polypharmacy, focusing on the patient's clinical needs. Importantly, treatment inertia can often occur, leading to a failure of clinicians to assess the ongoing needs of medication prescribing iteratively. For example, during a depressive episode, some patients may need a hypnotic prescription (e.g., suvorexant), but will not need the medication when the depressive episode resolves. However, continued medication prescribing may be common with the competing demands of the typical primary care visit.

Additional Considerations

Pharmacogenetics Pharmacogenetic testing is an emerging tool that aims to tailor medication choices to individual patients based on their genetic makeup. This type of testing evaluates how a person's genes will affect their response to various psychotropic medications, particularly regarding toxicity. Optimal use of genetic testing to treat BH conditions with common psychotropic medications is lacking, and its primary use is to identify potentially dangerous toxicities for populations at high genetic risk of severe reactions. For example, a clinician may order genetic testing for a patient of Southeastern Asian descent before starting Carbamazepine for bipolar disorder due to higher rates of HLA-B allotypes that could predispose to developing Stevens-Johnson syndrome. Of note, clinicians can refer to the medication and genetic guidance for certain medicines offered by the Clinical Pharmacogenetics Consortium through their website (Clinical Pharmacogenetics Implementation Consortium (CPIC), n.d.). Notably, the current state of evidence does not support the use of pharmacogenetic testing to determine the efficacy of medications, although this could be a future application of this technology (American Psychiatric Association (APA), 2019).

Ethical Considerations Ethical prescribing is foundational, extending beyond medication selection to encompass patient autonomy, informed consent, and confidentiality. Engaging patients in their treatment choices through shared decision-making respects their autonomy and significantly enhances treatment adherence and satisfaction.

Key Points

- PCPs are crucial in the evaluation and treatment of BH conditions, including the use of psychiatric medications.

- Utilizing evidence-based resources like *The Waco Guide to Psychopharmacology in Primary Care®* and measurement-based care empowers clinicians to prescribe psychiatric medications based on evidence.
- When starting medications for the treatment of BH disorders, clinicians should start low (low dosing range initiation), go slow (on titration upward), but go (ensure adequate trial dose and length).
- Use of good anticipatory guidance and collaborative prescribing principles are cornerstones of effective treatment.

References

American Psychiatric Association (APA). (2019). *Genetic testing to improve psychiatric medication choice*. American Psychiatric Association. https://www.psychiatry.org:443/news-room/apa-blogs/genetic-testing-to-improve-psychiatric-medication

Andrade, C. (2022). Psychotropic drugs with long half-lives: Implications for drug discontinuation, occasional missed doses, dosing interval, and pregnancy planning. *The Journal of Clinical Psychiatry, 83*(4). https://doi.org/10.4088/JCP.22f14593

Arroll, B., Macgillivray, S., Ogston, S., Reid, I., Sullivan, F., Williams, B., & Crombie, I. (2005). Efficacy and tolerability of tricyclic antidepressants and SSRIs compared with placebo for treatment of depression in primary care: A meta-analysis. *The Annals of Family Medicine, 3*(5), 449–456. https://doi.org/10.1370/afm.349

Cipriani, A., Furukawa, T. A., Salanti, G., Geddes, J. R., Higgins, J. P., Churchill, R., Watanabe, N., Nakagawa, A., Omori, I. M., McGuire, H., Tansella, M., & Barbui, C. (2009). Comparative efficacy and acceptability of 12 new-generation antidepressants: A multiple-treatments meta-analysis. *The Lancet, 373*(9665), 746–758. https://doi.org/10.1016/S0140-6736(09)60046-5

Clinical Pharmacogenetics Implementation Consortium (CPIC). (n.d.). Guidelines – CPIC. Guidelines—CPIC. https://cpicpgx.org/guidelines/

Coleman, K., Austin, B. T., Brach, C., & Wagner, E. H. (2009). Evidence on the chronic care model in the new millennium. *Health Affairs, 28*(1), 75–85. https://doi.org/10.1377/hlthaff.28.1.75

Committee on Quality of Health Care in America. (2001). *Crossing the quality chasm: A new health system for the 21st century*. National Academies Press.

Coulter, A., & Collins, A. (2011). *Making shared decision-making a reality*. The King's Fund. https://www.kingsfund.org.uk/insight-and-analysis/reports/making-shared-decision-making-reality

Curtin, F., & Schulz, P. (2011). Assessing the benefit: Risk ratio of a drug - Randomized and naturalistic evidence. *Dialogues in Clinical Neuroscience, 13*(2), 183–190.

Friedli, K., Guirguis, A., Almond, M., Day, C., Chilcot, J., Da Silva-Gane, M., Davenport, A., Fineberg, N. A., Spencer, B., Wellsted, D., & Farrington, K. (2017). Sertraline versus placebo in patients with major depressive disorder undergoing hemodialysis: A randomized, controlled feasibility trial. *Clinical Journal of the American Society of Nephrology: CJASN, 12*(2), 280–286. https://doi.org/10.2215/CJN.02120216

Hughes, P. M., Annis, I. E., McGrath, R. E., & Thomas, K. C. (2024, May 1). Psychotropic medication prescribing across medical providers, 2016–2019. *Psychiatric Services, 75*(5), 477–480.

Iosifescu, D. V., Jones, A., O'Gorman, C., Streicher, C., Feliz, S., Fava, M., & Tabuteau, H. (2022). Efficacy and safety of AXS-05 (dextromethorphan-bupropion) in patients with major depressive disorder: A phase 3 randomized clinical trial (GEMINI). *The Journal of Clinical Psychiatry, 83*(4), 14345. https://doi.org/10.4088/JCP.21m14345

Kesselheim, A. S., Misono, A. S., Lee, J. L., Stedman, M. R., Brookhart, M. A., Choudhry, N. K., & Shrank, W. H. (2008). Clinical equivalence of generic and brand-name drugs used in cardiovascular disease: A systematic review and meta-analysis. *JAMA, 300*(21), 2514–2526. https://doi.org/10.1001/jama.2008.758

Kroenke, K., Spitzer, R. L., & Williams, J. B. W. (1999). *Patient health questionnaire-9*. APA PsycTests. https://doi.org/10.1037/t06165-000

Laschober, R. D., Kelley, L. P., Sartor, Z. R., Johnson, S., & Griggs, J. O. (n.d.). *Waco guide to psychopharmacology in primary care*. https://wacoguide.org/

Mallya, M. M., Munoz, I. B., Liu-Zarzuela, J. A., Preble, R. G., Rajagopal, S., Reyna, A., Moy, M. I., Rowlinson, E. G., & Oorjitham, N. S. (2024). Implementation and evaluation of educational workshops to increase primary care provider and medical student comfort in psychiatric care. *Academic Psychiatry, 48*(3), 244–248. https://doi.org/10.1007/s40596-024-01960-4

Medic, G., Higashi, K., Littlewood, K. J., Diez, T., Granström, O., & Kahn, R. S. (2013). Dosing frequency and adherence in chronic psychiatric disease: Systematic review and meta-analysis. *Neuropsychiatric Disease and Treatment, 9*, 119–131. https://doi.org/10.2147/NDT.S39303

Posternak, M. A., & Zimmerman, M. (2007). Therapeutic effect of follow-up assessments on antidepressant and placebo response rates in antidepressant efficacy trials: Meta-analysis. *The British Journal of Psychiatry: the Journal of Mental Science, 190*, 287–292. https://doi.org/10.1192/bjp.bp.106.028555

Rush, A. J., Fava, M., Wisniewski, S. R., Lavori, P. W., Trivedi, M. H., Sackeim, H. A., Thase, M. E., Nierenberg, A. A., Quitkin, F. M., Kashner, T. M., Kupfer, D. J., Rosenbaum, J. F., Alpert, J., Stewart, J. W., McGrath, P. J., Biggs, M. M., Shores-Wilson, K., Lebowitz, B. D., Ritz, L., Niederehe, G., & STAR*D Investigators Group. (2004). Sequenced treatment alternatives to relieve depression (STAR*D): Rationale and design. *Controlled Clinical Trials, 25*(1), 119–142. https://doi.org/10.1016/S0197-2456(03)00112-0

Slade, M. (2017). Implementing shared decision making in routine mental health care. *World Psychiatry, 16*(2), 146–153. https://doi.org/10.1002/wps.20412

Spitzer, R. L., Kroenke, K., Williams, J. B. W., & Löwe, B. (2006). *Generalized anxiety disorder 7*. APA PsycTests. https://doi.org/10.1037/t02591-000

Tian, Y., Reichardt, B., Dunkler, D., Hronsky, M., Winkelmayer, W. C., Bucsics, A., Strohmaier, S., & Heinze, G. (2020). Comparative effectiveness of branded vs. generic versions of antihypertensive, lipid-lowering and hypoglycemic substances: A population-wide cohort study. *Scientific Reports, 10*(1), 5964. https://doi.org/10.1038/s41598-020-62318-y

Tolin, D. F., Frost, R. O., Steketee, G., & Muroff, J. (2015). Cognitive behavioral therapy for hoarding disorder: A meta-analysis. *Depression and Anxiety, 32*(3), 158–166. https://doi.org/10.1002/da.22327

U.S. Food and Drug Administration. (2021). *Generic drugs: Questions & answers*. U.S. Food & Drug; FDA. https://www.fda.gov/drugs/frequently-asked-questions-popular-topics/generic-drugs-questions-answers

Chapter 8
Behavioral Interventions for Mental Health Conditions in Primary Care

Katherine Bergs PhD, Adam Guck PhD, ABPP, Jessie Kao MD, and Meredith L. C. Williamson PhD, ABPP

It is increasingly recognized that a significant portion of a primary care clinician's workday involves chief complaints that include a behavioral health (BH) component. Within those complaints, primary care providers (PCPs) are most likely to see the "common colds" of the BH world—anxiety and depression—on a daily basis. Generally, the most common BH conditions that are managed in primary care fall into several categories: anxiety, depression, trauma/PTSD, and adjustment disorder. We fully encourage PCPs to feel confident in treatment of these conditions themselves, while also staying connected to BH providers and resources in their area.

Develop Your BH Team and Resources

We strongly recommend cultivating therapeutic resources for your patient panel in order to expand available treatment options. See Chap. 13 for a broader discussion about developing your team. For most BH concerns, the use of both medication and psychotherapy in some form yields the best outcomes. There are, of course, some scenarios where consultation with a psychiatrist, psychologist, or other BH provider is more likely. For example, while a PCP may choose to treat lower acuity or new onset depression in primary care, they may also choose to send more complicated, long-standing, or unique cases to BH colleagues when available. It is recommended that PCPs consider their referral resources and referral processes for complicated BH presentations depending on the context of the primary care practice and the training

K. Bergs PhD (✉) · A. Guck PhD, ABPP · J. Kao MD
John Peter Smith Hospital, Fort Worth, TX, USA
e-mail: kbergs@jpshealth.org

M. L. C. Williamson PhD, ABPP
Naresh K. Vashisht College of Medicine, Department of Primary Care and Rural Medicine, Texas A&M University, Bryan, TX, USA

M. L. C. Williamson and D. L. Terry (eds.), *Essentials for Treating Behavioral Health in Primary Care*, https://doi.org/10.1007/978-3-032-09558-9_8

of the PCP in BH. See Chap. 12 for discussion on models for integrating BH into primary care.

We recognize that there may be times when a PCP does not have easy access to specialty BH. In these cases, we recommend a complete medical workup, consultation with any available BH provider, and continued attempts to get the patient team-based care. In addition, we recommend getting to know local BH resources (in-person or via telehealth), as well as having proactive discussions with BH provider about how you collaborate, share information, and when or where they would like to be consulted.

Overview of Cognitive Behavioral Therapy for Common BH Conditions

Cognitive behavioral therapy (CBT) is one of the leading evidence-based psychotherapies for most BH conditions (Beck & Dozois, 2011; Coffey et al., 2015). CBT has been shown to be as effective or more effective than medications for a variety of BH conditions including depression, trauma disorders, and anxiety along with many other BH and health-related conditions. CBT is a time-limited and goal-oriented approach to BH conditions. The CBT model presumes that BH conditions arise due to an interrelationship between dysfunctional patterns of cognitions, behaviors, and emotions (see Fig. 8.1). The primary interventions include (1) identifying and understanding unhelpful or unrealistic cognitions (thoughts and beliefs) and developing strategies to modify these cognitions to be realistic and helpful (see Fig. 8.2 for a thought log example); (2) decreasing avoidance of beneficial behaviors and increasing engagement in these behaviors to create systems of positive reinforcement; and (3) increasing awareness of changes in emotional distress as cognitions and behaviors are modified. Descriptions of CBT interventions that can be employed by the PCP will be described throughout this chapter to treat common BH conditions.

Major Depressive Disorder

Approximately 10–20% of adult patients exhibit clinically significant symptoms of depression and, apart from generalized anxiety disorder (GAD), it is the most common BH issue seen in primary care patient populations (Kessler et al., 2003). Many primary care clinics and health systems have increased surveillance via universal screening with instruments like the PHQ-2/PHQ-9 (Kroenke et al., 2003). See Chap. 4 for complete discussion of screening tools. As such, the primary care encounter continues to be a common venue in which depression is first identified and where preliminary treatment is discussed (Olfson et al., 2014; Simon & VonKorff,

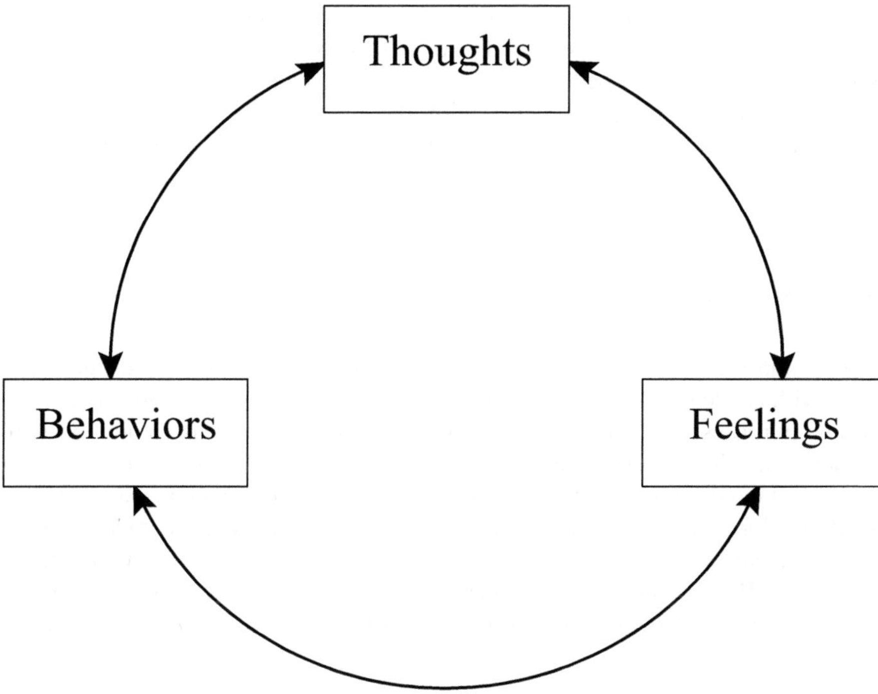

Fig. 8.1 Cognitive behavioral therapy model (Adapted from Coffey et al., 2015)

Anxiety Tracking Log

Day/Time	Situation	Thoughts	Physical Sensations	Anxiety Rating *1=low; 10=high*	What did I do?	What did I say to myself?	Second Rating *1=low; 10=high*
11/10 9:00am	Going to the grocery store, people were everywhere	"I am afraid something bad will happen to me because it is so crowded"	Heart racing, sweaty palms, difficult to breathe	10	Left the store	"This will never get better."	10
11/15 11:00am	Going to the grocery store, people were everywhere	"I am afraid something bad will happen to me because it is so crowded"	Heart racing, sweaty palms, difficult to breathe	10	Practiced breathing and spent time looking at store coupons on my phone	"I go to the grocery store all the time and nothing has ever happened."	5

Fig. 8.2 Thought log

1995). The psychological approach with by far the most supportive evidence in treatment of depression is CBT (Beck & Dozois, 2011; Newman et al., 2021). Patients show benefit from many aspects of CBT; however, the intervention with the strongest supportive evidence is behavioral activation (BA), a behavioral strategy focused on increasing engagement in meaningful activities (Dimidjian et al., 2006; Dobson et al., 2008; Ekers et al., 2014; Jacobson et al., 2001).

Psychoeducation

In the primary care setting, any discussion of treatment for depression generally begins with an element of brief psychoeducation (Fig. 8.3). Psychoeducation serves multiple purposes simultaneously: De-stigmatizing depression as a common issue by addressing the perception of personal failings or "weakness," underscores the risks of leaving depression untreated by prolonging suffering and increasing risk of suicide, explores the driving factors that contribute to depression, and instills hope by noting that depression tends to be both treatable and encourages active participation in treatment. Psychoeducation on depression may emphasize one or several different talking points, and should include discussion of the so-called depressive cycle.

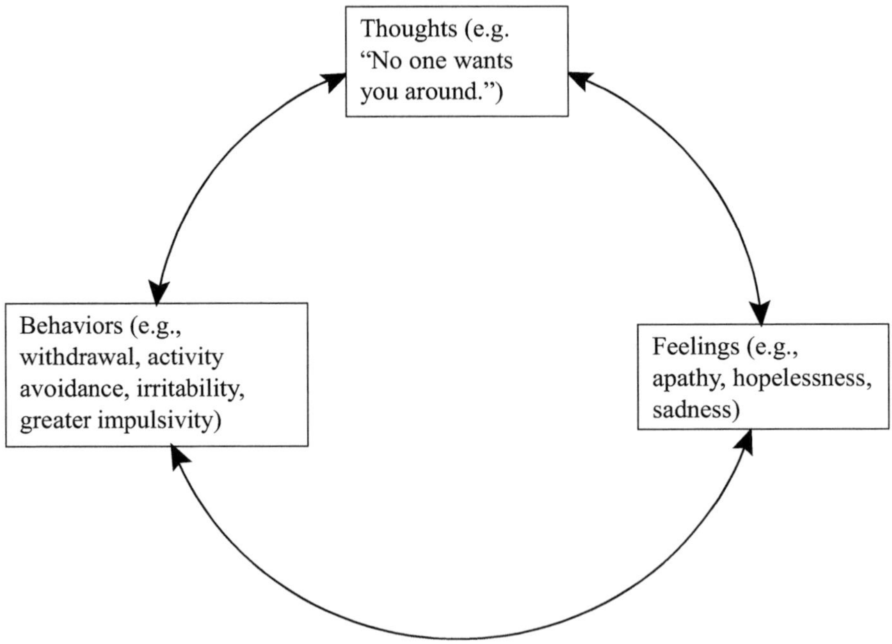

Fig. 8.3 CBT example for depression (Adapted from Coffey et al., 2015)

In the context of major depression, inactivity or activity avoidance plays a role in perpetuating the depressive cycle by reinforcing negative mood states, maintaining maladaptive behavioral patterns, and reducing or removing patients from activities, environments, and coping resources that might otherwise have reduced depressive symptoms (Martell et al., 2010). Patients with low activity have fewer social interactions, miss out on opportunities for positive reinforcement and activities that might allow for pleasure or accomplishment. This further contributes to feelings of guilt, worthlessness, isolation, and hopelessness. Emphasizing the central role of activity in the maintenance of depressive symptoms during the provision of psychoeducation tends to both resonate with patients and serves as a useful segue into behavioral activation (BA) as an intervention.

Behavioral Activation for Depression

Behavioral activation (BA) is a therapeutic approach rooted in behavioral psychology (Lewinsohn et al., 1976; Lewinsohn & Libet, 1972) and aims to reduce depressive symptoms in favor of positive mood and adaptive coping by encouraging individuals to increase engagement in rewarding and meaningful activities (Martell et al., 2010). At its core, BA operates on the principle that behaviors play a significant role in influencing mood and can either contribute to depressive pathology or lead to alleviation of symptoms. The supportive evidence, taken in combination with the relative ease and efficiency with which it can be delivered in a brief encounter, make BA the behavioral treatment of choice for depression within primary care.

BA is the development of a plan to engage in daily structured activities irrespective of the presence or absence of depressive symptoms (see Table 8.1). This goes against patient preference to be inactive due to depressive symptoms. That is, they engage in tasks or activities according to a daily structure, goal or treatment plan, not just "if they feel like it." Some clinicians and patients find it helpful to think of BA as a kind of "behavioral antidepressant" wherein specific, goal-directed or mood-enhancing activities are "prescribed" to address depression. Much like antidepressant medications, the patient is encouraged to do activities every day to see optimal benefit, and to "take" them irrespective of their subjective mood on that particular day. While some immediate symptom improvement may be expected, it may take time (i.e., a few weeks) to experience optimal benefit (Martell et al., 2010).

Table 8.1 Behavioral activation activity selection and planning

Mood-enhancing	Collaboratively selecting activities that uplift mood is crucial. Experimentation may be needed to find what works best for the individual. For instance, if it is discovered that socializing during breaks at work boosts mood, scheduling similar social activities after work could be beneficial
Active vs. passive	While passive activities like watching TV or playing video games can provide short-term enjoyment, they may not contribute to long-term mood enhancement or well-being. Evidence has shown that time spent on technology tends to give a distorted sense of both time and experience, wherein patients may not feel or accurately perceive the time spent on activities, suggesting it may be more closely associated with activity avoidance than activity engagement (Rosen et al., 2013). Patients should be encouraged to pursue activities which involve movement and, where possible, independence from technology
Social vs. solitary	Social interaction can provide powerful reinforcement while patients attempt to increase their self-care activities and may simultaneously provide other therapeutic benefits by helping the patient feel less isolated, put them in contact with those in their social support network and, where motivational factors may interference with task completion, boost accountability by recruiting a trusted support
Values-consistent	Understanding the personal significance of an activity, such as cooking for the family, can guide selection. While time constraints during the medical encounter may not allow for in-depth discussion of values (e.g., values clarification), aligning tasks with personal value can inform effective choices
Practical considerations	Assess the feasibility of activities across various domains, taking into account physical ability, time constraints, cost, and transportation to name a few. It is important to note that often these need not be insurmountable obstacles, but rather opportunities for the patient to think practically and creatively to achieve a similar activity goal
Behavioral tracking form	Patient and PCP should write out weekly goals (see Fig. 8.3). The tracking form serves to clarify goals, increases accountability, allows patients to keep track of "wins." reviewing the form with a PCP at follow ups allows the patient to capitalize on success, identify stuck points, and determine if revisions are needed
Small and high frequency behaviors	Especially early in treatment, patients are advised to implement goals that can be completed within 15–20 min and are done with greater frequency throughout the week. This can be as simple as taking a shower or brewing a cup of coffee on a morning schedule. The example tracking form breaks up the day into "morning, afternoon, and evening" but this can be further divided as needed

(continued)

Table 8.1 (continued)

Integrate into pre-existing daily routine	BA activities can be implemented with the greatest success if they are integrated alongside existing daily routines
Values-consistent	Unforeseen setbacks, waning motivation, and lack of buy-in are normal and expected components of BA implementation. A motivational interviewing (MI) framework is advised. Clinicians should avoid the temptation of playing the role of "coach" or "cheerleader" in the face of obstacles and should instead maintain an empathic stance which is evocative and reflective (see Miller et al., 2011) Understanding the personal significance of an activity, such as cooking for the family, can guide selection. While time constraints during the medical encounter may not allow for in-depth discussion of values (e.g., values clarification), aligning tasks with personal value can inform effective choices. There is benefit to patients selecting value-consistent tasks as this allows the clinician to ask the patient "who or what is important in your life?" and reflect on the role the target behavior plays in that context. Even if values are not salient to the task itself, clinicians may query about the role that management of depression plays in the patient's life. Beyond "feeling better" what important roles or values does depression detract from in the patient's life, and what would it mean to them to continue attempts to manage?

Selecting a Behavioral Activation Activity It is important that selection of the activity/activities be a collaborative process between patient and clinician. Activities can continue to be modified as needed and increased as the patient improves to restore functioning and hope during a depressive episode. Exercise can be included as a BA activity and has been found to reduce depressive symptoms alone without additional activities (Cooney et al., 2013). Following selection of the activity, it is important to work with the patient to develop an implementation plan (See Fig. 8.4) The Mood Tools application can be utilized to track BA along with cognition or thought tracking. As part of discussion of activity selection, PCPs may describe the following elements of an effective BA activity: (Rosen et al., 2013).

Behavioral Activation

Engaging in activities you enjoy or feel successful completing can help decrease depression.

List three activities you enjoy:

1.

2.

3.

List three responsibilities you need to take care of:

1.

2.

3.

Try doing at least 1 activity each day. Use the following scale to rate your depression and sense of achievement before and after the activity. You can also use the scale to rate any pleasant emotions you experience after you complete an activity.

0	1	2	3	4	5	6	7	8
None				Moderate				Extreme

Weekly schedule for Behavioral Activation

Create a schedule of activities you have enjoyed in your life. If you are down or lack motivation then it might be difficult to complete complicated tasks. Start small and for brief periods of time.

Day	Morning	Afternoon	Evening
Example	*Take a shower at 7:30am*	*Call a friend*	*Make Dinner*
Monday			
Tuesday			
Wednesday			
Thursday			
Friday			
Saturday			
Sunday			

Fig. 8.4 Behavioral activation

Anxiety Disorders

Generalized Anxiety Disorder While the overall prevalence of GAD is roughly 3% in the American population (American Psychiatric Association, 2022), PCPs may expect to see a higher prevalence of GAD in their exam room, as it often prompts patients to seek care (worries about concerning symptoms, distress about level of worry, etc.). GAD treatment in primary care starts with adequate assessment and detection. See Chap. 4 for common screening measures. For many patients, the most successful outcomes will be achieved via the use of CBT (see Fig. 8.5) alongside psychotropic medications. The most useful, primary care appropriate psychological treatments for GAD consist of psychoeducation and behavioral interventions.

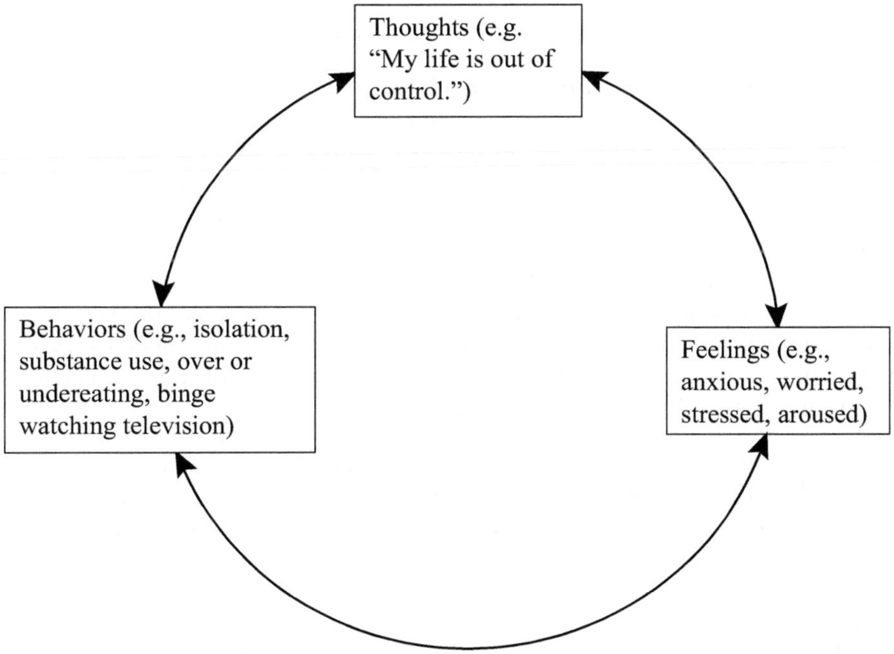

Fig. 8.5 CBT example for anxiety (Adapted from Coffey et al., 2015)

Psychoeducation

For many patients with GAD, one of the key questions that prompts them to seek help is worry about something being "wrong with them" or "going crazy." Additionally, many interventions for anxiety management may seem counterintuitive at face value. Thus, an important first step to successful anxiety treatment is psychoeducation about the physical and behavioral nature of anxiety (see Table 8.2). Here are some options of ways clinicians might frame key topics for psychoeducation about anxiety to patients, which can be tailored and adjusted to meet their needs:

Behavioral Interventions for GAD

The majority of behavioral interventions for GAD are aimed at both tolerance and reduction of unpleasant symptoms of anxiety (see Table 8.3). We suggest starting with short, time-limited behavioral interventions and then moving to cognitive interventions, such as cognitive restructuring if needed.

Autogenic Coping Skills Training Since much of the discomfort of anxiety is a response to uncomfortable (but not dangerous) physical or emotional symptoms, skills to both tolerate and alleviate these symptoms can be useful for patients to feel more in control of their anxiety. The top three skills in this arena are diaphragmatic breathing, progressive muscle relaxation, and mindfulness/grounding.

Implementation of Interventions for GAD When asking patients to avoid avoidance, and engage with anxious feelings, clinicians ask them to do things that may be overtly unpleasant. As a result, getting buy-in to both the model of understanding and practicing exercises is extremely important. Patients need to trust that clinicians have their best interests at heart. Additionally, we recommend a gym workout metaphor in this situation, enhancing the concept of working hard and feeling sore to increase function and strength. For example, anxiety treatment is like a new workout (or any activity) regimen, it is appropriate to feel anxious or even frustrated or distressed as one learns new skills. Often, we are "sore" as we grow, and we may not look forward to something, but we do it for the purpose of improving. Over time, we can increase the intensity of workouts without feeling sore.

At the outset of anxiety treatment, it is important to emphasize that an appropriate workup has been completed. This is especially true for patients with health anxiety. For trust to be established, clinicians will want to discuss the following with patients: what they have ruled out, why they are not worried about more dire differentials, and when they might begin to worry. Finally, we almost universally recommend having patients engage in some sort of behavioral tracking about the behavior (worrying, etc.) that they are trying to change and the intervention they are engaging in (diaphragmatic breathing, etc.). Sometimes just the act of recording with a behavioral tracker (See

Table 8.2 Psychoeducation for Anxiety

Topic	Brief script
Normal physiological reactions to anxious stimuli	As humans, we are built to react to scary or threatening stimuli with an anxious response. This response includes three main options: fight, flight, or freeze. Let's discuss how these three reactions look and feel. When you encounter something scary, your brain is primed to send signals for how the rest of the body should react in order to help keep you safe. In fight or flight modes, when there is an emergency, the body might need more oxygen in order to run or fight and therefore breathing and heart rate will increase. There are many physical sensations of anxiety that might feel scary, like jitteriness, fast breathing, rapid heart rate, etc., but these are all your body sending the signal to fight or flee. There is also a third option where your body might just press pause if your brain doesn't see a way out of the threat. This is what we call freeze, where you might feel stuck or unable to think straight. Any of these reactions to a scary situation are normal. In addition, they are normal reactions to what your body perceives as a scary situation, even if there is no major threat. So, when we feel anxious symptoms it is really our body just telling us to gear up because there is a threat. The good news is that there are ways to help input signals to our body and brain that there is no threat, and we can begin to work on feeling less anxious
Avoid avoidance	When we feel the (sometimes) unpleasant symptoms of anxiety, it can be tempting to avoid the trigger for these symptoms, whether it's a physical trigger or something you think about. However, avoiding these negative experiences makes it more likely that you'll avoid them in the future, starting a vicious cycle (akin to avoiding the dentist for long periods of time makes it scarier to eventually go). When you avoid something scary/negative, you get a rush of good brain chemicals telling you that was good for safety—you made it out! However, if we avoid something that is not actually scary, we really just make it more likely that the experience seems scary in the future, leading to more avoidance. Are there things you think of that you might be avoiding?
Working with (not against) medication	If using medication, it is important to have appropriate expectations about what medication can and can't do. While we might wish it was case, medications for anxiety are not magic and do not wipe away anxiety long term. Instead, what they do is help you feel a little calmer and give you more mental space to be able to think through your options. They might also help you physically feel more relaxed, but it is important to also think about things that contribute to relaxation. For instance, we can work with medications for anxiety by getting exercise and avoiding things that make us jittery, like too much caffeine

Table 8.3 Behavioral interventions for anxiety

Intervention	Brief description
Diaphragmatic breathing	The goal for patients is to slow breathing down and increase blood oxygenation, in direct opposition to the fight or flight responses. There are several key points regarding diaphragmatic breathing when teaching it to patients, including tying it back into previous psychoeducation about anxiety responses. When using DB, there are two most important things to focus on with patients: the "way" of breathing and the rate of breathing. Regarding the "way" of breathing, the goal is for patients to breath in such a way that they are able to see their belly rise/extend on the inhale and fall on the exhale. This often takes coaching and we recommend having patients practice this in vivo during office visits for correction. The goal is to slow breathing and increase mindfulness on the patient's breathing patterns. Second, it is important to focus on the rate of breathing where patients should be exhaling for twice as long as the inhale. It does not matter if patients choose a 3/6 cadence or a 4/8 cadence, but we encourage patients to count in for several seconds and out for 2 times that amount of seconds. Finally, we recommend reiterating that this skill is best practiced when calmer, so that the skill can develop and be "ready for use" when anxiety occurs. We recommend assigning 10 reps, twice as day for practice during initial treatment. The Breathe2Relax application from the U.S. Department of Veterans Affairs is available for patients to practice with their PCP in the office or practice at home (U.S. Department of Veterans Affairs, 2024a)
Progressive muscle relaxation	Progressive muscle relaxation (PMR) is another tool for patients to reduce the subjective experience of anxiety, which centers on tensing muscles as a means of ultimately relaxing those same muscles. Simply thinking about an instruction to "relax muscles" can be challenging, and patients may not even be aware of places where they hold muscle tension. Instead, the provision of a guided method for initially tensing muscles as a means of identifying tension as well as targeting sensation of muscle groups can then help patients intentionally relax those muscles. Instruction in PMR includes a guide to patients to tense up muscle groups in a set order (typically starting either shoulders down or feet up) and ending with head/face. Instructions to patients typically involve the instruction to focus on each muscle group and hold tension as much as is reasonably comfortable, for 10 s. Then, focus immediately on relaxation of that muscle as much as possible. The "Muscle relaxation" tool through the U.S. Department of Veterans Affairs PTSD Coach application is available for patients to practice with their PCP in the office or practice at home (U.S. Department of Veterans Affairs, 2024b)

(continued)

Table 8.3 (continued)

Intervention	Brief description
Grounding	For acute episodes of anxiety, patients may do well with the behavioral/mindfulness approach known as "grounding." Grounding involves the use of the five senses to bring the patient out of the anxious/panic state into feeling more in control. It is especially important to set the stage for this exercise that nobody is expecting magical results, but that the use of grounding can help give the brain a moment to catch up and realize that the emergency is not actually happening. This can put a slight pause in the fight or flight (or freeze) response. At its simplest form, instructions for the patient in grounding involve asking them to report something that they experience with each of the senses. You might ask for three things the patient sees, three things they hear, etc. You may also offer them the chance to describe what they are experiencing out loud. This is especially useful for acute anxiety when the anxiety symptoms feel overwhelming or out of control. The "Grounding" tool through the U.S. Department of Veterans Affairs PTSD Coach application is available for patients to practice with their PCP in the office or practice at home (U.S. Department of Veterans Affairs, 2024b)
Exercise and physical activity	We almost always recommend exercise (or some form of physical activity) for its benefits for both health and mental well-being. However, with anxiety we are especially clear about the benefits. Key benefits of exercise for anxiety include having a way to discharge nervous energy as well as increasing odds of getting sleep at night (as for many patients, insomnia and anxiety go hand-in-hand)
Resiliency training	As an adjunctive to behavioral interventions, we also suggest some very brief stress inoculation/resilience training. It might be helpful to help patients reframe some of the relationship to uncertainty. Often, an intolerance of uncertainty is noticeable in highly anxious patients. This makes sense given the relationship of anxiety symptoms to the brain's attempt to find safety. Patients can benefit from psychoeducation about embracing uncertainty and how to know when there is risk (when any situation is dangerous; e.g., "being sexually assaulted at a party") versus ways to tolerate uncertainty without risk ("e.g., talking to someone you don't at a party")

Fig. 8.2) alone can help spur patients toward change in addition to providing much needed information for PCP.

Specific Anxiety, Phobias, and Panic Disorder

Psychoeducation

When it comes to anxiety conditions, it is important to educate the patient that fear is natural and that the stress reaction is protective (Poulton & Menzies, 2002). When the specific phobia impedes performance or patients determine there is a negative consequence of the specific phobia, therapy can be helpful to address the concern. It may be helpful to identify where the patient first learned of the specific fear. Traumatic conditioning develops after a direct negative experience (McCabe & Antony, 2008). Information transmission is when fear is transmitted from parents or close friends.

It can be helpful to educate patients with panic attacks or panic disorder that there are biological and psychological systems at play contributing to the disorder. Biologically, patients typically have overly sensitive aspects of their nervous systems while psychologically, patients may believe that the physical symptoms (racing heart, shortness of breath, dizziness) are an immediate threat to life (Clark, 1986). Patients feel physical symptoms, leading to anxiety about the symptoms and interpret them as dangerous. This creates even more symptoms which eventually evolves into a panic attack. Exposure interventions as part of CBT are utilized as behavioral interventions for anxiety disorders.

Anxiety often comes in "waves" and when one has an anxiety disorder they often try to avoid intensifying anxiety which leads to increased fear that anxiety cannot be controlled (See Fig. 8.6). Exposure interventions for anxiety disorders teach patients that they have control over anxious thoughts and behaviors by exposing them to anxiety provoking stimuli in safe environments by helping patients "ride the wave" of anxiety until their physiological arousal begins to dissipate by staying in anxiety provoking situations for an extending period of time repeatedly and learning that the situation does not need to be feared because it is safe.

Exposure Therapy

The primary way to help individuals over the anxiety wave is to engage in these exposure interventions (See Fig. 8.7). Graded exposure is an intervention that has been the most extensively studied for treatment of specific phobia (Wolitzky-Taylor et al., 2008). Exposure therapy can be started in the PCP's office by helping the patient create a fear ladder (Antony & Swinson, 2000). To create an exposure hierarchy, the patient's goal is placed at the top. The bottom of the ladder consists of tasks that are not anxiety provoking. For example, if the ultimate goal for a patient with social phobia is to go to a concert with thousands of people in attendance, this goal is placed on top. The bottom of the hierarchy could be the task of staying inside a bedroom alone. Next, create steps to the top. Each step should include an activity that produces an incremental increase in stress. For example, the next step could be stepping outside to grab the mail, eating dinner with family or friends, or going to the grocery store and talking to the cashier. The goal of each step is to think of increasingly challenging activities that are still achievable for the patient. Each activity should be brainstormed by the patient. Generally, in vivo (live experiences) activities are preferred compared to imaginary activities, however, imagined activities may be required as first steps to gain confidence. It may be impractical to have in vivo exposure for some specific phobias (e.g.: thunderstorms or flying), for which case, imagined activities may be best (Choy et al., 2007).

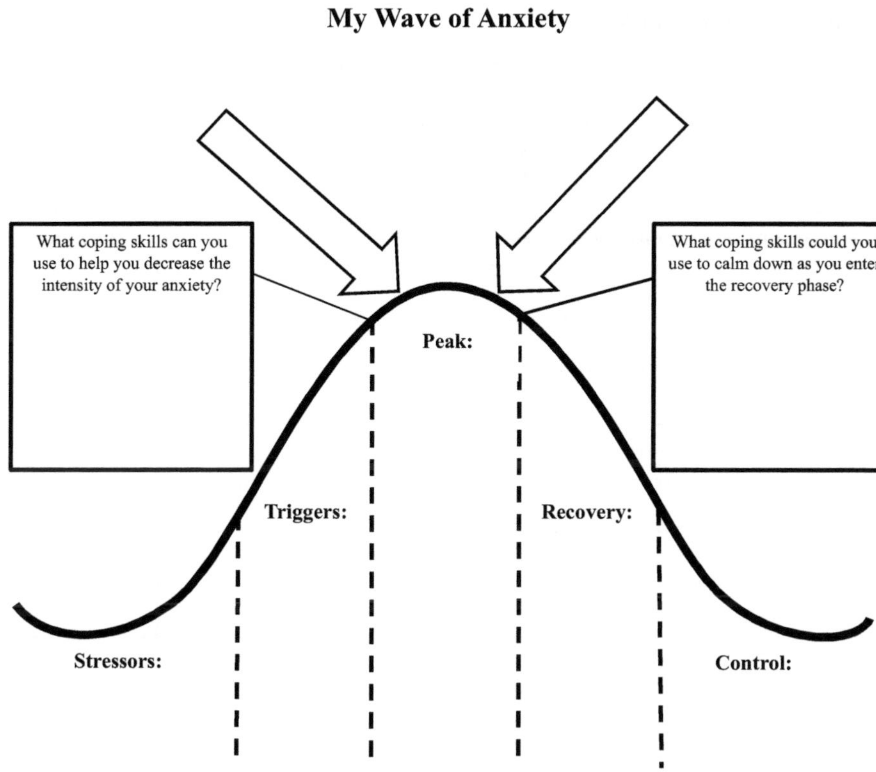

Fig. 8.6 Anxiety wave (Adapted from Hub for Helpers https://www.hubforhelpers.com/product/riding-the-wave-of-anxiety/)

When implementing the exposure hierarchy (See Fig. 8.7), it is important to emphasize regular repetition for each step. The first exposure activity chosen through collaborative partnership between the PCP and the patient should be chosen based on its evoking *some* fear (subjective unit of distress between 30–50) but not being so anxiety provoking that the patient will never be successful at repeated exposure practice. Once successful at repeated practice (and generally with a reported reduction in SUDS), the patient can continue to move up to more challenging exposure activities. Exposure therapy is most effective when patients repeat activities enough times that they learn whatever they are most worried about rarely occurs and, most importantly, patients realize they are able to cope with their fears (Craske et al., 2014). It is important to implement self-monitoring by writing down which activity is attempted and rating the distress before, during, and after the activity (create a scale of 1–100, often termed subjective units of distress scale [SUD]). A decrease in distress can assist with determining when a patient feels comfortable moving up to the next activity. Patients typically move up to the next activity when fear is meaningfully reduced. Setbacks are expected during this practice. Some common setbacks

Exposure Hierarchy

Make a list of anxiety-provoking situations. Include situations where SUDS = 0 and SUDS = 100 in addition to a list of situations with SUDS between 0-100. Be as detailed as possible.

Subjective Units of Distress Scale (SUDS)

100 = extreme anxiety
50 = significant anxiety
0 = no anxiety

Describe specific anxiety-provoking situations:	SUDS (0-100)

Fig. 8.7 Exposure hierarchy

that patients may include the feeling that fear is not decreasing, or that fear returns on the next attempt. Acute anxiety management techniques such as diaphragmatic breathing, grounding, or progressive muscle relaxation may be used in conjunction with exposure therapy (Wolitzky-Taylor et al., 2008). Discomfort during practice is expected and it is important to emphasize self-efficacy by encouraging patients that they have the ability to persevere. With enough repetition of activities that do not produce adverse effects, patients eventually have a decreased fear response to these events (Bouton et al., 2006).

As an example, school refusal is typically seen in younger children and is often due to anxiety. Providers can approach school refusal by trying to fill out a school refusal exposure hierarchy with the help of the parent (Pina et al., 2009; Williamson et al., 2023). Coordinating with school counselors and teachers can be especially helpful. Finally, as PCPs talk about how the tasks are going, it may be helpful to notice common cognitive errors that patients endorse that contribute to anxiety (Craske et al., 2006). PCPs may hear about patients overestimating the fear or catastrophizing the situation. It is helpful to encourage patients to treat each fear as a hypothesis to be tested instead of a fact to determine if the fear is helpful or realistic.

Panic Disorder

Reducing Maladaptive Coping with Panic It is important to identify how patients deal with panic attacks since the majority of episodes subside with time. It is crucial to not correlate improvement in symptoms with a safety behavior such as calling 911, going to the emergency room, or taking medication. In fact, in one study, 77% of patients who have had panic attacks have visited the emergency department for non-cardiac chest pain (Foldes-Busque et al., 2019). Many times, the panic attack subsides by the time the patient arrives at the emergency room. It is not the emergency room that improved the symptoms, rather the symptoms reduce as a function of the passage of time (see Fig. 8.7 for example of the anxiety wave). It is equally important to determine if the patient is avoiding situations that cause panic, as this contributes to long-term anxiety. Avoidance interrupts the process of deconditioning fear of the bodily sensation that causes the panic attack (Salkovskis et al., 1996). Finally, it is beneficial to identify any medications that patients take for panic attacks. There may be a role for de-prescribing benzodiazepines since these medications do not provide lasting benefits and interfere with cognitive behavioral therapy and exposure therapy (Otto et al., 2000; Otto & Henin, 2007). Patients may even become dependent on benzodiazepines if they continue to take them every time there is a panic attack.

Increasing Adaptive Coping with Panic Cognitive behavioral therapy including exposure interventions are more efficacious for the treatment of panic disorder/panic attacks compared to placebo and treatment gains are maintained long term (Butler et al., 2005; Carpenter et al., 2018). PCPs can teach brief behavioral techniques during the clinic visit such as diaphragmatic breathing or grounding for when the patient is in an acute panic episode. These exercises help patients endure panic and allow time for the symptoms to subside. As patients successfully work through panic episodes, they grow in self-efficacy and it becomes easier to work through subsequent episodes. Ultimately, treatment goals for the PCP include identifying and correcting maladaptive coping strategies while introducing the strategies described above. Referral to a BH provider could be beneficial if available to begin the process of interoceptive deconditioning, where patients begin purposefully inducing previous anxiety provoking symptoms in order for their bodies to adapt and acclimate to those symptoms.

Post-Traumatic Stress Disorder (PTSD)

For many patients, the PCP relationship is an ongoing, trusted continuity relationship that may span years or even decades. This relationship, coupled with increase in screening for trauma and/or adverse childhood experiences (ACES) makes it increasingly likely that contact with patients may occur in both the immediate aftermath of a psychological trauma, or serve as the setting for patients to divulge a trauma from earlier in the lifespan (See Chap. 11 for further discussion on ACES). It is highly recommended that PCPs and healthcare organizations adopt trauma-informed care (TIC) practices such as those advised by Substance Abuse and Mental Health Services Administration (SAMHSA) (2023) at the organizational/institutional level as a means of supporting patients who have experienced trauma and to facilitate timely access to treatment. Of those recommendations, it is advised that primary care treatment settings adopt practices that emphasize physical and emotional safety, screening for trauma and ACES as indicated, patient-centered practices, culturally-informed care, and workforce training and development on service to patients with trauma (Substance Abuse and Mental Health Services Administration (SAMHSA), 2014).

Caution on Premature/Overtreatment in Acute Stress

For PCPs, the urge to mobilize a timely and empathic response in the wake of acute trauma should be tempered by a few considerations. Literature examining outcomes of treatments such as critical incident stress debriefing (CISD) and others shows the very real possibility of poor outcomes and, in some instances, psychological harm caused from treatment that was either delivered too quickly, in a mandatory manner, and by untrained/non-licensed professionals (Bisson & Lewis, 2009; Roberts et al., 2009; Rose et al., 2002; van Emmerik et al., 2002). In any event, the risks associated with overtreatment and/or poorly conceived treatment should not be taken lightly. Clinicians should bear in mind that the presence of a traumatic event, recent or distant, is not sufficient alone to warrant a PTSD diagnosis or recommendation for treatment. Effective screening (e.g., PC-PTSD-5) and diagnostic clarity are key in avoidance of misdiagnosis and overtreatment (Prins et al., 2015; Weathers et al., 2013; Williamson et al., 2022). While estimates vary, approximately 10–30% of those experiencing emotional trauma go on to be diagnosed with PTSD. Therefore, unless behavioral health treatment is specifically requested by patients, it is advised that clinicians engage in watchful waiting of symptoms until they reach the requisite one-month symptom duration to both make a diagnosis of PTSD and discuss the possibility of treatment.

Psychoeducation and Supportive Interventions for Trauma

Psychoeducation for trauma and PTSD should focus on de-stigmatizing and normalizing the occurrence of trauma and any residual emotional distress experienced. Many themes such as guilt, self-blame, anger, resentment, loss of identity, and focus on unfairness are common. Clinicians should attempt to reassure patients that the medical encounter is a safe and supportive venue, and that their desire to discuss (or not discuss) elements of the trauma will be respected. Clinicians should be mindful that patients open up at their own pace, so active, empathic listening should take priority over any desire to collect details or induce patients to "process" the event.

Referral for PTSD Treatment

For patients who express a desire for treatment for trauma or PTSD, particularly where they wish to address the intrusive thoughts/memories related to the trauma, referral to evidence-based trauma treatment is recommended. Trauma-focused cognitive behavioral approaches show the most evidence for successful outcomes. This includes treatment modalities such as Prolonged Exposure (PE), Cognitive Processing Therapy (CPT), and Eye Movement Desensitization and Reprocessing (EMDR) (Bisson et al., 2013; Coventry et al., 2020; Roberts et al., 2016). Completion of the treatment protocols generally occurs over the span of 10–13 sessions, however more sessions may be deemed necessary. For those in low-resource or rural settings, PCPs and patients can seek resources on PTSD and treatment resources from The National Center for PTSD (U.S. Department of Veterans Affairs, 2024d) and the PTSD Coach Mobile app (U.S. Department of Veterans Affairs, 2024c).

For sites with onsite BH support, brief exposure-based protocols have been developed which are tailored to the primary care setting and may be delivered by BH professionals (Cigrang et al., 2017; Rauch et al., 2023). Similarly, a brief protocol for Written Exposure Therapy (WET) has been developed which comprises approximately five sessions and could be delivered by BH professionals in the primary care setting (Sloan & Marx, 2019). In either case, it may benefit patients for their PCP to outline a course of intervention with patients to assist with treatment planning, increase referral adherence, and reduce dropout. It may be of benefit to set the expectation that, early in treatment, patients may see a short-term increase in PTSD symptoms (within the first 3 sessions). This is a normal and predictable aspect to treatment. Generally, patients see improvement in symptoms after this brief interval. Lastly, it is expected that patients with PTSD may show reluctance to engage in

Table 8.4 Four "Rs" of trauma-informed care (Substance Abuse and Mental Health Services Administration (SAMHSA), 2014)

Realize	Understand trauma is everywhere and it affects systems and individuals
Recognize	Understand signs of trauma. Know how to screen for trauma and trauma disorders
Respond	Consider clinic and organization wide policies and procedures for employing trauma-informed approaches to all medical care
Resist Retraumatization	Be on the lookout for how organizational and systemic practices may result in retraumatizatio.

treatment and, even when delivered by competent BH professionals, treatment drop out is common. In these instances, PCPs should be encouraged to lean on trauma-informed care best-practices of fostering trust, support, safety, and patient autonomy (see Table 8.4). Within this framework, referral to treatment and treatment completion are best conceptualized as "process" rather than direct outcome.

Special Considerations for Other BH Disorders

Adjustment Disorders Adjustment disorders often present first to primary care and are frequently due to contextual stressors (See Chap. 2 for discussion of contextual interviewing). Often symptoms will either remit after the stressor is resolved, or the patient will go on to develop a diagnosable BH condition. The PCP will benefit from utilizing empathy to discuss current contextual stressors and encourage self-care when possible to cope with stressors. The BH interventions discussed throughout this chapter can be beneficial for adjustment responses as well as diagnosed BH conditions.

Eating Disorders Eating disorders are often first identified within primary care settings (see Table 8.5). Over 8% of the US population will have an eating disorder at some point in their lifetime (Deloitte Access Economics, 2020). Special medical and BH considerations are needed when treating individuals with eating disorders (Harrington et al., 2015). Treatment is most effective when an interdisciplinary team is a part of the care including the PCP, BH providers, dietician, and other specialty medical providers as needed due to medical complications from the eating disorder. Eating disorders include avoidant restrictive food intake disorder, anorexia nervosa, bulimia nervosa, binge eating disorder, along with other specified eating disorders that do not meet criteria for the predominant patterns of disordered eating behavior. The National Eating Disorder Association (NEDA) and the Academy of Eating Disorders provides detailed information on assessment and treatment of eating disorders for PCPs (Academy for Eating Disorders, 2021; National Eating Disorders Association, 2024). The goals for treatment include medical stabilization, restoration of nutritional

Table 8.5 PCP considerations when an eating disorder is identified (Adapted from Academy for Eating Disorders, 2021)

Weighing patients	Continuous weight checks are necessary for tracking weight restoration. However, patients should be weighed backwards when possible with limited discussion of specific weight data during PCP visits
Caloric tracking	Caloric recall can be helpful to assess calorie intake for patients by asking them what they consumed in the last day along with any engagement in eating disorder behaviors (binging/purging/excessive exercise). Photos of food and traditional behavioral tracking can be utilized. It is recommended that individuals with eating disorders are not asked to track specific caloric intake by calories but instead asked to track diabetic exchanges or specific food items and size/amount
Avoidance or lack of awareness of the eating disorder	Most patients will minimize, hide, or rationalize their eating disorder behaviors. Social support will likely be necessary to assist individuals with eating disorders in recovery at any age
Avoid blame	Help the patient and any social support understand that this is BH diagnosis and the patient did not choose to have it nor did any specific family members cause the eating disorder
Monitor physical and BH concerns	Patients should regularly be monitored for acute and chronic complications, but understand that physical exam and laboratory test may not reveal any diagnostic concerns despite individuals suffering from life threatening eating disorders Assess for BH concerns when an eating disorder is identified due to the high comorbidity of eating disorders and other BH diagnoses. Suicide is the cause of death for up to half of individuals with eating disorders

deficits, normalization of eating patterns, and treatment for co-occurring BH concerns (Academy for Eating Disorders, 2021).

Personality Disorders Personality disorders are common in primary care. Individuals with these diagnoses can cause significant emotional responses with PCPs and struggle to consistently respond to medical guidance (Ward, 2004). PCPs knowledge of personality disorders is important in order to consider strategies for developing collaborative partnerships for medical care in spite of the challenges in interpersonal interactions. The most important intervention for these individuals is empathy and assurance of your care for the patient while maintaining clear communication and boundaries. Despite being challenging to treat and chronic in nature, dialectical behavior therapy for borderline personality disorder has been one treatment that has shown benefit (Koerner et al., 2021).

Bipolar and Schizophrenia Spectrum and Other Psychotic Disorders The PCPs role with these BH conditions is primarily identification of symptoms and support in maintenance of medication adherence to reduce symptoms of these BH conditions. Recommendations for collaborative support for medication adherence include utilization of psychoeducation about the BH diagnosis and need for medication to reduce symptoms, motivational interviewing (See Chap. 9), behavioral reinforcement with reminders such as alarms and checklists, along with social support (Loots et al., 2021; Marzani & Neff, 2021). PCPs will benefit from knowledge of medication utilized to treat these BH conditions and monitoring for BH crisis situations (See Chap. 5 for crisis information and Chap. 7 for psychopharmacology). BH interventions can be utilized as adjunctive treatment for these conditions (Marzani & Neff, 2021). Care coordination with specialty BH if often essential for treating these BH conditions.

Key Points

- The most common BH conditions that are managed in primary care fall into several categories: anxiety, depression, trauma/PTSD, and adjustment disorder.
- It is recommended that PCPs consider their referral resources and referral processes for complicated BH presentations depending on the context of the primary care practice and the training of the PCP in BH.
- For most BH concerns, the use of both medication and psychotherapy in some form yield the best outcomes.

Appendix A: Behavioral Activation Tracking Form—BLANK

	MON	TUE	WED	THR	FRI	SAT	SUN
Morning							
Afternoon							
Evening							

Appendix B: Behavioral Activation Tracking Form—SAMPLE

	MON	TUE	WED	THR	FRI	SAT	SUN
Morning	Go for morning walk		Go for morning walk		Call a friend to catch up	Go for morning walk	
Afternoon		Meet friend for coffee	Sit with a friend at lunch			Walk in the park	
Evening	Read a book before bed	Listen to music	Read a book before bed	Watch a favorite movie	Listen to music		

References

Academy for Eating Disorders. (2021). *Eating disorders: A guide to medical care (AED report 2021-4th).* https://www.aedweb.org/resources/publications/medical-care-standards

American Psychiatric Association. (2022). *Diagnostic and statistical manual of mental disorders* (5th ed.). American Psychiatric Publishing. https://doi.org/10.1176/appi.books.9780890425787

Antony, M. M., & Swinson, R. P. (2000). *Phobic disorders and panic in adults: A guide to assessment and treatment.* American Psychological Association. https://doi.org/10.1037/10348-000

Beck, A. T., & Dozois, D. J. A. (2011). Cognitive therapy: Current status and future directions. *Annual Review of Medicine, 62*, 397–409. https://doi.org/10.1146/annurev-med-052209-100032

Bisson, J. I., & Lewis, C. (2009). Systematic review of psychological first aid. *The British Journal of Psychiatry, 195*(1), 5–16.

Bisson, J. I., Roberts, N. P., Andrew, M., Cooper, R., & Lewis, C. (2013). Psychological therapies for chronic post-traumatic stress disorder (PTSD) in adults. *Cochrane Database of Systematic Reviews, 2013*(12), CD003388. https://doi.org/10.1002/14651858.CD003388.pub4

Bouton, M. E., Westbrook, R. F., Corcoran, K. A., & Maren, S. (2006). Contextual and temporal modulation of extinction: Behavioral and biological mechanisms. *Biological Psychiatry, 60*(4), 352–360. https://doi.org/10.1016/j.biopsych.2005.12.015

Butler, A. C., Chapman, J. E., Forman, E. M., & Beck, A. T. (2005). The empirical status of cognitive-behavioral therapy: A review of meta-analyses. *Clinical Psychology Review, 26*(1), 17–31. https://doi.org/10.1016/j.cpr.2005.07.003

Carpenter, J. K., Andrews, L. A., Witcraft, S. M., Powers, M. B., Smits, J. A. J., & Hofmann, S. G. (2018). Cognitive behavioral therapy for anxiety and related disorders: A meta-analysis of randomized placebo-controlled trials. *Depression and Anxiety, 35*(6), 502–514. https://doi.org/10.1002/da.22728

Choy, Y., Fyer, A. J., & Lipsitz, J. D. (2007). Treatment of specific phobia in adults. *Clinical Psychology Review, 27*(3), 266–286. https://doi.org/10.1016/j.cpr.2006.10.002

Cigrang, J. A., Rauch, S. A., Mintz, J., Brundige, A. R., Mitchell, J. A., Najera, E., Litz, B. T., Young-McCaughan, S., Roache, J. D., Hembree, E. A., Goodie, J. L., Sonnek, S. M., Peterson, A. L., & STRONG STAR Consortium. (2017). Moving effective treatment for posttraumatic stress disorder to primary care: A randomized controlled trial with active duty military. *Families, Systems & Health, 35*(4), 450–462. https://doi.org/10.1037/fsh0000315

Clark, D. M. (1986). A cognitive approach to panic. *Behaviour Research and Therapy, 24*(4), 461–470. https://doi.org/10.1016/0005-7967(86)90011-2

Coffey, S. F., Banducci, A. N., & Vinci, C. (2015). Common questions about cognitive behavior therapy for psychiatric disorders. *American Family Physician, 92*(9), 807–812.

Cooney, G. M., Dwan, K., Greig, C. A., Lawlor, D. A., Rimer, J., Waugh, F. R., McMurdo, M., & Mead, G. E. (2013). Exercise for depression. *Cochrane Database of Systematic Reviews, 9.* https://doi.org/10.1002/14651858.CD004366.pub6

Coventry, P. A., Meader, N., Melton, H., Temple, M., Dale, H., Wright, K., Cloitre, M., Karatzias, T., Bisson, J., Roberts, N. P., Brown, J. V. E., Barbui, C., Churchill, R., Lovell, K., McMillan, D., & Gilbody, S. (2020). Psychological and pharmacological interventions for posttraumatic stress disorder and comorbid mental health problems following complex traumatic events: Systematic review and component network meta-analysis. *PLoS Medicine, 17*(8), e1003262. https://doi.org/10.1371/journal.pmed.1003262

Craske, M. G., Barlow, D. H., & Antony, M. M. (2006). *Mastery of your specific phobia: Therapist guide* (2nd ed.). Oxford University Press.

Craske, M. G., Treanor, M., Conway, C. C., Zbozinek, T., & Vervliet, B. (2014). Maximizing exposure therapy: An inhibitory learning approach. *Behaviour Research and Therapy, 58*, 10–23. https://doi.org/10.1016/j.brat.2014.04.006

Deloitte Access Economics. (2020). *The social and economic cost of eating disorders in the United states of America: A report for the strategic training initiative for the prevention of eating disorders and the academy for eating disorders.* https://www.hsph.harvard.edu/striped/report-economic-costs-of-eating-disorders/

Dimidjian, S., Hollon, S. D., Dobson, K. S., Schmaling, K. B., Kohlenberg, R. J., Addis, M. E., Gallop, R., McGlinchey, J. B., Markley, D. K., Gollan, J. K., Atkins, D. C., Dunner, D. L., & Jacobson, N. S. (2006). Randomized trial of behavioral activation, cognitive therapy, and antidepressant medication in the acute treatment of adults with major depression. *Journal of Consulting and Clinical Psychology, 74*(4), 658–670. https://doi.org/10.1037/0022-006X.74.4.658

Dobson, K. S., Hollon, S. D., Dimidjian, S., Schmaling, K. B., Kohlenberg, R. J., Gallop, R. J., Rizvi, S. L., Gollan, J. K., Dunner, D. L., & Jacobson, N. S. (2008). Randomized trial of behavioral activation, cognitive therapy, and antidepressant medication in the prevention of relapse and recurrence in major depression. *Journal of Consulting and Clinical Psychology, 76*(3), 468–477. https://doi.org/10.1037/0022-006X.76.3.468

Ekers, D., Webster, L., Straten, A. V., Cuijpers, P., Richards, D., & Gilbody, S. (2014). Behavioural activation for depression; an update of meta-analysis of effectiveness and sub group analysis. *PLoS One, 9*(6), e100100. https://doi.org/10.1371/journal.pone.0100100

Foldes-Busque, G., Denis, I., Poitras, J., Fleet, R. P., Archambault, P., & Dionne, C. E. (2019). A closer look at the relationships between panic attacks, emergency department visits and non-cardiac chest pain. *Journal of Health Psychology, 24*(6), 717–725. https://doi.org/10.1177/1359105316683785

Harrington, B. C., Jimerson, M., Haxton, C., & Jimerson, D. C. (2015). Initial evaluation, diagnosis, and treatment of anorexia nervosa and bulimia nervosa. *American Family Physician, 91*(1), 46–52.

Jacobson, N. S., Martell, C. R., & Dimidjian, S. (2001). Behavioral activation treatment for depression: Returning to contextual roots. *Clinical Psychology: Science and Practice, 8*(3), 255–270. https://doi.org/10.1093/clipsy.8.3.255

Kessler, R. C., Berglund, P., Demler, O., Jin, R., Koretz, D., Merikangas, K. R., Rush, A. J., Walters, E. E., & Wang, P. S. (2003). The epidemiology of major depressive disorder: Results from the National Comorbitiy Survey Replication (NCS-R). *JAMA, 289*(23), 3095–3105. https://doi.org/10.1001/jama.289.23.3095

Koerner, K., Dimeff, L. A., & Rizvi, S. L. (2021). Overview of DBT. In *Dialectical behavior therapy in clinical practice: Applications across disorders and settings* (2nd ed., pp. 3–20). The Guilford Press.

Kroenke, K., Spitzer, R. L., & Williams, J. B. W. (2003). The patient Health Questionnaire-2: Validity of a two-item depression screener. *Medical Care, 41*(11), 1284–1292. https://doi.org/10.1097/01.MLR.0000093487.78664.3C

Lewinsohn, P. M., Biglang, A., & Zeiss, A. M. (1976). Behavioral treatment of depression. In *The behavioral management of anxiety, depression, and pain* (pp. 91–146). Brunner/Mazel.

Lewinsohn, P. M., & Libet, J. (1972). Pleasant events, activity schedules, and depressions. *Journal of Abnormal Psychology, 79*(3), 291–295. https://doi.org/10.1037/h0033207

Loots, E., Goossens, E., Vanwesemael, T., Morrens, M., Van Rompaey, B., & Dilles, T. (2021). Interventions to improve medication adherence in patients with schizophrenia or bipolar disorders: A systematic review and meta-analysis. *International Journal of Environmental Research and Public Health, 18*(19), 19. https://doi.org/10.3390/ijerph181910213

Martell, C. R., Dimidjian, S., & Herman-Dunn, R. (2010). *Behavioral activation for depression: A clinician's guide.* The Guilford Press.

Marzani, G., & Neff, A. P. (2021). Bipolar disorders: Evaluation and treatment. *American Family Physician, 103*(4), 227–239.

McCabe, R. E., & Antony, M. M. (2008). Anxiety disorders: Social and specific phobias. In *Psychiatry* (3rd ed., pp. 1409–1442). John Wiley & Sons. https://doi.org/10.1002/9780470515167.ch70

Miller, B. F., Teevan, B., Phillips, R. L., Jr., Petterson, S. M., & Bazemore, A. W. (2011). The importance of time in treating mental health in primary care. *Families, Systems & Health, 29*(2), 144–145. https://doi.org/10.1037/a0023993

National Eating Disorders Association. (2024). National Eating Disorders Association (NEDA). https://www.nationaleatingdisorders.org/national-eating-disorders-association/

Newman, M. G., Agras, W. S., Haaga, D. A., & Jarrett, R. B. (2021). Cognitive, behavioral, and cognitive behavioral therapy. In *Bergin and Garfield's handbook of psychotherapy and behavior change* (pp. 469–506). John Wiley & Sons.

Olfson, M., Blanco, C., Wang, S., Laje, G., & Correll, C. U. (2014). National trends in the mental health care of children, adolescents, and adults by office-based physicians. *JAMA Psychiatry, 71*(1), 81–90. https://doi.org/10.1001/jamapsychiatry.2013.3074

Otto, M. W., & Henin, A. (2007). Combined pharmacotherapy and cognitive-behavioral therapy for anxiety disorders: Medication effects, glucocorticoids, and attenuated treatment outcomes. *Clinical Psychology: Science and Practice, 14*(2), 160–173.

Otto, M. W., Pollack, M. H., & Gould, R. A. (2000). A meta-analytic review of the efficacy of benzodiazepines and cognitive behavioral therapies in the treatment of panic disorder. *Journal of Anxiety Disorders, 14*(4), 275–292.

Pina, A. A., Zerr, A. A., Gonzales, N. A., & Ortiz, C. D. (2009). Psychosocial interventions for school refusal behavior in children and adolescents. *Child Development Perspectives, 3*(1), 11–20. https://doi.org/10.1111/j.1750-8606.2008.00070.x

Poulton, R., & Menzies, R. G. (2002). Non-associative fear acquisition: A review of the evidence from retrospective and longitudinal research. *Behaviour Research and Therapy, 40*(2), 127–149. https://doi.org/10.1016/s0005-7967(01)00045-6

Prins, A., Bovin, M. J., Kimerling, R., Kaloupek, D. G., Marx, B. P., Pless Kaiser, A., & Schnurr, P. P. (2015). *The primary care PTSD screen for DSM-5 (PC-PTSD-5).* National Center for PTSD.

Rauch, S. A. M., Venners, M. R., Ragin, C., Ruhe, G., Lamp, K. E., Burton, M., Pomerantz, A., Bernardy, N., Schnurr, P. P., Hamblen, J. L., Possemato, K., Sripada, R., Wray, L. O., Dollar, K., Wade, M., Astin, M. C., & Cigrang, J. A. (2023). Treatment of posttraumatic stress disorder with prolonged exposure for primary care (PE-PC): Effectiveness and patient and therapist factors related to symptom change and retention. *Psychological Services, 20*(4), 745–755. https://doi.org/10.1037/ser0000783

Roberts, N. P., Kitchiner, N. J., Kenardy, J., & Bisson, J. I. (2009). Systematic review and meta-analysis of multiple-session early interventions following traumatic events. *American Journal of Psychiatry, 166*(3), 293–301. https://doi.org/10.1176/appi.ajp.2008.08040590

Roberts, N. P., Roberts, P. A., Jones, N., & Bisson, J. I. (2016). Psychological therapies for post-traumatic stress disorder and comorbid substance use disorder. *Cochrane Database of Systematic Reviews, 4*(4), CD010204. https://doi.org/10.1002/14651858.CD010204.pub2/full

Rose, S. C., Bisson, J., Churchill, R., & Wessely, S. (2002). Psychological debriefing for preventing post traumatic stress disorder (PTSD). *Cochrane Database of Systematic Reviews, 2*(2), CD000560.

Rosen, L. D., Whaling, K., Rab, S., Carrier, L. M., & Cheever, N. A. (2013). Is Facebook creating "iDisorders"? The link between clinical symptoms of psychiatric disorders and technology use, attitudes and anxiety. *Computers in Human Behavior, 29*(3), 1243–1254. https://doi.org/10.1016/j.chb.2012.11.012

Salkovskis, P. M., Clark, D. M., & Gelder, M. G. (1996). Cognition-behaviour links in the persistence of panic. *Behaviour Research and Therapy, 34*(5–6), 453–458. https://doi.org/10.1016/0005-7967(95)00083-6

Simon, G. E., & VonKorff, M. (1995). Recognition, management, and outcomes of depression in primary care. *Archives of Family Medicine, 4*(2), 99–105. https://doi.org/10.1001/archfami.4.2.99

Sloan, D. M., & Marx, B. P. (2019). *Written exposure therapy for PTSD: A brief treatment approach for mental health professionals* (p. 115). American Psychological Association (APA). https://doi.org/10.1037/0000139-000

Substance Abuse and Mental Health Services Administration (SAMHSA). (2014). *SAMHSA's concept of trauma and guidance for a trauma-informed approach.* Substance Abuse and Mental Health Services Administration. https://ncsacw.acf.hhs.gov/userfiles/files/SAMHSA_Trauma.pdf

Substance Abuse and Mental Health Services Administration (SAMHSA). (2023). *Practical guide for implementing a trauma-informed approach. SAMHSA Publication No. PEP23–06–05-005.* National Mental Health and Substance Use Policy Laboratory.

U.S. Department of Veterans Affairs. (2024a). *Device review: Breathe2Relax [general information].* Rehabilitation and Prosthetic Services. https://www.prosthetics.va.gov/AssistiveTechnology/reviews/2017-Breathe2Relax.asp

U.S. Department of Veterans Affairs. (2024b). *PTSD coach.* VAMobile. https://mobile.va.gov/app/ptsd-coach

U.S. Department of Veterans Affairs. (2024c). *PTSD coach.* PTSD: National Center for PTSD. https://www.ptsd.va.gov/appvid/mobile/ptsdcoach_app.asp

U.S. Department of Veterans Affairs. (2024d). PTSD: National Center for PTSD [Program Homepage]. https://www.ptsd.va.gov/

van Emmerik, A. A., Kamphuis, J. H., Hulsbosch, A. M., & Emmelkamp, P. M. (2002). Single session debriefing after psychological trauma: A meta-analysis. *The Lancet, 360*(9335), 766–771. https://doi.org/10.1016/S0140-6736(02)09897-5

Ward, R. K. (2004). Assessment and management of personality disorders. *American Family Physician, 70*(8), 1505–1512.

Weathers, F. W., Litz, B. T., Keane, T. M., Palmieri, P. A., Marx, B. P., & Schnurr, P. P. (2013). *The PTSD checklist for DSM-5 (PCL-5).* National Center for PTSD.

Williamson, M. L. C., Roberman, S., Sopchak, K., & Mosley, T. M. (2023). School avoidance: How to help when a child refuses to go. *Journal of Family Practice, 72*(7), 304–319. https://doi.org/10.12788/jfp.0653

Williamson, M. L. C., Stickley, M. M., Armstrong, T. W., Jackson, K., & Console, K. (2022). Diagnostic accuracy of the primary care PTSD screen for DSM-5 (PC-PTSD-5) within a civilian primary care sample. *Journal of Clinical Psychology, 78*(11), 2299–2308. https://doi.org/10.1002/jclp.23405

Wolitzky-Taylor, K. B., Horowitz, J. D., Powers, M. B., & Telch, M. J. (2008). Psychological approaches in the treatment of specific phobias: A meta-analysis. *Clinical Psychology Review, 28*(6), 1021–1037. https://doi.org/10.1016/j.cpr.2008.02.007

Chapter 9
Behavioral Interventions for Health Behaviors in Primary Care

Kaylee Jackson PhD, Mariah Montgomery PhD, Rebecca M. Daniel PsyD, Rolando Botello MEd, Giannina Mixco MEd, Taliyah Mosley MEd, Danielle Porter MS, Morgan Sekula MEd, Jennifer Swanson MEd, Susan Roberman MD, FAAFP, and Meredith L. C. Williamson PhD, ABPP

Chronic Health Conditions and Physical Health Concerns in Primary Care

Individuals with chronic health conditions have poorer overall health, use more healthcare services, and have higher healthcare expenditures than those without (Buttorff et al., 2017). An estimated 129 million people in the US, or six in ten adults, have at least one chronic disease (Benavidez, 2024; Buttorff et al., 2017). While primary care physicians (PCPs) are well versed in medical interventions for these physical health concerns, many of these conditions have behavioral components that also can be addressed with patients. This chapter will provide an overview of skills and pharmacotherapy that PCPs can use when addressing behavioral components of chronic disease management and health behaviors, as well as disease-specific behavioral interventions for PCPs to utilize in their practice.

Rolando Botello, Giannina Mixco, Taliyah Mosley, Danielle Porter, Morgan Sekula and Jennifer Swanson contributed equally to this publication.

K. Jackson PhD (✉) · S. Roberman MD, FAAFP · M. L. C. Williamson PhD, ABPP
Naresh K. Vashisht College of Medicine, Department of Primary Care and Rural Medicine, Texas A&M University, Bryan, TX, USA
e-mail: kayleejanae@tamu.edu

M. Montgomery PhD
Dell Medical School, The University of Texas at Austin, Austin, TX, USA

R. M. Daniel PsyD
Wake Forest University School of Medicine, Winston-Salem, NC, USA

R. Botello MEd · G. Mixco MEd · T. Mosley MEd · D. Porter MS · M. Sekula MEd · J. Swanson MEd
Texas A&M University, College Station, TX, USA

M. L. C. Williamson and D. L. Terry (eds.), *Essentials for Treating Behavioral Health in Primary Care*, https://doi.org/10.1007/978-3-032-09558-9_9

The Role of Psychosocial and Behavioral Factors in the Maintenance or Worsening of Physical Health and Chronic Disease

Patients may engage in behaviors that enhance or impede their overall health. For example, diet and exercise habits, medication adherence, and substance use impact chronic diseases (Hacker, 2024). Psychosocial factors and social determinants of health such as finances, transportation to clinic, ability to take time to attend appointments, access to medications, and comorbid behavioral health (BH) and physical health conditions may also maintain or worsen a patient's health conditions (Hacker, 2024). Chronic diseases disproportionately affect socioeconomically disinvested communities and people, and effective management of these health conditions requires addressing individual behaviors and psychosocial factors (Benavidez, 2024). When PCPs treat chronic health conditions without considering the broader context of their patients, attempts to help patients manage their health may be unsuccessful. In primary care clinics with integrated BH services (IBH), BH providers can aid PCPs in identifying and addressing health behaviors impacting disease. In clinics without BH support, PCPs can utilize the following skills to address these behaviors within the context of their visits.

Importance of Holistic Care

Even when health behaviors are interfering with disease management, it is still imperative to screen for and treat medical conditions as appropriate. When the first-line treatment for a condition is a medical intervention that should be the PCPs primary recommendation. However, for some diagnoses first-line recommendations are behavioral (e.g., insomnia; Qaseem et al., 2016). Additionally, even when first-line interventions are pharmacological or procedural in nature, there may be important behavioral factors that are impeding patients' overall health that PCPs have an opportunity to address. PCPs also want to be careful not to dismiss patient concerns as exclusively behavioral in nature and miss potential underlying medical causes. For example, PCPs may ascribe a patient's concerns about their weight or pain exclusively to their management of diet and exercise, rather than considering a potential underlying health condition. PCPs should aim for *whole-person* care that takes the patient's entire context into consideration.

Overview of Macro Skills for Assessment and Intervention

The 5 A's model of assess, advise, agree, assist, and arrange has been used for assessment and intervention for a range of presenting problems within primary care (Bosworth et al., 2017; Carroll et al., 2016; Fehily et al., 2020; Goldstein et al., 2016). PCPs can utilize this framework across a variety of problems to help encourage health behavior changes in their patients.

Assess This phase involves gathering information about symptoms, risk factors, behaviors, barriers, and attitudes (Goldstein et al., 2004; Hunter et al., 2024). This phase may be done briefly at the start of a visit with a patient, available family members, and from multiple sources, such as routine health screenings done at the beginning of encounters, information gathered from electronic health records (EHRs), focused screening measures based on presenting concerns, or from support staff who assist during visits. PCPs are encouraged to rely on their teams to help gather information to help reduce burnout and improve clinical flow (Kim et al., 2018).

One framework for gathering psychosocial information from patients is the contextual interview (See Table 9.1), which allows for understanding the patient's life context and helps them tailor practical interventions to match (Cahill et al., 2024; Robinson et al., 2011; see Chap. 2 for additional information). Contextual interviewing involves questions across domains of love, work, play, and health behaviors (see Table 9.1 for more details). PCPs can use contextual interviewing to guide subsequent questions during their visit, as well as to assess social determinants of health, barriers, risk factors, and stages of change (see below). It can be applied generally or to specific presenting concerns, information can be collected over multiple visits and can help inform treatment planning.

Managing chronic diseases requires significant lifestyle changes for most patients (e.g., changing diet or exercise habits, changing substance use, etc.). While gathering information, PCPs can assess readiness and motivation to change using the *Transtheoretical Model of Change,* also known as the Stages of Change Model (see Fig. 9.1) as a framework (Prochaska & Velicer, 1997), in addition to motivational interviewing (MI) strategies (see Rollnick et al., 2022 for complete discussion of motivational interviewing in healthcare settings). Through employment of MI strategies, PCPs may ask patients how important it is to change, or if they would like things to be

Table 9.1 Contextual interviewing domains (Cahill et al., 2024; Robinson et al., 2011)

Domain	Content of questions to ask
Love	Relationships, social supports, living situation
Work	Education, work, finances
Play	Hobbies, values, enjoyment
Health behaviors	Can be focused on presenting concerns

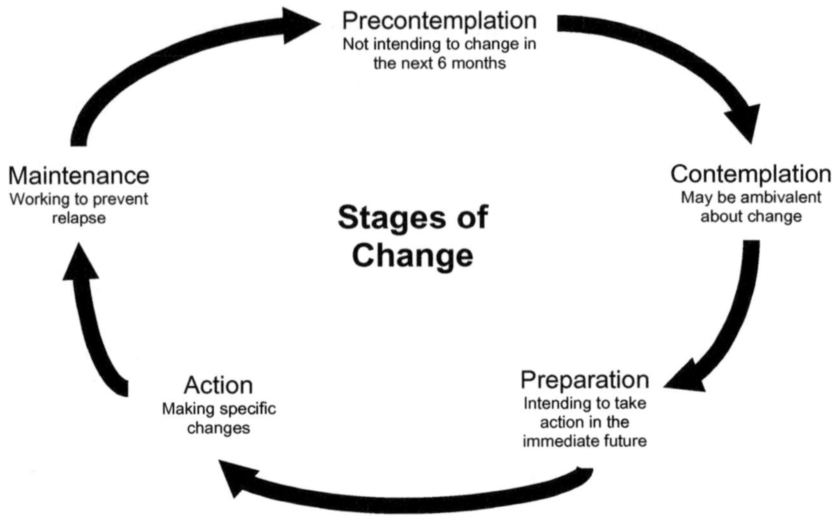

Fig. 9.1 Stages of change model (Prochaska & Velicer, 1997)

different than they currently are to assess where the patient is at in the change process. MI can assist providers in selecting appropriate interventions that allow the patient to be successful in their attempts at health behavior change. Rather than convincing patients to change, which may feel frustrating and be ineffective, PCPs can help patients transition throughout the stages of change (Zimmerman et al., 2000).

Utilizing behavior tracking can provide several benefits in moving patients closer to change. For instance, using a behavior tracking sheet can aid patients in understanding the extent to which their behaviors are impacting their health (positively and negatively), aid in goal setting, and inform providers about adherence to the treatment plan. Patients may already be tracking behavior without realizing it in the form of smart devices that monitor physical activity, sleep, and more. When introducing tracking, PCPs should ensure patients have a plan for *how* to track their behavior, whether that is through a specific phone app, smart device, or paper and pen. A script for introducing behavior tracking, also referred to as self-monitoring, could look like this:

> PCP: To better understand how your physical activity is impacting your chronic pain I would like for you to keep track of your daily movement. This will help us tailor your treatment plan and better understand what your body needs. I will show you the tracking sheet I would like you to use, and we can also problem solve ways to help you remember. Some people find that they remember best when they pair it with an activity that they already have a habit of doing each day, like eating breakfast or brushing their teeth. Others find alarms helpful. Where do you think this would best fit into your routine?

Example self-monitoring form

Day	Activity and duration	Sleep quality	Next day functioning	Notes
Tues, 10/1/24	Walking, 1 mile	7/10	4/10	I slept better but am very sore today and was not able to garden. Maybe I need to start smaller and build up my walks.

Providers may find it helpful to be mindful of patient bias toward the negative or tendencies to select unattainable goals and to choose tracking goals accordingly (see the Agree section below for help selecting goals). For example, if a patient is strongly focused on their pain try shifting the focus to improvements in functioning. Functioning should be collaboratively defined with the patient and will be unique to each person. For example:

> PCP: I would like for us to focus on the activities you want to do that your pain has gotten in the way of recently. What are three things we can look at this month that you would like to do more of?
> Patient: I would really like to garden more. My friends have also been wanting me to call and make plans, but I am always so tired. I would also like to keep my sink clean and not wait so long to do the dishes.
> PCP: Wonderful! What great ideas. How might we make those easily trackable for you?
> Patient: I guess I can just write down if I did them?
> PCP: Sure! We can change it later if we find that doesn't work. Based on our conversation today, it sounds like you tried limiting your physical activity due to pain but it hasn't helped. This is also consistent with what research tells us. For the next month, I really just want you to be curious about how the amount of activity your body is getting impacts your ability to do these things you enjoy. Remember what we talked about regarding pacing!

In this example the PCP collaborated with the patient on goals, invited the patient to problem solve potential barriers, demonstrated that they were listening to the patient's previous strategy of reducing movement and its impact, and provided education on evidence-based treatment. While this example is specific to chronic pain, these principles can be applied to each health condition discussed in this chapter.

Advise In this phase providers should provide personalized recommendations based on the information gathered in the Assess phase. MI techniques are the most effective strategies for moving patients from precontemplation and contemplation to preparation (DiClemente & Velasquez, 2002; Zimmerman et al., 2000). For patients in preparation or action phases, providers may choose to focus on options that provide the patient choices for how to minimize symptoms and bolster quality of life. Providers should give patients the rationale for their recommendations and ensure patients have all necessary information to make an informed choice. PCPs can avoid "preaching" at patients by asking permission to share advice (e.g., "Is it okay if I share some information about better managing your diabetes with you?") or filling in gaps in patients' existing knowledge.

Example Conversation with Patient

"From your lab work today we see that your A1C has gone up since your last visit, which is an indicator of how well you are controlling your blood sugar. From what we've just discussed *[gathered during the "assess" part of the visit]*, it sounds like you have been eating a lot more fast food lately due to working longer hours at work and having less time and energy to cook well-balanced meals at home. Do you know how stress and your diet may be impacting your diabetes? *[allow patient to provide their knowledge, ask if it would be okay to share your knowledge, and if patient agrees then fill in any gaps]*

"Eating a well-balanced diet, getting exercise, and managing stress are all helpful strategies to manage your diabetes, and I know that work can make these things difficult to do at times. I wonder if we can come up with some goals together that can help you do even one of these things?" *[move into agreement phase]*

Agree Selection of goals will ideally be a collaborative process. In this phase, providers work with their patients to select goals and treatment(s) based on the patient's motivation, circumstances, and readiness for change. The patient may not be ready to commit to any of the treatment options, in which case providers should continue to engage with the patient from a place of curiosity, to aid the patient in the shared decision-making process.

If patients are experiencing significant ambivalence regarding changing their behaviors, PCPs may utilize MI techniques to help increase patients' readiness for change. While it can be frustrating or saddening to see patients make decisions that negatively affect their physical health, PCPs can provide information about the consequences of decisions while respecting patient's decision-making autonomy regarding their healthcare.

PCPs can utilize the SMART (Specific, Measurable, Attainable, Relevant, Time-bound; See Fig. 9.2) goal-setting method to set agreed upon goals with their patients (Doran, 1981). Figure 9.2 outlines the components of SMART goals.

Assist After setting goals, PCPs want to ensure that patients know *how* to reach their goals. PCPs will assist patients in meeting their agreed upon goals by providing education, teaching skills, or addressing problem-solving barriers together. Research suggests that less may be more, so PCPs may choose to provide fewer numbers of interventions that the patient feels confident they can follow up on, rather than providing a laundry list of changes to make (Nigg & Long, 2012). Cognitive functioning can also affect patients' abilities to follow treatment plans; considering

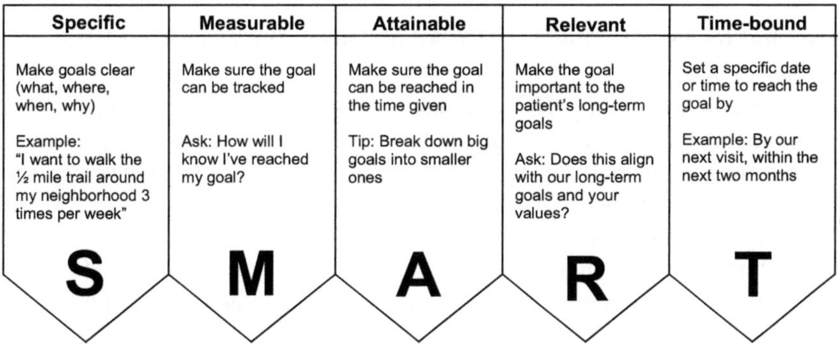

Fig. 9.2 SMART Goals (Doran, 1981)

patients' functioning will be important in formulating a plan that is achievable and the best fit for their needs.

PCPs may also find that patients need assistance in problem-solving barriers that they face when making behavior changes. Engaging in step-by-step problem-solving with patients may assist them in reaching the agreed upon goals. These steps can include defining the problem, brainstorming solutions, evaluating solutions, selecting the best solution, implementing the chosen solution, and assessing the outcome (usually at follow-up visits; Hunter et al., 2024). Providers can also utilize MI to explore patient ambivalence to medication adherence and help them articulate their own rationale for increasing adherence. Additional strategies include simplifying dosing regimens (Claxton et al., 2001), encouraging use of pill organizers or automatic dispensers (Kripalani et al., 2007), electronic monitoring devices that display the date last opened (Velligan et al., 2010), and phone applications that patients can track medication adherence and set reminders in (Morrissey et al., 2016). When barriers relating to the patient's BH, such as anxiety and depression, are causing significant interference to adherence, a referral to a BH provider may be warranted.

Arrange During the last phase, the patient and provider will arrange for any follow-up care (e.g., next office visit, phone calls, etc.). This may include reminding patients what to bring into their next visits (e.g., tracking information or progress toward goals) or helping coordinate referrals to specialty care as needed. PCPs may find that information may need to be gathered over multiple visits, or that some behavior changes may not be solved in one single visit.

Some visits may be focused on moving patients into the contemplation or preparation stage of change, or PCPs may choose to implement one behavior change at a time and schedule more frequent follow-ups with patients until target goals are met. If PCPs have BH services available to them in their clinic, they may choose to include them in follow-up care, or as an adjunct to help the patients in their behavior changes.

Tips and tricks - Or How Do I Do All of This in the Time That I Have?

Targeted questions

PCPs can utilize targeted questions to keep conversations on track (e.g., "you mentioned to the nurse that you have been having some stomach issues, tell me more about that"). They can also employ compassionate redirection to patients to help refocus conversations.

Stick to the principles

PCPs may not have time to fully engage with the 5As at every visit. However, they can employ principles of shared decision making and respect for patient autonomy care in every encounter, regardless of time.

Use your team and data

It is imperative that PCPs utilize their clinic team and resources to gather information prior to seeing the patient (e.g., medical assistants, medical records, etc.) to prevent burnout (Kim et al., 2018).

Good documentation

Thorough documentation to keep track of progress on shared goals will also be helpful in making the most of the time that PCPs have in the room with patients. PCPs may choose to utilize goal setting worksheets that they scan into patient charts to help or develop their own strategies to help remember what goals and strategies they have discussed with patients.

Beginning follow up sessions with a recap

PCPs may save time, and help patients feel heard, by beginning each follow up visit with a brief recap of what was covered in the previous visit. This may be especially useful to avoid reiterating information that was previously gathered, and to make efficient use of time during brief visits.

Health Behavior Specific Interventions

Diabetes and Cardiovascular Disease Management

A major contributing factor to the development of chronic diseases such as diabetes and cardiovascular disease (CVD) is modifiable health behaviors that serve as risk factors. It is important for providers to be mindful that chronic health disparities also commonly exist in marginalized populations including individuals of low socioeconomic status, lower educational attainment, and racial/ethnic minority groups partly because of systemic policies that favor certain groups (Remington et al., 2011).

Assess Psychosocial factors have a significant influence on the management of diabetes and CVD, and the effective management of these require significant lifestyle changes which may impact multiple domains of a patient's life (Benavidez, 2024). A contextual interview can provide insight into these domains and guide intervention planning. For example, for patients who are used to connecting with others over food, having to make the significant dietary changes required of diabetes and CVD may negatively affect their relationships. Further, contextual interviewing can provide insight into barriers that might otherwise be missed, such as limited access to fresh foods due to financial concerns, transportation issues, or proximity to grocery stores. Patients requiring increased physical activity may lack access to a safe environment or have limited time due to the demands of their occupation (e.g., working multiple jobs) or caregiving responsibilities. When inquiring about patient's baseline dietary and movement habits, asking for most recent 24-hour food and beverage recall is a useful tool.

Individuals with diabetes and CVD demonstrate higher rates of depression, anxiety, and overall stress (Hunter et al., 2024). Experiencing such distress can negatively affect one's successful management of their chronic disease and overall quality of life. Brief assessments exist that can be utilized as an adjunct to evaluate distress (time permitting), such as the Diabetes Distress Scale 2 (Fisher et al., 2008).

Advise Intervention options for patients with diabetes and CVD should emphasize changes in lifestyle to target modifiable risk factors, such as poor dietary habits, tobacco use, physical inactivity, and severe alcohol use (Ketola et al., 2000; Knowler et al., 2002). While exploring intervention options, a patient may feel overwhelmed by the thought of making various changes to one's life. It is therefore important to provide support to the patient by demonstrating empathy and understanding. A provider can do so by remaining aware of their patient's feelings and any nonverbal communication that is demonstrated, while normalizing their experience. Advice is most effective when tailored to the patient and their circumstances, which may help the patient feel empowered and motivated for change (Glasgow et al., 2003; Goldstein et al., 2004). It is critical to have buy-in from the patient, or an openness to adhere to the provided advice, as the majority of health outcomes are determined by a patient's management of their symptoms (Glasgow et al., 2003). MI strategies are useful in helping patients make the lifestyle changes necessary to manage these chronic conditions (Morton et al., 2015).

Agree During the Advise phase, presenting patients with a wide variety of lifestyle changes and intervention options can be overwhelming. It is recommended that the patient be guided to select one or two areas they would like to target. For example, providers may need to give support in increasing medication adherence, making changes in healthy diets, or discussing ways to add more physical activity to a patient's life. It is not recommended to encourage change in all three areas at once. Additionally, a regular assessment of motivation for change will assist with ongoing treatment planning. Specifically, providers will need to assess once the patient has made changes in a specific area (e.g., medication adherence) whether they are ready to make other lifestyle changes (e.g., dietary habits, physical activity). See below for an example conversation with a patient.

It is common for PCPs to have big goals for patients navigating chronic disease and for providers to feel urgency regarding the necessity of change in their patients' lives. A common mistake is to start patients on goals that are too large and use fear as a motivator (e.g., "If you do not do this, you will die"). Unfortunately, this strategy is often unhelpful (Glasgow et al., 2003; Kok et al., 2018; van't Riet & Ruiter, 2013). A more helpful approach is providing patients with information on how they can cope with their conditions (Milne et al., 2000). This can be done by utilizing the SMART goals (see Fig. 9.2) method and intentionally choosing the first steps that are likely to give the patient a win. For example, PCPs may guide the patient to increase physical activity by only 5 min a day in the first visit. In the next visit, PCPs and patients can continue to increase the goal behavior as their patients build confidence in their ability to change.

PCP: I know you we have discussed many possible target areas that will help you reach your goal of feeling better. I heard you mention wanting to be able to keep up with your grandchildren and be there for them throughout their lives. With these goals in mind, which area would you like to target first?
Patient: I honestly just don't know; I am overwhelmed with everything I need to do. It just seems like so much.
PCP: That is really common. You are not alone in feeling overwhelmed at all the options. Based on your specific goals, I recommend we start with either increasing movement or adjusting your nutrition. Which of these two would you like to start with?
Patient: Probably movement.
PCP: Great! Earlier in our visit, you mentioned that you don't get much movement due to working a desk job and feeling tired when you get home. We might start with a 5 minute walk each day or taking a short movement break between each meeting at work. Which of these, if any, would be most doable?
Patient: Surely 5 minutes isn't enough and how could a couple minutes between meetings make a difference?
PCP: At this stage, we just want to help your brain and body start building a new habit. This first goal should feel almost "too easy." That's a sign that we are on the right track! We also want to monitor your progress by documenting your movement. Some patients like to use the self-monitoring forms we provide while others like to make a sticker chart or use their phones.
Patient: Ok, I see. I think I will do the movement breaks at work. I'll put a star on my desk calendar for each day that I do them. That could actually be pretty motivating. Maybe I can even get some colleagues to join in.
PCP: That sounds perfect! Maybe you can take a picture at the end of the month before you come for your next visit so we can look at your progress together and plan the next steps. How does that sound?

Assist PCPs are likely aware that patients with diabetes or CVD will benefit from self-monitoring (e.g., blood pressure, A1C), engaging in physical activity, changing

Table 9.2 Barriers and solutions for implementing lifestyle changes

Barrier	Potential solution
Patient often eats out with important others, disrupting their dietary goals	• Counsel patient on small changes they can make at common restaurants • Brainstorm other ways patient can connect others (e.g., meeting to go on a walk, book clubs, or other shared interests)
Patient has limited access to fresh food	• Work with clinic staff to provide resources for food insecurity (e.g., food pantry, SNAP benefits) • Counsel patient on nutritious options when utilizing SNAP
Patient has difficulty increasing physical activity	• Counsel patient on small changes they can make to their daily routine (e.g., setting alarms to take movement breaks, involve those they are caregiving for in the movement activity) • Develop SMART goals to slowly increase activity over time (e.g., start with 5–10 min/day of movement)

dietary habits, and adhering to treatment regimens. PCPs can encourage patients with diabetes to use digital health apps to support self-monitoring such as Diabetes:M (Sirma Medical Systems, 2024), mySugr (mySugr GmbH, 2024) or Glucose Buddy (Ali Sherazi et al., 2023; Azumio Inc, 2024). Patients with CVD can be encouraged to monitor blood pressures at home with reminders set at certain times of the day on their phones. It may be beneficial for PCPs to encourage intuitive eating practices such as increasing recognition of physical hunger cues and identifying a comfortable fullness level to stop eating at mealtimes (Warren et al., 2017). PCPs have likely experienced frustrations or barriers when helping patients engage in these lifestyle changes. By utilizing information gathered in the Assess phase, PCPs may have a better understanding of the barriers that their patients face and can help problem solve strategies to overcome them (See Table 9.2). MI strategies to assist patients who may be experiencing ambivalence around changes will also be useful. See examples below for how this can be done in practice. PCPs may recommend disease-specific self-management support in the community, such as Chronic Disease Self-Management Programs (Brady et al., 2011). PCPs are also encouraged to utilize creative solutions such as prescribing 90-day medication supplies to reduce patient pharmacy trips for diabetes or CVD-related medications.

Gastrointestinal Disorders

Gastrointestinal (GI) disorders affect more than 40 million people in the United States and these disorders account for a significant number of clinical visits and healthcare expenditures annually (Peery et al., 2022). Individuals with GI disorders often report substantial declines in their daily functioning, and increased prevalence of depression and anxiety (Bryant et al., 2011; Roohafza et al., 2016). Further, for those with functional GI disorders, such as irritable bowel syndrome (IBS), studies have shown that unnecessary surgeries are common (Black et al., 2020; Longstreth, 2007).

Assess Given the stigma associated with GI disorders, inquiring about patients' thoughts and feelings in addition to their GI symptoms may allow them to feel more comfortable discussing their symptoms (Black et al., 2020). It is also important for providers to evaluate the quality of life of their patients, including how severe the patient's symptoms are and the level of functional impairment they experience (Keefer et al., 2018). This can be assessed through a contextual interviewing framework that focuses on how GI symptoms influence patients' overall functioning in different areas of their lives. General quality of life questionnaires, such as the Gastrointestinal Quality of Life Index (GIQLI; Eypasch et al., 1995), along with specific diagnostic questionnaires, such as the Short Inflammatory Bowel Disease Questionnaire (SIBDQ; Irvine et al., 1996), the Irritable Bowel Syndrome Quality of Life (IBS-QOL; Patrick et al., 1998), or GERD-Health-Related Quality of Life Questionnaire (GERD-HRQL; Velanovich, 2007) also exist as adjunct assessments should providers want to incorporate them when time permits. PCPs can also assess their patient's quality of life by asking simple, relevant, and open-ended questions. For example, asking "How are you most affected by your bowel symptoms?" or "What activities do you modify due to pain?" can allow the patient to express distress and offer providers additional context to the patient's complaints (Keefer et al., 2018). Providers should also utilize recall or tracking to assess when patients are experiencing GI symptoms. This can help tie physical symptoms to stress or triggers and guide intervention.

Advise A strong patient-provider relationship is key for successful GI symptom management, and it is important to help patients understand they can make changes that might help them feel better (Liu et al., 2020; Rollnick et al., 2022). Providers should highlight that although factors such as quality and quantity of sleep, eating patterns, and exercise may not have caused the patient's disorder, the patient can still try implementing healthier habits to reduce symptoms (Keefer et al., 2018).

Psychoeducation on the brain-gut pathway (i.e., the bidirectional relationship between stress and GI symptoms) is often helpful for patients to understand their condition and the treatment plan. Providers may find it easier to explain information to patients by using diagrams or images that simplify these complex topics. Not only can this allow patients to be more knowledgeable, independent, and confident about their symptoms, but it will also reduce the likelihood of seeking answers from unreliable sources (Black et al., 2020; Halpert et al., 2007).

When discussing dietary changes, PCPs should note that children and adolescents tend to have less control over their diets and may require collaboration with parents/caregivers to identify realistic adjustments that can be maintained. Food insecurity can also contribute significantly to patients' ability to manage their GI symptoms.

Additionally, special considerations should be made for patients with a history of eating disorders or avoidant/restrictive food intake disorder. These patients may have challenges avoiding relapse, interpreting physical hunger cues, or consuming sufficient calories (Chey et al., 2021).

Agree Patients experiencing significant pain or discomfort may be reluctant to engage in behavioral changes or treatments if they feel their physical distress is ignored. They might also not want to make behavioral changes if they do not understand brain-gut interactions, do not have enough time or resources to make changes, or lack awareness of how their own stress and anxiety contribute to their symptoms (Black et al., 2020; Keefer et al., 2018). PCPs can use evaluative open-ended questions (e.g., "Tell me what you know about how stress affects your symptoms?" or "What resources would help you make changes to improve your symptoms?") to see what factors or limits in their understanding may be barriers. With disorders such as IBS, patients are most likely to experience relief from multifaceted, individualized treatment plans that are tailored to their individual capacities, resources, symptoms, and needs (Liu et al., 2020). Consider the case example below.

Case Example

Louisa is a 34-year-old mother of two elementary aged children with IBS. Since the school year started, she has gotten a promotion at work, and her children are both involved in weekend sports and after school activities. She presents to the office because she is experiencing more frequent flare ups of her IBS, especially when she is rushing between activities or events for work or her children.

PCP: From what you have shared today, it sounds like you have been really busy these days! Has that been causing you more stress than usual?

Louisa: Yeah, running around all the time has been stressful, plus with my IBS acting up more, that is adding to the stress of everything.

PCP: Sometimes stress can create a vicious cycle for IBS symptoms. Stress can make symptoms worse, but worse symptoms also adds to our stress. Does that sound like what may be happening for you these days?

Louisa: When you put it that way, yeah. I know I have heard before about managing my stress can help with my IBS, but it feels like it is causing most of my stress these days.

PCP: That makes a lot of sense, it feels like your IBS is your main stressor these days?

Louisa: Yeah, I mean work has been stressful, and getting the kids to all their things on time is also chaotic. But it always feels like I have a flare up at the most inconvenient time, right on the days when I'm running late or trying to get the kids to their practices.

PCP: It sounds like on some of these days when all of these other obligations feel the most pressing, that's when your IBS shows up. I wonder if you were able to better manage your stress on these busy days it might help your IBS symptoms? Is there anything with the kids or at work that you think could be adjusted to help those feel more manageable?

Louisa: I have noticed that the days my kids have after school practice are particularly bad because I am rushing from work to pick them up to make it everywhere on time, but I seem to always have a flare-up. I think I could maybe start leaving work 30 minutes early on those days to see if that helps.

PCP: Great! Let's make a game plan for what that will look like for you, and you can start tracking your symptoms to see if making this change helps with your symptoms.

Assist GI disorders are typically not resolved with only one behavioral or medical change, and patients have often tried to resolve symptoms on their own prior to seeking treatment (Keefer et al., 2018; Lenhart et al., 2018). Providers can support patients in selecting the most feasible and preferred treatments based on information gathered in the assess and agree phase of the visit.

Psychoeducation: Many GI diseases are chronic and progressive, and patients will benefit from education about what to expect from their diseases, potential for developing cancers, how the disease may impact their quality of life (including sexual or reproductive functioning; Gikas & Triantafillidis, 2014). This information can be provided with care and sensitivity, while giving the patient realistic expectations for the course of their disease.

Lifestyle Changes and Treatment Adherence: PCPs can utilize MI techniques and SMART goal setting (see Fig. 9.2) to encourage patients to reduce or manage stress and change dietary habits (e.g., reduce acidic foods with GERD, eat slowly and consistently, adhere to a low-FODMAP diet for IBS). MI and problem-solving strategies can be utilized to help patients adhere to medication regimens or engage in preventative cancer screenings or referrals to specialists. Patients can also be encouraged to track their symptoms and track how implementing changes influences these symptoms using trackers or phone applications specifically tailored to GI symptoms. Tracking apps, such as Bowelle (Bowelle, 2024) and Cara Care (HiDoc Technologies GmbH, 2020), are tailored for tracking GI-related symptoms (Tresca, 2023).

Stress Management and Reduction: Patients with IBS may experience elevated attentional bias toward sensations in their gut, higher levels of stress hormones and hypervigilance (van Tilburg et al., 2013). Strategies such as mindfulness, yoga, and relaxation training can help patients distract from these sensations and reduce symptoms (see Table 9.3; Chey et al., 2021; Keefer et al., 2018). Applying relaxation and mindfulness strategies prior to or during the onset of gut pain or other symptoms can provide prompt reductions in GI symptoms (Chey et al., 2021). Patients can be directed to utilize YouTube videos or phone applications such as Mindfulness Coach to practice these skills on their own (Veteran Affairs National Center for PTSD, 2024). More exercises can be found in Table 9.5 later in this chapter.

Table 9.3 Mindfulness exercises

Skill	Brief description
Guided imagery	The patient will find a comfortable position imagining themselves in a calm environment. Patients should close their eyes and try to engage as many senses as possible to make it feel as if they were there. For imagining being at the beach, the patient can try to feel the sand, see the waves, smell the breeze, and hear seagulls
Meditation	Patients will try to enter a state of awareness that allows them to experience their thoughts and emotions in the present. Patients find a comfortable position to sit or lay and focus on their breathing. As they focus on the feeling of them inhaling and exhaling, the patients allow any thoughts to exist without giving them too much attention. Remind the patient, they are not trying to quiet their mind, but to focus in on the present moment and their breathing
Body scanning	As an addition to meditation, body scanning has the patient bring awareness to different parts of their body. Once in a meditative state (as above), the patient will systematically scan their body from toes to their head. Patients will focus on textures, temperature, and any aches. It is important they only become aware of the sensations and do not try to change these feelings

CBT and Hypnotherapy: Cognitive behavior therapy (CBT) has been found to be effective in both children and adults in reducing negative emotionality in IBS, Crohn's disease, gastroesophageal reflux disease (GERD), and functional GI disorders (Ballou & Keefer, 2017; Ford et al., 2014; Szigethy et al., 2007; Thompson et al., 2012). CBT for IBS has been shown to be effective when self-administered by patients in as little as four sessions (Lackner et al., 2008). Research on hypnotherapy also supports its use in children and adults, particularly with reducing hypervigilance, hypersensitivity, and somatic symptoms (Ford et al., 2014; Keefer et al., 2018; Szigethy, 2015). During visits, PCPs can offer brief training on simple cognitive strategies and encourage patients to use self-help guides to manage their emotional symptoms or unhelpful thoughts around their GI symptoms. PCPs can encourage patients to use positive self-talk and affirmations when feeling overwhelmed. Also, providers can review thought-challenging worksheets with the patient to teach and practice the technique. A common strategy is to ask the patient to review evidence for and against distressing thoughts. Once the evidence is reviewed, the provider can help to develop a thought that is more likely to happen (e.g., "these situations are always bad for me" to "these situations feel bad at times, but this one can be different"). This can support self-management, acceptance of, and reduction of symptoms for the patient (Keefer et al., 2018; Naliboff & Mayer, 2006; Tran & Mulligan, 2019). Phone applications designed for self-administration of CBT or hypnotherapy for IBS or GI symptoms have also been developed (though some are paid or require a prescription; Aubrey, 2022). Examples include Nerva (Mindset Health Pty Ltd, 2024) and Mahana (Mahana Therapeutics, Inc, 2024).

Psychotherapy Referral: Providers may refer patients to brief counseling when the patient presents with elevated stress or emotional symptoms that appear to impact their ability to cope with gastrointestinal symptoms, or when symptoms do not alleviate within 3 to 6 months (Palsson & Whitehead, 2013).

Chronic Pain

Many Americans suffer from chronic pain that limits daily activities, the majority of which is managed in the primary care setting (Fink-Miller et al., 2014). Chronic pain is complex, biopsychosocial in nature, and often co-occurs with BH concerns, including depression, anxiety, and substance use disorders (Rikard, 2023). These factors make chronic pain difficult for many PCPs to manage, a picture further complicated by lack of access to non-opioid treatments and training in pain care.

Assess Assessing chronic pain is challenging due to its complex nature and the restrictions in time and resources that often exist in the primary care setting. In addition to assessing the severity, impact, and type of pain the patient is experiencing, the PCP's goal is to utilize contextual interviewing skills to best understand the unique factors influencing their patients' ability to manage their chronic pain. In the domain of "work," providers may uncover that their patient is employed in a position that requires manual labor, which exacerbates their pain, or conversely, that their patient's pain has led to an inability to maintain work. Discussing their patients' hobbies can aid in better understanding the impact of pain on their quality of life and allow the PCP to empathize with difficult emotions, such as hopelessness. For example, patients may express that engagement in hobbies that once brought them joy now seems unattainable due to their pain.

Advise The biopsychosocial framework for pain defines the interactions between biological, psychological, and social aspects of pain as bidirectional, with substantial evidence supporting the influence of biopsychosocial factors (see Table 9.4) in the development and maintenance of chronic pain (Bevers et al., 2016). Ensuring patients have a strong understanding of the biopsychosocial framework of pain is foundational for future interventions, including incorporation of non-pharmacological methods of pain management.

Discussion of non-pharmacological pain management options should be included at the onset of treatment. These suggestions, such as exercise or psychotherapy,

Table 9.4 Biopsychosocial model facts for patients (Meg Foundation for Pain, 2024)

Biological	• When there is physical damage to our body, we receive pain signals to let us know • The state of our bodies (e.g., how tired, sick, hungry we are) influences our perception of pain signals • Treating pain requires us to take care of our bodies holistically
Psychological	• Thoughts, feelings, and mood can all influence our bodies' experience of pain • Our pain also influences our thoughts, feelings, and mood • This bidirectional connection allows us to use our thoughts and feelings to help us gain better control over our pain experience
Social	• Just like when children look to their parents after a fall or accident to gauge how they should react, how others respond to us changes our experience of pain

may bring up common misconceptions for patients living with chronic pain (e.g., "Does this mean my pain is all in my head?"; Becker et al., 2017). Because of this, pain-validation and education about chronic pain (e.g., activity pacing) will be an essential aspect of the early stages of managing chronic pain. Pain-validation is defined as the belief of the provider that the patient's pain is true, acceptance of the patient's expression of their pain, and communication from the provider of belief and acceptability to the patient (Nicola et al., 2022). Adherence to behavioral pain management strategies is difficult, and pain-validation in early stages of treatment can enhance patient motivation and compliance (Nicola et al., 2022). The *Pain Coach* phone application is one resource that can assist PCPs with education on chronic pain (U.S. Department of Veterans Affairs, 2024a).

Agree PCPs should continue to highlight the biopsychosocial factors and how emotions and cognitions play a role in maintaining patients' pain experiences, making sure to set realistic goals with their patients. Patients often have high expectations regarding pain reduction and report feeling unsatisfied with treatment (Geurts et al., 2017). For example, they may expect to be fully pain free, to not have pain flare ups, or to be able to resume former activity levels right away for the treatment to be "working." Exploring patient expectations and setting manageable goals that patients can incrementally work toward will help maintain engagement and aid patients in gaining better understanding of their chronic pain. Notably, patient satisfaction is associated with physician empathy and clear communication regarding treatment expectations (Licciardone et al., 2023).

Assist *Breathing and relaxation exercises.* Breathing and relaxation exercises (See Table 9.5) help patients manage pain by reducing their stress level and regulating their nervous system (Schaffer & Yucha, 2004). There are a wide variety of exercises for patients to try with videos and guided options available online. Having handouts of common exercises for patients to try is helpful; practicing together during the visit is ideal. Several common exercises include color breathing, box breathing, and progressive muscle relaxation.

Connection: Studies have demonstrated that social support is associated with reduced emotional distress and better treatment outcomes for those with chronic pain (Franqueiro et al., 2023). Supportive individuals may still provide physical comfort (e.g., hugs, holding hands, back rubs) and pain-validation, but their most important role is encouraging the patient to engage in helpful activities and distractions.

Sleep and Diet: Sleep and diet play a critical role in the management of chronic pain (Nijs et al., 2020). Maintaining a regular sleep schedule with adequate quantity and quality of sleep helps regulate patients' bodies and improve their experience of pain (Finan et al., 2013; Nijs et al., 2020). Similarly, regular consumption of a balanced meal helps patients feel less stressed and improves their pain experience.

Movement: Movement is both vital to the management of chronic pain, and exceptionally difficult for many patients. Existing studies show that physical activity both reduces pain severity and improves physical functioning when incorporated appropriately (Geneen et al., 2017). It is natural for patients to believe that their pain is

Table 9.5 Breathing and relaxation exercises

Skill	Brief description[a]
Color breathing	The patient will identify a color to represent stress/tension/pain and a color representing relaxation. Each inhale, the patient will visualize the relaxation color filling their body. Each exhale, they will imagine the stress color leaving their body
Box breathing	Patients will inhale for 4 s, hold the inhale for 4 s, exhale for 4 s, and then pause for 4 s before the next breath. Cue patients to keep their neck and shoulders relaxed and focus on *slow relaxed* breathing rather than deep breathing
Progressive muscle relaxation (PMR)	Patients will systematically tense and relax muscle groups (e.g., left foot, left calf, left thigh, etc.) moving from their feet to their head. Pair tensing the muscle group with the patients inhale and relaxing with their exhale. Providers can skip injured muscle groups or areas of the body associated with trauma. Guided PMR videos are widely available online and can also aid patients with sleep

[a] To practice trauma-informed care providers should provide a description of the skill and ask the patient's consent to practice together

a signal that they either should not, or cannot, engage in movement. However, this makes pain worse (Vlaeyen & Linton, 2000). Patients may also struggle with moderation and enter a cycle of extreme movement on days with less pain, followed by exhaustion and being sedentary to recover. This cycle is often referred to as boom and bust. The concept of *pacing* encourages patients to identify manageable movement that does not put them into a boom-and-bust cycle. Referral to physical therapy can also aid patients in identifying what is considered manageable for their bodies.

Example Script for Discussing Pacing:
PCP: I am hearing you describe what we call boom-and-bust, on good days you really push your body to do a lot because you aren't sure when you will feel good again. It also sounds like the consequences of pushing your body so much is that you spend several days in bed in a lot of pain and feel afraid to try new forms of movement like physical therapy. Does that sound right?
Patient: Yes! I am so mad at my body. I can't do what people want me to do, no one understands what it is like.
PCP: I think a tool called pacing will be helpful for you. It will take some time for us to figure out a good balance of rest and movement, but this will help you stay out of the boom-and-bust cycle. The goal of pacing is to stay closer to the middle, on days when you have more pain you still push yourself to have some movement and on days when you feel really good, you intentionally hold back a bit to leave some energy "in the tank." over time, this will help you feel more in touch with your body's needs and help you do more of what you enjoy. Let's make an activity plan based on what you can remember about your activity

for the last few weeks. You can use the self-monitoring forms we discussed previously to track your progress between now and our next appointment.

Psychotherapy: Multiple modalities of psychotherapy have demonstrated efficacy in treating chronic pain, including cognitive behavioral therapy, acceptance and commitment therapy, operant-behavioral therapy, and mindfulness-based stress reduction (Sturgeon, 2014). Psychotherapy aims to shift patients' perspective and experience of their pain, reduce stress, increase adaptive coping, and improve functioning. Referral to a BH provider specializing in treatment of chronic pain may be beneficial for patients who are having difficulty adhering to treatment or need more focused time than can be provided in the primary care setting.

Sexual Functioning

Sexual health is an important aspect of quality of life for many people, even among older adults and people with poor health (Flynn et al., 2016). Sexual problems can affect people of all genders at multiple stages in their lives and can cause a deficit in sexual response or problems in experiencing sexual pleasure. Sexual disorders are more common among people with chronic diseases or history of cancer and the risk may increase as patients age and encounter normal aging transitions such as menopause (Ramlachan & Naidoo, 2024). The US Preventive Services Task Force (USPSTF) has put forth recommendations for screening for sexually transmitted diseases, but not sexual dysfunctions (Meyers et al., 2008). However, the Academy of American Family Physicians (AAFP) recommends that PCPs be *proactive* in identification and management of sexual dysfunctions that may arise with chronic illness. Thus, PCPs may want to incorporate routine sexual functioning assessment for individuals with chronic diseases (Nusbaum et al., 2003).

Assess PCPs want to become comfortable in assessing sexual history, including problems in patients of all ages. When conducting a sexual history, following the five Ps (partners, practices, protection from sexually transmitted diseases, history of sexually transmitted diseases, and pregnancy plans) can serve as a guide (Savoy et al., 2020). While physical factors may contribute to the initial etiology of the problem, psychological factors may maintain the problem, and intervention here can be valuable for the patient.

The Ex-PLISSIT model can be used for assessing and intervening with patients regarding their sexual health (Faubion & Rullo, 2015; Taylor & Davis, 2006). In the Ex-PLISSIT model, permission giving is incorporated throughout the assessment and treatment of sexual health, as well as the initial intervention. The Ex-PLISSIT model provides interventions of escalating intensity. First, give the patient *permission* to speak about sexual health and what they wants to do or are doing sexually, and validate the patient for sharing information. This can be done through questions or signage in the office inviting patients to talk about their sexual health. Next, provide *limited information* on basic and accurate sex education, or expected medication side effects. For example, informing patients that some medications may modify sexual desire. Depending on the patient presenting problem, the PCP gives *specific suggestions* to increase sexual function. Finally, validate symptoms and provide resources for *intensive therapy* as appropriate. Intensive therapy can include changes in medications, lifestyle changes, or other interventions discussed in this section.

The AAFP recommends that PCPs are trained in the use of sensitive terminology with patients, utilization of cultural humility, and that they undertake an assessment of their own personal internal biases to facilitate improved patient interactions (Savoy et al., 2020). Some patients may be sensitive to discussions on sexual dysfunction due to social, cultural, and religious factors. These direct recommendations should be considered within the context of the patient. It is important when assessing sexual health, that PCPs do not assume their patient's gender identity or sexual orientation. The following table provides some helpful language for assessing gender identity and sexual partners (see Table 9.6).

Commonly cited barriers to inquiring about sexual health in PC include time, awareness of sexual dysfunction, knowledge of treatment options, cultural barriers, and comfort addressing the topic (Barnhoorn et al., 2022). Data suggests that most patients prefer an active inquiry about their sexual health, especially when done with sensitivity and in the context of a good patient-provider relationship (Ryan et al., 2018).

Across all sexual dysfunctions, PCPs want to inquire about arousal, orgasms, and libido. PCPs may also want to assess menopausal and perimenopausal aged women for changes associated with menopause, including hot flashes, sleep problems, and hormonal changes. The Arizona Sexual Experience Scale (ASEX; McGahuey et al., 2000) is a brief, 5-item self-report questionnaire that has shown to be reliable for quantifying sexual dysfunction across clinical settings and populations (Elnazer & Baldwin, 2020). Tools such as the ASEX, along with disorder screeners as outlined in the table below (see Table 9.7), may help PCPs assess for sexual dysfunctions, time permitting.

Advise Across sexual dysfunctions, discussing the importance of cognitions and emotions involved in the sexual response can help patients engage in behavioral recommendations (Fischer et al., 2022; Hunter et al., 2024). Additionally, involving

Table 9.6 Inclusive language recommendations (Centers for Disease Control and Prevention (CDC), 2024a)

Sex vs. gender identity	"What was your sex assigned at birth?" "What is your current gender identity (and correct pronouns)?"
Sexual history	Are you currently having any kind of sex (vaginal, oral, anal)? What are the genders of your sex partners?

Table 9.7 Screening questionnaires for sexual dysfunctions

Sexual dysfunctions	Screening questionnaires
Male sexual dysfunctions (erectile disorder and premature ejaculation)	Erectile performance anxiety index (Telch & Pujols, 2013) Premature ejaculation severity index (Metz & McCarthy, 2003)
Female sexual dysfunctions (hypoactive sexual arousal, female orgasmic disorder, vaginismus, dyspareunia, vaginal dryness)	Female sexual functioning index (Meston, 2003)

patient's partners in treatment is recommended (Crowe, 2012; Hunter et al., 2024; Li et al., 2016).

It can be helpful to share with patients that even if their sexual dysfunction has a physical etiology, behavioral interventions can be effective for managing their symptoms (Hunter et al., 2024). Providing psychoeducation on normal aging transitions and normative sexual responses may help patients feel more comfortable talking about their sexual health. Discussing healthy lifestyle changes, adjusting medications, and reducing anxiety around sex can be important places to start to improve a patient's sexual well-being.

Agree With a variety of treatments available for sexual dysfunctions, especially for men, patients may be more hesitant to engage in BH interventions (Hunter et al., 2024). PCPs may highlight the biopsychosocial factors and how emotions and cognitions play a role in maintaining patients' experiences, while making sure to set realistic goals with their patients. For example, patients may expect to be fully erect during every sexual encounter, or that their partners are solely responsible for bringing them to orgasm, and helping to adjust these beliefs to find realistic and helpful goals will set patients up for success.

Assist Lifestyle changes (e.g., quitting smoking, losing weight, reducing alcohol consumption) have been shown to be effective for improving sexual wellness, especially for erectile dysfunction, and patients may want to focus on these changes as a first line for improving sexual health (Maiorino et al., 2015). Specific behavioral interventions include sensate focus, start-stop-squeeze, sexual communication, and masturbation training. While these interventions are evidence based for sexual dysfunction, some may be off putting for some patients (e.g., directed masturbation) or go against their cultural belief systems. PCPs should be sensitive of patient contexts when making recommendations.

Cognitive Restructuring and Anxiety Management: Worries about sex, performance anxiety, and unhelpful thoughts or expectations around sex can maintain sexual problems (Tavares et al., 2020). PCPs may elicit unhelpful thoughts or beliefs around sex from patients during the assessment phase of the visit. Encouraging patients to focus on behaviors and sensations rather than their unhelpful thoughts, as well as helping patients to challenge these thoughts can help to decrease anxiety surrounding sex and improve sexual functioning (see Chap. 8 for information on cognitive restructuring; Hunter et al., 2024).

Sensate Focus: Sensate focus is designed to help improve intimacy and decrease anxiety around sexual performance (Masters & Johnson, 1970). It has been used in a variety of contexts and sexual dysfunctions (Avery-Clark et al., 2019). Patients and their partners are encouraged to dedicate at least 1 h in a comfortable space where they engage in non-sexual touching (e.g., massaging, fondling, caressing) and focus on the sensations of being touched. Partners are encouraged to provide direct feedback about what feels good and what does not during the exercise.

Stop-Start and Squeeze: The stop-start and squeeze technique is intended to help patients with premature ejaculation recognize sensations of impending ejaculation and do something different to increase their control (Polonsky, 2000). Patients are instructed to first masturbate without lubrication until they feel close to ejaculating, then stop and allow the sensation to subside. Squeezing the penis where the shaft meets the head or at the base can help delay ejaculation. After sensations dissipate, patients can resume masturbation, repeating the cycle several times before allowing themselves to ejaculate. Patients can practice this several times per week, and then, once they have gained more control, progress to varying the types of stimulation rather than stopping, then adding lubrication, then intercourse with a partner.

Sexual Communication: Communication between partners surrounding expectations about sex and the meaning assigned to sexual dysfunction may need to be addressed (e.g., "If he really loved me, he would be able to maintain an erection"). Patients will also benefit from communicating with their partners about sexual preferences, such as what they like and don't like, or what feels good and what does not. This type of communication may feel new and unfamiliar to patients; PCPs can help them utilize assertive communication skills and encourage patients to both elicit and give feedback.

Masturbation Training: Guided masturbation training can help patients learn about their own sexual preferences and discover which sensations may lead to orgasm (Marchand, 2021; McMullen & Rosen, 1979). Patients can be encouraged to incorporate sexual fantasies, vibrators, relaxation strategies, and experiment with different rhythms, speeds, or pressures.

Cancer

In the United States there are over 1,700,000 new cases of cancer annually (U.S. Department of Health and Human Services, Centers for Disease Control and Prevention, and National Cancer Institute, 2024). Each year, PCPs are estimated to diagnose between 4 and 12 patients with cancer (Hamilton, 2010; Kiernan & Frame, 1996; Wilkinson, 2021). Over half of all patients with cancer will develop distress as a result of their cancer diagnosis (Mehnert et al., 2018). This results in a significant need for supportive communication within medical encounters and attention to psychosocial concerns when treating this population (Institute of Medicine (US) Committee on Psychosocial Services to Cancer Patients/Families in a Community Setting [IOM], 2008).

Assess It is recommended that PCPs assess the level of distress among patients that they identify as having cancer or regularly treat throughout their cancer journey (National Comprehensive Cancer Network, 1999). Cancer-related pain, depression, and fatigue are often underdiagnosed and undertreated, but are critical points of intervention for PCPs managing patients with cancer in their practice (Smith & Toonen, 2007).

Tools that assess distress such as The National Comprehensive Cancer Network Distress Thermometer and Problem List can be utilized as a free and brief assessment method to assist PCPs in their visit (Riba et al., 2019). Contextual interviewing (See Chap. 2) will help PCPs understand the broad impact that cancer may have on their patients' lives.

Advise When delivering the news of a possible cancer diagnosis it can be helpful to consider the SPIKES protocol (See Table 9.8) for delivering bad news (Baile et al., 2000; Smith & Toonen, 2007). This will allow the PCP to assess what information will be most beneficial to the patient. Following the initial disclosure, it is important to continually assess the level of distress the patient is experiencing and consider treatment recommendations not only for their physical health concerns, but also their psychosocial needs (IOM, 2008). The IOM (2008) outlined the most common psychosocial needs and strategies to address these needs within medical encounters. These needs include (1) information about the diagnosis, treatment, and services; (2) assistance with coping with emotions elicited following the diagnosis and/or treatment; (3) assistance managing the illness including changing behaviors to decrease negative side effects from the disease; (4) logistical barriers and disruptions to work, family and school obligations; and (5) financial concerns (IOM, 2008).

Agree It is important to be mindful in collaborative decision-making and treatment planning that a cancer diagnosis can result in significant personal growth and not just grief or loss for individuals and their social networks (PDQ® Supportive and Palliative Care Editorial Board, 2004). PCPs will need to rely on shared decision-making and patient autonomy to prioritize which symptoms are most distressing, or what the patient would like for their treatment goals to be.

Assist Patients with cancer will likely have teams of providers helping to manage their care. The role of the PCP may be to coordinate care and manage symptoms of the cancer and treatment such as nausea, fatigue, and psychosocial changes (see Table 9.9).

Table 9.8 SPIKES protocol for delivering bad news (Adapted from Baile et al., 2000)

S = setting up the interview	Arrange for some privacy; sit down; manage time constraints and interruptions; involve significant others; make a connection with the patient
P = perception	Before you tell, ask what the patient knows
I = invitation	Explore the patient's wishes for receiving information
K = knowledge and information given to the patient	Warn the patient that bad news is coming
E = addressing the patient's emotions with empathetic responses	Continue empathetic statements and gestures until the patient is calm
S = strategy and summary	Discuss treatment options if the patient is ready; a clear plan for the future will reduce anxiety; confirm the patient's understanding of the discussion

Table 9.9 Behavioral interventions for cancer-related concerns

Cancer-related concern	Intervention
Fatigue	Exercise prescription, support groups, and stress management
Pain	Psychoeducation, pharmacotherapy, mindfulness (see above for interventions for pain)
Depressive symptoms	Antidepressants, behavioral interventions for depression (see Chap. 8)

Sleep

Over one-third of adults and children, and over 75% of adolescents do not get sufficient sleep (Centers for Disease Control and Prevention (CDC), 2023, 2024; Child and Adolescent Health Measurement Initiative, 2023). Sleep disorders also affect quality of sleep (Graci, 2021). An estimated 50–70 million Americans have a sleep disorder (i.e., insomnia, obstructive sleep apnea, restless legs syndrome/periodic limb movement, parasomnias, and narcolepsy; (Colten et al., 2006; Graci, 2021). Sleep disorders increase risk for the development of additional medical and psychiatric diagnoses and are associated with increased healthcare costs (Yamamoto et al., 2023). Despite their prevalence, sleep disorders often go undetected in primary care settings (Senthilvel et al., 2011).

Differential BH diagnoses for disordered sleeping include depression, anxiety, bipolar disorder, trauma stress, and substance use (Yamamoto et al., 2023). Medical concerns including restless leg syndrome, chronic pain, or obstructive sleep apnea can also present as insomnia. Understanding the source impeding progress will direct the provider in recommending an appropriate behavioral/cognitive modification, prescription medication, or referral.

Assess PCPs can initiate sleep discussions by simply and directly asking the patient if they are having any trouble with sleep (Yamamoto et al., 2023), as well as using contextual interviewing to explore how disrupted sleep is impacting functioning. Follow-up questions should explore the details of the sleep problem, a typical sleep schedule, sleep health, and duration of the problem (Yamamoto et al., 2023). Brief screening tools, such as those outlined below (See Table 9.10), may be useful in diagnosing chronic sleep problems or tracking improvements in sleep over time.

Advise PCPs can share with patients that sleep disorders are common, can impact quality of life, and there are effective treatments for improving sleep. For instance, research has demonstrated that behavior therapy is as effective as pharmacotherapy in treating insomnia (Rossman, 2019; Weir, 2022). The American College of Physicians recommends Cognitive Behavioral Therapy for Insomnia (CBT-I) as a first-line treatment for insomnia (Qaseem et al., 2016). Providers conduct CBT-I over 4–8 sessions, aiding patients in addressing sleep interfering behaviors and cognitions. Additional behavioral treatments may include brief behavioral therapy for insomnia (BBTi; Troxel et al., 2012), Imagery Rehearsal Therapy (IRT) for nightmares, and behavior therapy for hypersomnia (Weir, 2022). While CBT-I is generally administered by BH providers, BBTi is designed to be briefer, and delivered in the primary care setting without extensive training. PCPs should also provide tailored education on sleep health (i.e., consistent sleep and wake times, reducing blue-light screen time, reducing nicotine and caffeine use at night). PCPs may consider developing a sleep health educational handout for patients to take home with them or utilizing the free BBTi step-by-step guide that is available at http://sleepprimarycareresources.org.au/ (Sweetman et al., 2021).

The CBT-I Coach phone application is an additional resource that providers may encourage patients to use to increase understanding of their sleep patterns and effectively intervene (U.S. Department of Veterans Affairs, 2024b). This app enables patients to engage with psychoeducational material at their own pace, maintain a

Table 9.10 Screening tools for sleep functioning

Screening tools	What they assess
Patient health Questionnaire-9 (PHQ-9)	General depression screener. Item 3 assesses how frequently the patient is struggling with falling asleep, staying asleep, or sleeping too much (Kroenke et al., 1999)
Insomnia severity index	A seven-item self-report that explores insomnia symptoms (Morin, 1993)
STOP-bang questionnaire	Assess for obstructive sleep apnea using eight yes or no questions (Chung et al., 2016)
Epworth sleepiness scale (ESS)	Uses eight items to assess general daytime sleepiness to inform providers on common symptoms of obstructive sleep apnea, narcolepsy, limb movement disorder, and insomnia (Johns, 1991)

sleep diary, calculate their sleep efficiency, and receive a personalized wake/sleep time. However, sleep health or hygiene recommendations alone will not resolve sleep concerns among those with a diagnosis of insomnia. Thus, BBTi or CBT-I interventions will be required in most cases.

Agree A collaborative and empathetic clinical interviewing style is particularly useful when broaching use of behavioral therapy to improve disordered sleeping, decreasing resistance to treatment, and setting goals to decrease dysfunction. Introducing behavioral intervention for sleep at the first visit (including discussion of self-monitoring with a sleep diary) before or in conjunction with prescribing medications is crucial to the acceptance of behavioral interventions as first line options for the treatment of insomnia. Examples of motivational interviewing prompts for engaging patients in behavioral interventions for sleep:

1. Can you help me better understand the difficulty that you are experiencing with sleep?
2. How has your disordered sleep affected you?
3. What are some methods that you have used to improve your sleep?
4. It sounds like your previous strategies for managing your sleep have been less helpful lately. Would you be open to learning some new skills to improve your sleep?

Assist While PCPs will not likely conduct CBT-I with their patients, they can employ strategies of CBT-I and BBTi to help their patients achieve better quality sleep. This includes psychoeducation on sleep health, stimulus control, relaxation therapy, and sleep restriction (Rossman, 2019; Troxel et al., 2012; Walker et al., 2022).

PCPs should have patients identify their sleep patterns through the creation and maintenance of a sleep diary. Through the utilization of the patient's self-report and the maintenance of a sleep diary the provider will be able to evaluate sleep concerns and measure intervention progress. When sleep improvements are stagnant and progress is not being made, the provider should interview the patient to determine the cause. Barriers to progress may include lack of treatment adherence, difficulty tracking sleep, excessive resting in bed, napping, not engaging in an activity when experiencing difficulty sleeping, distractions in the sleeping space, and an alternating work schedule (Walker et al., 2022). An example of a sleep diary is below, if patients do not want to or are unable to use the CBT-I app or prefer to keep a paper copy. Patients should be reminded to complete the diary in the morning to the best of their ability, and not to worry about being accurate to the exact minute, so as not to create more anxiety around sleep.

Today's date	1/1/2020	1/2/2020	1/3/2020
Did you nap or doze yesterday?	Yes; 20 min	No	Yes; 45 min
What time did you get into bed yesterday?	9 pm	11:30 pm	10 pm

(continued)

(continued)

Today's date	1/1/2020	1/2/2020	1/3/2020
What time did you try to go to sleep?	10 pm	11:30 pm	10:30 pm
How long did it take you to fall asleep?	1 hour	20 min	45 min
How many times did you wake up, not counting your final awakening?	2×	1×	1×
How long did these last?	15 min	5 min	30 min
What time was your final awakening?	5:30	6:15 am	8 am
Did you wake up earlier than you wanted to?	Yes	No	No
What time did you get out of bed today?	6 am	6:15 am	8:30 am
How would you rate the quality of sleep?	Fair	Poor	Fair

Psychoeducation on sleep health contributes to a foundational understanding of the bidirectional impact of behaviors on sleep and functioning. This foundational knowledge is imperative to provide a rationale for adhering to the treatment plan and understanding the factors that facilitate healthy sleep (Edinger & Carney, 2014; Walker et al., 2022).

Stimulus control helps re-establish the bed as a cue for sleep by limiting bed-related activities to sleep and sex. It involves going to bed only when sleepy, exiting bed if unable to sleep after brief period (10–15 min) with attempts at reinitiation of sleep once drowsy, maintaining a consistent wake-up time, and avoiding naps (Edinger & Carney, 2014; Rossman, 2019; Troxel et al., 2012). This reconditioning reduces anxiety and wakefulness associated with the bed, leading to better sleep quality.

Sleep restriction is a technique that involves restricting time in bed without successful sleep onset (Edinger & Carney, 2014; Rossman, 2019; Troxel et al., 2012). This intervention involves tracking the patient's sleep (using a sleep diary) and utilizing the tracking information to develop a bedtime and wake time that compresses the time in bed to the time the patient has reported being asleep. For example, if the patient reports that they are only sleeping for six hours, restrict the time in bed to six hours total (it is not recommended to restrict time to less than five and ½ hours hours). Once the patients sleep efficiency is increased (e.g., the time they spend in bed is time spent *asleep*, the time in bed can be increased by 15 min. The CBT-I app will calculate restriction times for patients based on their completed sleep diary in the app. This intervention is imperative to acquire and maintain a regular sleep schedule that allows the patient to increase their sleep efficiency.

Relaxation and anxiety management techniques help patients relax their mind, regulate emotions, and prepare for sleep. Scheduling a time to write down anxieties or worries earlier in the day, creating a calming pre-sleep routine, and learning specific relaxation strategies can calm the nervous system and promote sleep (Rossman, 2019). Additional behavioral intervention with a BH clinician may be needed to address negative thoughts or cognitions surrounding sleep initiation and maintenance.

Special Populations with Sleep Sleep impacts everyone; however, providers may notice a heightened prevalence of presenting concerns regarding sleep in infancy, children with neurodevelopmental disorders, and older adults. Providing sleep training and support for parents during infancy is crucial, as establishing healthy sleep patterns early on can have lasting benefits for both the child and the family (Meltzer & Mindell, 2007). Individuals with neurodevelopmental disorders often struggle with sleep, which can impact their overall functioning and quality of life as well as exacerbate challenges associated with their primary diagnoses (Cortese et al., 2020). Similarly, older adults frequently experience difficulties with sleep, including insomnia and fragmented sleep patterns (Tatineny et al., 2020). Those with dementia and Alzheimer's disease are particularly affected (Zhang et al., 2022).

Providers may also see heightened concerns for sleep disorders in special populations, including people experiencing homelessness, refugees, individuals who are incarcerated, and individuals working nights/shift work (Al-Khalil et al., 2024; Jehan et al., 2017). Understanding the context of the patient's environment can help inform which sleep interventions are effective, or if sleep should be the first concern targeted.

Weight Management

In the United States, an estimated 41.9% of adults have obesity, which can be associated with a variety of other chronic health conditions and early mortality (Centers for Disease Control and Prevention (CDC), 2024b; Di Angelantonio et al., 2016). Obesity disproportionately affects certain populations (e.g., non-Hispanic Black and Hispanic adults) and can develop due to a variety of modifiable (e.g., poor access to healthcare, exposure to adverse childhood experiences, poverty, lack of access to safe places to exercise, chronic stress, poor sleep) and non-modifiable (e.g., genetics) risk factors (Hunter et al., 2024; Petersen et al., 2019). Gender differences in the development of obesity are also observed, such that more women than men are classified as having obesity (particularly in individuals age 50 and older; Cooper et al., 2021; Knight et al., 2021; Ogden et al., 2012; Petersen et al., 2019; Seamans et al., 2015). Studies suggest that those who belong to sexual minority populations, particularly women, report higher BMIs than their heterosexual counterparts (Bowen et al., 2008; Calzo et al., 2017; Gordon et al., 2023). This may be in part due to weight-based discrimination on top of other psychosocial stressors unique to that population, contributing to poorer health outcomes (Gerend et al., 2023). Despite the growing prevalence of obesity, many patients do not receive adequate diagnosis or referral to services to help manage this manageable chronic illness (Hunter et al., 2024; Wolfgang et al., 2022). While the development and management of obesity can be complex, proper assessment and treatment by the PCP can lead to meaningful change (Masood & Moorthy, 2023).

It is also important to note that not all individuals with obesity have disordered eating, just as not all individuals with eating disorders have a particular body size;

however, for individuals pursuing weight loss, between 9 and 29% endorse binge episodes (with 1–2% meeting criteria for binge eating disorder; McCuen-Wurst et al., 2018). It is also possible that the engagement in traditional self-directed restrictive dieting approaches (including those recommended by the popular media or healthcare providers) may predispose an individual to a binge episode and thereby undermine weight loss efforts, lead to weight gain, and impact self-esteem. When considering a referral to weight management services, PCPs should always screen for disordered eating patterns so that interventions prescribed to the patient do not reinforce pre-existing unhelpful behaviors, and so patients can be referred to specialty treatment if-needed (Cardel et al., 2022).

Working with Children and Adolescents

Rates of excess weight and obesity are on the rise for children as well with obesity being the most prevalent in Hispanic children (26.2%) and non-Hispanic Black children (24.8%; Centers for Disease Control and Prevention (CDC), 2024a). As it pertains to supporting children with excess weight, it is important to note that most of the interventions will be *parent focused* and must be delivered with sensitive, non-weight focused, compassionate language. It may be helpful to discuss a child's health metrics and potential weight concerns without the child present to avoid inadvertently influencing a child/adolescent's self-esteem or introducing weight bias. In fact, a significant number of individuals who later develop an eating disorder note that a precipitating factor was language and/or stigma used in the primary care clinic office (Braddock et al., 2023). Similarly, roughly 25% of parents who perceive their children as being victims of weight discrimination in the office are likely to avoid future visits altogether (Puhl et al., 2011). As such, it is of the utmost importance that PCPs consider their language and audience while navigating these sensitive topics with youth and adolescents.

Integrating Patient Cultural Values into Treatment

When discussing weight, health, eating habits, and recommendations, it is imperative that providers consider the patient's cultural background (Dao et al., 2020; Lindberg et al., 2012). For example, individuals in Hispanic cultures may tend to prefer carbohydrate-dense meals (e.g., rice, beans, tortillas) and food-focused family gatherings. As such, providers should consider taking time to understand how patient cultural background may influence their relationship with food, weight, and dietary changes.

Provider Weight Bias and Language

Weight bias is not only a concern with the broader population, but with providers themselves. For many well-meaning healthcare professionals, bias toward individuals in larger bodies can exist outside of their immediate awareness and have a direct impact on the care they deliver to their patients. Studies have shown that judgmental, critical, and shaming language may indeed be a contributing factor to the growing rates of obesity, as the emotional toll of the above can lead to increased cortisol levels, thereby impacting a person's hunger and fullness hormones as well as metabolic functioning. See Table 9.11 for current person-first language recommendations and other discussion-based considerations (Albury et al., 2020; Obesity Action Coalition, 2024).

Assess Body mass index (BMI) is the most common screening tool to identify individuals who have excess weight or obesity. In addition to BMI, assessment may include a brief biopsychosocial history along with some brief screening measures that can be administered in minutes (if not already completed). The following screeners are free, publicly available, and quick to administer (See Table 9.12). The following measures are not meant to be diagnostic in nature; rather, they are for treatment planning and general clinical decision-making. For a comprehensive list of assessment tools for obesity from psychological, dietary, activity level, and body composition perspectives, please see Beechy et al. (2012).

Advise After a patient has screened positive for either having excess weight or obesity via BMI, the PCP should consider how to approach the topic of weight and/

Table 9.11 Language recommendations for conversations about weight (Albury et al., 2020; Obesity Action Coalition, 2024)

Language to avoid	Current language recommendations
"Fat"	"Adiposity" "excess adiposity"
"An obese person"	"A person with obesity; a person with excess adiposity"
"Weight loss surgery"	"Bariatric surgery"
"Non-compliant"	"Non-adherent"
"Exercise" (this is patient dependent)	"Movement" "enjoyable physical activity"
Focus on percentage of weight loss and specific pounds lost	Focus on values and meaningful behavioral topics; focus on small patient successes irrelevant to weight loss
Avoiding blame and causality when discussing development of obesity and/or complications	Speaking broadly about obesity-related patterns and exploring how patient may or may not relate
Avoiding assumptions about a patient's weight gain/loss trajectory	Individual curiosity surrounding a patient's history, ability to engage in ADLs, interests, hopes, and goals

Table 9.12 Screening and tracking tools for weight and eating-related concerns

Screener	What they assess
24 h food/beverage recall	Specific food and beverage choices, quantity of food, timing of food and beverage intake, estimate of caloric intake and disordered consumption patterns (PCP can suggest patient's take pictures of their food before and after a meal as well for recall information)
Brief biopsychosocial assessment	Onset of weight concerns, co-occurring conditions, medications, weight trajectory, previous diets/lifestyle change attempts, how helpful (or not) previous attempts have been, use of weight loss medications, biggest barriers to lifestyle changes, helpers to lifestyle change, family culture around food, impact of weight on quality of life, current stressors, coping skills, value-based goals (e.g., hiking with children, grocery shopping without a scooter, traveling), current eating habits, current activity level
Modified YFAS (adults; Schulte & Gearhardt, 2017)	13-item screener assessing addictive-like behaviors toward eating
SCOFF (adults; Morgan et al., 1999; Perry et al., 2002)	5-item screener assessing for disordered eating symptoms
YFAS 2.0 For Children (Gearhardt et al., 2013)	25-item screener assessing addictive-like behaviors and distress toward eating
My Fitness Pal (Lee, 2024)	A free app that can help patients self-monitor weight, nutrition, and physical activity. Note: this resource should be considered only for those without active disordered eating patterns

or weight management with the patient. Some patients have no concerns with directly discussing weight and weight loss interventions, while other patients (particularly ones with a history of disordered eating, weight-based discrimination, or poor body image) may find conversations related to weight to be particularly challenging and potentially reinforcing of unhelpful patterns or beliefs. By this step, the PCP's brief assessment of the patient's history should help determine the language used to advise the patient on their personal health status and recommendations. If it is not clear how to navigate this conversation, PCPs can also simply ask the patient how they would prefer to have these discussions (e.g., "I would like to take a few minutes to talk about your overall health. Some patients do not mind directly discussing weight or BMI as it relates to their well-being, while others prefer to focus on specific health markers with less emphasis on specific weight-related numbers. How would you like to have this discussion?") In either case, the PCP should aim to strike a balance between respecting a patient's autonomy to discuss what they would find the most helpful during the visit with the PCP's weight-related medical concerns for the patient. For those who may not benefit from direct discussion regarding specific body weight numbers, weight loss, or BMI expectations, the PCP may want to focus on providing clear and compassionate feedback regarding a patient's health status (e.g., elevated A1C, hypertension, nonalcoholic fatty liver disease) and associated helpful interventions (e.g., increased physical activity, opting for sugar free foods, reducing dietary fat intake), all of which may ultimately influence weight as well.

Along with individual health status, it would be helpful to provide education regarding the complexity and individualized nature of weight loss and weight gain to reduce any potential shame the patient may experiencing due to body weight or shape. Additionally, advising that it does not take extraordinary amounts of weight loss (i.e., 5–10%) to lead to significant improvements in health outcomes such as blood pressure, energy, sleep, and pain can make behavior change seem less intimidating (Hunter et al., 2024). If applicable, provide the patient with information regarding the difficulty in sustaining health behavior change while coping with untreated BH concerns (e.g., major depressive disorder, posttraumatic stress disorder, bulimia, etc.). Patients with significant and untreated co-occurring BH concerns would likely benefit from an improvement in psychological symptoms before engaging in an active weight management program.

For interested patients (and for those who qualify), advice on appropriate weight loss medications could be beneficial, alongside other recommended health behavior changes.

Agree After gathering patient data from the brief biopsychosocial screener (and any others), along with providing the patient with individualized education regarding their current circumstances, it would be helpful to briefly summarize the patient's concerns and goals. Here, you want to see if the patient is still on board with making changes compatible with weight loss and/or lifestyle changes to improve their health status. Assuming the patient is willing to make a change, proceed with identifying appropriate interventions below.

Assist While there may be many different treatment targets (e.g., weight loss, lowered blood pressure, improving A1C, improving mobility), it is often the most helpful for patients to identify a single goal that they feel equipped to do and motivated to target. Patients who are already actively making and sustaining lifestyle changes may benefit from a scaffolding approach, where new goals are added on top of existing helpful behaviors. As noted in earlier chapters, use of motivational interviewing questions can help enhance a patient's motivation for change and identify what has already worked for them before (and can help resolve barriers before they occur). Overwhelming patients with multiple lifestyle changes to make at once, or by giving vague advice (e.g., "eat less and move more") may feel discouraging and overwhelming to the patient, which may interfere with goal attainment, thereby reducing the effectiveness of the intervention and reducing motivation. Also, avoid "weight loss" as a single goal; rather, work with the patient to identify behaviors consistent with weight loss and work to improve those areas.

Weight Loss Specific Interventions Below are some specific behavioral interventions that may be helpful to the patient. Again, use the patient's personal goals to identify which intervention may help them meet their needs. Remember to help the patient problem solve any foreseeable barriers to successful intervention and emphasize their strengths/previous successes in goal attainment.

Psychoeducation: Patients are inundated with information from many sources about what is or is not helpful with weight loss. Getting a general sense of what the patient understands about nutrition, weight gain, weight loss, and dieting can be helpful, particularly through that patient's cultural lens. Additionally, offering information regarding the relationship between weight loss, sleep, and BH is often quite helpful for patients, as patients often view psychological and physical functioning as separate.

Self-monitoring: Patients are often unaware of how much (or how little) they are eating. Encouraging patients to monitor their food intake via paper or mobile applications can be enlightening. Because food tracking can be tedious, some patients also benefit from keeping a photo diary of their meals. Encourage patients to keep a diary for 1–2 weeks and then plan to have a follow-up visit to discuss and make goals (e.g., prioritizing regular eating episodes, reduced sugar intake, increasing protein, drinking more water). It is important to note that if you have any concerns that a patient is experiencing disordered eating or has a history of significant restrictive patterns, calorie tracking may actually reinforce unhelpful behaviors (Simpson & Mazzeo, 2017). For the reasons stated above, assessment of disordered eating history can help guide this recommendation.

Many patients also benefit from practicing intuitive eating and monitoring eating patterns from a weight-neutral approach. Intuitive eating traditionally rejects traditional dieting behaviors (i.e., caloric restriction, unless dictated by specific health concerns) and encourages mindfulness, self-respect, awareness, and intention (Van Dyke & Drinkwater, 2014). Intuitive eating can help patients to reduce binge behaviors, increase awareness of the use of food as a coping skill and enhance the patient's ability to use alternate coping skills, improve the patient's awareness of hunger/fullness cues, and overall improve their relationship with food (Babbott et al., 2023; Grider et al., 2021; Warren et al., 2017). Notably, intuitive eating may not lead to weight loss (and is not intended to); however, this can be useful for patients who prefer a reduced emphasis on calories and weight and improved satisfaction and relationship with food. Use of a Hunger-Satiety scale can help patients monitor and ultimately rebuild their internal hunger/fullness cues. Additionally, utilizing a free mobile application such as Recovery Record can help patients track meals (without emphasis on calories), thoughts, coping skills, and any disordered eating behaviors (Recovery Record, 2024). Recovery Record also has a partner application that the PCP can download to monitor patient's logs (cost associated), although as with the above, encouraging the patient to log their Hunger-Satiety cues with meals along with any other relevant data from Recovery Record for at least 1–2 weeks with a planned follow-up visit would be helpful. For more information on the background and practice of intuitive eating, see Intuitive Eating (Tribole & Huber, 2021) and the Intuitive Eating Workbook: 10 Principles for Nourishing a Healthy Relationship with Food (Tribole & Resch, 2017).

Using Reminders: Many patients do not eat or drink water at regular intervals, so utilizing their cell phone, digital calendars, physical calendars, and visual reminders can be helpful to establish new patterns.

Encouraging Regular Meal Spacing and Fluid Intake: Eating regularly helps patients to keep from getting hungry, which can make it easier to make healthy choices (vs. making impulsive food choices while hungry). Additionally, regular meal spacing helps to encourage the patient's metabolism and ensures that they are eating enough throughout the day.

Stimulus Control:

- Encourage patients to eat only at the table and not in front of the television or while surfing the web to reduce mindless eating or eating past satiety.
- Encourage patients to place their fork down between bites to slow down eating, which helps to develop more internal awareness of hunger/fullness cues.
- Remove unhelpful foods from the home or move them to different cabinets that are not as easily or readily seen.
- Place healthy snacks in easily observable locations.
- Pack up leftovers after serving dinner.
- Leave the table after eating.

Mobilizing Social Support: Encouraging the patient to open up to trusted peers or family members can be extremely helpful, especially as it pertains to making social plans, asking for help with meal prep, finding an exercise buddy, or just having someone to talk to about the challenges of weight loss.

Schedule Pleasant Activities: If food is serving the purpose of providing emotional comfort, or the patient is generally struggling with low mood, scheduling pleasant non-food-related activities can be helpful. Examples could include going for a walk/exercise, calling a loved one, reading a book, playing with a puppy, etc.

Weight Loss Medications: Several medications have been approved by the FDA to reduce weight that can be used along with dietary and activity modifications (National Institute of Diabetes and Digestive and Kidney Diseases, 2024). These medications have different recommendations for BMI levels and should not be used in patients who are pregnant or those with certain eating disorders. Medications should be monitored closely and discontinued if weight loss is not seen. Not all insurance companies cover these medications and costs can be prohibitive for many patients.

Orlistat is a lipase inhibitor and works in the intestines to prevent the fat in foods from being absorbed in the intestines. It is available by prescription (Xenical) for ages 12 years and up and at a lower dose (Alli) over the counter. It commonly causes diarrhea, especially after fatty meals and should not be used by people who have trouble absorbing nutrients from their food. The medication is dosed 3 times a day and patients may adjust the dosing to fit activities.

Phentermine-topiramate (Qsymia) is a combination medication that is also approved for ages 12 years and older. Phentermine is a stimulant that decreases the appetite. Topiramate is an anticonvulsant that decreases appetite by causing feelings of fullness. Although the combination is approved for long-term use, phentermine when used alone is only approved for use for 12 weeks. Blood pressure and heart rate should be monitored when this medication is used. The medication is dosed once a day and dosage can be adjusted as needed. Sleep can be affected if taken late in the day. This medication should be avoided in patients with glaucoma and hyperthyroidism.

Naltrexone-bupropion (Contrave) is another combination medication and can be taken once or twice a day. Naltrexone is also used for alcohol and drug dependence and bupropion is used for depression and tobacco cessation. The combination helps decrease appetite and reduce cravings. This medication should not be used in patients with uncontrolled high blood pressure, patients with seizures, patients taking opioids, patients with anorexia or bulimia, patients who are already taking one of the ingredients, or patients who have recently taken an MAOI.

Liraglutide (Saxenda) and semaglutide (Wegovy) are glucagon-like peptides-1 (GLP-1) injections and mimic hormones that target areas of the brain that regulate appetite and food intake. They were both initially approved to treat type 2 diabetes and should not be used in patients with a personal or family history of medullary thyroid cancer or multiple endocrine neoplasia syndrome. Similarly, tirzepatide (Zepbound) contains a glucose-dependent insulinotropic polypeptide (GIP) in addition to the GLP-1 and has been found to be helpful for weight loss.

Food for thought: What are some questions that you learned from motivational interviewing that can help you to explore a patient's history with weight and assess their readiness for change? What are some common SMART goals that you may want to set with your patients? How can you incorporate brief screening measures into your clinic flow in a way that is efficient, yet clinically informative?

Tobacco Cessation

Tobacco use is the leading cause of preventable death in the United States (Centers for Disease Control and Prevention (CDC), 2024c). Although the overall rate of tobacco use has decreased over the past decades, ethnic and racial minority groups, those with low socioeconomic status, those with BH disorders, and sexual minority groups experience increased rates of tobacco-related disease and illnesses; this may be due to social and environmental stressors, discrimination, or targeted marketing (Arrazola et al., 2023; Hall & Prochaska, 2009; Simmons et al., 2016). On average, people who smoke die 10 years earlier than those who do not, and those with BH diagnoses who smoke die 15 years earlier than those without BH diagnoses who do not smoke (Jha et al., 2013; Tam et al., 2016). Approximately two-thirds of people who smoke say that they would like to quit, and patients who have been advised to quit smoking by their doctors have a higher rate of success (Van Frank et al., 2024).

Assess The USPSTF recommends that clinicians treat tobacco use as a vital sign and ask all adults about their tobacco use (United States Preventative Services Task

Force, 2021). During a contextual interview, PCPs should inquire how tobacco use impacts patients' relationships with others or their ability to engage in leisure or work activities. PCPs can also ask how tobacco is currently serving the patient (i.e., helps to relieve stress, form of social connection, a habit they would like to quit). Since many people who use tobacco products are aware of the negative health consequences of their use, there are likely other reasons that seem bigger than the health risks that are keeping them using. PCPs can also assess whether patients have tried to quit tobacco in the past and how successful they were. PCPs should ask whether patients are currently thinking about changing their tobacco use, and any reasons they may have to change to assess what stage of change the patient is at.

Advise After assessing the patient's history with tobacco products, why and how they are currently using, and what stage of change the patient is at, PCPs can provide tailored information on changing the patient's tobacco use. For patients who are in the precontemplation stage of change and are not interested in quitting, providers should increase awareness of the need to change without criticizing or shaming the patient. PCPs can personalize the risks or consequences of tobacco use based on the information provided by the patient and inform them that they are available when the patient is ready to make a change. While patients may be aware of the broad negative consequences of tobacco use, they may be unaware of the immediate effects of quitting, and that quitting at any age can enhance quality of life and improve their health status (U.S. Department of Health and Human Services, 2020). Patients who are in the precontemplation stage will benefit from motivational interviewing strategies that help them explore the benefits of change, barriers to quitting, and engage them in change talk. An example conversation could go as follows:

> *Patient:* I've been smoking for as long as I can remember, what would it matter if I stop now.
> *Provider:* Since you've been smoking for so long, you don't see how quitting might make a difference in your health?
> *Patient:* I mean, I know that smoking is bad for me, but isn't the damage already done?
> *Provider:* It sounds like you've heard before about the health risks of smoking, and considered how your smoking has impacted your own health. I wonder if it would be helpful if I shared how quitting even after smoking for years can improve your health?
> *Providers should be mindful of approaching these conversations by asking for permission and having a genuinely curious tone and approach to avoid sounding "judgy" or "preachy" towards patients.

For patients who are in the preparation stage of change, providing them with resources, motivation, and support to take action will be helpful. This can problem solving barriers to quitting, providing Quitline and counseling referrals, or discussing pharmacotherapy for cessation.

Agree If the patient is willing to make a change, PCPs can work with them to agree upon feasible next steps to begin changing their tobacco use. PCPs can encourage patients to select a quit date and begin tracking their use over time to work toward being tobacco free by that date. Patients can track their tobacco use using apps, such as the quitSTART app, or paper journals (U.S. Department of Veterans Affairs, 2024a). Tracking use will help to identify situations and triggers when patients are more likely to use tobacco and help in identifying goals for cutting back on use. Providers can help patients set personalized SMART goals to change their tobacco use over time. If patients are not ready to fully quit, reduction of tobacco use should be considered as a target goal (Odorico et al., 2019). See Table 9.13 for an example tracking sheet and example conversation with a patient.

Provider: Great job tracking your cigarettes over the past week! It looks like waking up and mealtimes are most of your triggers, with the middle of the day at work the time that you most desperately need a cigarette.
Patient: Yeah, I was a little surprised that it wasn't later in the day, but I was pretty easily able to distract myself in the evening and not have a cigarette. But lunch time at work I am used to going outside with my coworkers, smoking, and talking to relieve the stress of the morning, so it has been really hard to not have that cigarette.
Provider: That makes a lot of sense that it has been hard to give up those lunch time cigarettes. I wonder if we can problem solve and make a plan together for these situations when you are most likely to have a cigarette to help you have something else to do?
Patient: Sure we can try. I'm not really sure where to start though.
Provider: That's ok! You've mentioned that you like to relieve stress at lunch time, one idea could be taking a short walk at lunch instead of smoking a cigarette with a friend who doesn't smoke. Or we can talk about other ideas that might work well for you.

Table 9.13 Excerpt from patient's cigarette tracking log

Date	Time of Day	Activity	Need for Cigarette (1–3)[a]
1/1/24	7 am	Waking up	2
1/1/24	8 am	Drinking coffee	3
1/1/24	12 pm	Lunch break	1

[a] Key: 1 = Cigarette needed desperately; 2 = Cigarette wanted but not needed; 3 = Cigarette smoked out of habit (American Academy of Family Physicians, 2015)

Assist Problem solving and skills training counseling, and social support are especially effective, and most effective when combined with medications (Tobacco Use and Dependence Guideline Panel, 2008). The AAFP has developed multiple resources for providers and patients, including a Quit Smoking Guide (available at: https://www.aafp.org/family-physician/patient-care/care-resources/tobacco-and-nicotine/tobacco-tools.html; American Academy of Family Physicians (AAFP), 2024), which provides patients with skills and resources to help them quit.

Problem solving and skills training. Patients and providers can work together to identify triggers for smoking and problem solve strategies to overcome these triggers. Additionally, patients can be encouraged to take small steps to decrease their tobacco use, such as decreasing by one cigarette per day, rather than trying to quit "cold turkey." Patients can also be given strategies to manage their stress without tobacco, such as physical exercise, relaxation breathing, and social support from important others.

Distractions and changing routines. Patients can be encouraged to change their routines around smoking, such as going for a walk at lunch, chewing gum after breakfast, or changing to a non-preferred brand of tobacco. Patients should also be encouraged to avoid others who smoke or taking "smoke breaks" until they feel confident in their ability to resist tobacco use.

Utilizing electronic health records (EHRs), teams, and quitlines. PCPs may consider building quitline referrals into their (EHRs) for patients who screen positive for tobacco use, and utilizing medical assistants or staff to help assess tobacco use at every visit. Staff may also help follow-up with patients who begin to make changes in their tobacco use, and can help encourage patients to continue to make healthy changes. Quitlines can offer free counseling for individuals who are trying to quit, and some programs may also offer free nicotine replacement therapy products to individuals who engage in their services.

Medications for tobacco dependence. Due to the addictive nature of the nicotine in tobacco products many patients find that medication to help with nicotine withdrawal can be helpful in tobacco cessation. Medications can be helpful with irritability, nervousness, headaches, sleep disturbances, depressive symptoms, and cravings that can accompany tobacco cessation (Centers for Disease Control (CDC), 2024). To aid with tobacco cessation the FDA has approved 3 medications-nicotine replacement, bupropion and varenicline (U.S. Department of Health and Human Services, 2020; U.S. Food and Drug Administration, 2018).

Nicotine replacement therapy (NRT) (common brand names include Nicorette, NicoDerm and Nicotrol) comes in 5 forms. Nicotine patches, gum, and lozenges are available over the counter and sometimes free from cessation programs. Nicotine oral and nasal inhalers are available by prescriptions only. NRT can be helpful in tapering patients off cigarettes and can be used by combining different forms as well as in conjunction with other tobacco cessation medications. NRT use is approved for adults, but caution should be used in pregnancy, breast feeding, and patients with heart disease (U.S. Department of Health and Human Services, 2020). Dosing tables are available online at the National Institute of Health (NIH) website (Theodoulou et al., 2023).

Bupropion SR (common brand names are Zyban and Wellbutrin) can be helpful with combatting weight gain and depressive symptoms associated with tobacco cessation (U.S. Department of Health and Human Services, 2020). It is available by prescription only for adults and should be started 1–2 weeks prior to the quit date and is typically continued for 12 weeks total but may be given longer. On the first 3 days, 150 mg should be given in the mornings only. After day 3, the dosage should be increased to 150 mg twice a day and should be taken at least 8 hours apart. Bupropion should not be given to patients with a history of a seizure disorder, anorexia, bulimia, or patients currently or have recently taken MAO inhibitors. Bupropion should be used with caution in patients who are pregnant or breastfeeding, have liver disease or use alcohol or other sedating medications. Side effects include nausea, irritability, mood disturbances, constipation, dry mouth, and seizures (U.S. Department of Health and Human Services, 2020).

Varenicline is available for adults with a prescription and has been found to be the most effective medication to aid in tobacco cessation when used alone but is also the costliest (U.S. Department of Health and Human Services, 2020). Varenicline (common brand name is Chantix) should be started 8–35 days prior to the quit date by taking a 0.5 mg tablet daily for days 1–3. On days 4–7 a 0.5 mg tablet should be taken in the morning and in the evening. On day 8 and afterward a 1 mg tablet should be taken in the morning and the evening for 12 weeks. All doses should be taken with food or a full glass of water. Side effects include nausea, mood or behavior changes, constipation, somnolence, and sleep disturbances, particularly vivid dreams. Caution should be used in patients who are pregnant or breastfeeding, have seizure disorders, heart disease, mood disorders, or kidney problems. Concomitant use with alcohol may cause increased toxicity (U.S. Department of Health and Human Services, 2020).

Key Points

- Chronic health conditions have a strong biopsychosocial component to effective management in primary care.
- PCPs can utilize a 5As approach, contextual interviewing, and patient-centered strategies to help patients engage in behavior changes to better manage their chronic health conditions.
- There are effective behavioral strategies to help patients manage their chronic health conditions that PCPs can help patients engage in.

References

Albury, C., Strain, W. D., Le Brocq, S., Logue, J., Lloyed, C., & Tahrani, A. (2020). The importance of language in engagement between health-care professionals and people living with obesity: A joint consensus statement. *The Lancet Diabetes and Endocrinology, 8*(5), 447–455.

Ali Sherazi, B., Laeer, S., Krutisch, S., Dabidian, A., Schlottau, S., & Obarcanin, E. (2023). Functions of mHealth diabetes apps that enable the provision of pharmaceutical care: Criteria development and evaluation of popular apps. *International Journal of Environmental Research and Public Health, 20*(1), 64. https://doi.org/10.3390/ijerph20010064

Al-Khalil, Z., Attarian, H., Dunietz, G. L., Gavidia Romero, R., Knutson, K., & Johnson, D. A. (2024). Sleep health inequities in vulnerable populations: Beyond sleep deserts. *Sleep Medicine: X, 7*, 100110. https://doi.org/10.1016/j.sleepx.2024.100110

American Academy of Family Physicians. (2015). *Quit smoking guide.* American Academy of Family Physicians. https://www.aafp.org/dam/AAFP/documents/patient_care/tobacco/stop-smoking-guide.pdf

American Academy of Family Physicians (AAFP). (2024). *Tobacco cessation tools & resources.* https://www.aafp.org/family-physician/patient-care/care-resources/tobacco-and-nicotine/tobacco-tools.html

Arrazola, R. A., Griffin, T., Lunsford, N. B., Kittner, D., Bammeke, P., Courtney-Long, E. A., & Armour, B. S. (2023). U.S. cigarette smoking disparities by race and ethnicity—Keep going and going! *Preventing Chronic Disease, 20*, E45. https://doi.org/10.5888/pcd20.220375

Aubrey, A. (2022). *For stomach pain and other IBS symptoms, new apps can bring relief*. NPR. https://www.npr.org/sections/health-shots/2022/10/16/1129325699/ibs-irritable-bowel-syndrome-symptoms-treatment

Avery-Clark, C., Weiner, L., & Adams-Clark, A. A. (2019). Sensate focus for sexual concerns: An updated, critical literature review. *Current Sexual Health Reports, 11*(2), 84–94. https://doi.org/10.1007/s11930-019-00197-9

Azumio Inc. (2024). *Glucose buddy diabetes tracker* (version 5.430) [Mobile app]. App store. https://apps.apple.com/us/app/glucose-buddy-diabetes-tracker/id294754639

Babbott, K. M., Cavadino, A., Brenton-Peters, J., Consedine, N. S., & Roberts, M. (2023). Outcomes of intuitive eating interventions: A systematic review and meta-analysis. *Eating Disorders, 31*(1), 33–63. https://doi.org/10.1080/10640266.2022.2030124

Baile, W. F., Buckman, R., Lenzi, R., Glober, G., Beale, E. A., & Kudelka, A. P. (2000). SPIKES—A six-step protocol for delivering bad news: Application to the patient with cancer. *The Oncologist, 5*(4), 302–311. https://doi.org/10.1634/theoncologist.5-4-302

Ballou, S., & Keefer, L. (2017). Psychological interventions for irritable bowel syndrome and inflammatory bowel diseases. *Clinical and Translational Gastroenterology, 8*(1), e214. https://doi.org/10.1038/ctg.2016.69

Barnhoorn, P. C., Prins, I. C., Zuurveen, H. R., Oudsten, B. L., Ouden, M. E. M., Numans, M. E., Elzevier, H. W., & van Ek, G. F. (2022). Let's talk about sex: Exploring factors influencing the discussion of sexual health among chronically ill patients in general practice. *BMC Primary Care, 23*(1), 49. https://doi.org/10.1186/s12875-022-01660-8

Becker, W. C., Dorflinger, L., Edmond, S. N., Islam, L., Heapy, A. A., & Fraenkel, L. (2017). Barriers and facilitators to use of non-pharmacological treatments in chronic pain. *BMC Family Practice, 18*(1), 41. https://doi.org/10.1186/s12875-017-0608-2

Beechy, L., Galpern, J., Petrone, A., & Das, S. K. (2012). Assessment tools in obesity—Psychological measures, diet, activity, and body composition. *Physiology & Behavior, 107*(1), 154–171. https://doi.org/10.1016/j.physbeh.2012.04.013

Benavidez, G. A. (2024). Chronic disease prevalence in the US: Sociodemographic and geographic variations by zip code tabulation area. *Preventing Chronic Disease, 21*. https://doi.org/10.5888/pcd21.230267

Bevers, K., Watts, L., Kishino, N. D., & Gatchel, R. J. (2016). The biopsychosocial model of the assessment, prevention, and treatment of chronic pain. *US Neurology, 12*(2), 98–104. https://doi.org/10.17925/USN.2016.12.02.98

Black, C. J., Drossman, D. A., Talley, N. J., Ruddy, J., & Ford, A. C. (2020). Functional gastrointestinal disorders: Advances in understanding and management. *The Lancet, 396*(10263), 1664–1674. https://doi.org/10.1016/S0140-6736(20)32115-2

Bosworth, H. B., Fortmann, S. P., Kuntz, J., Zullig, L. L., Mendys, P., Safford, M., Phansalkar, S., Wang, T., & Rumptz, M. H. (2017). Recommendations for providers on person-centered approaches to assess and improve medication adherence. *Journal of General Internal Medicine, 32*(1), 93–100. https://doi.org/10.1007/s11606-016-3851-7

Bowelle AB. (2024). *Bowelle—The IBS tracker* (version 1.24.8) [Mobile app]. App store. https://apps.apple.com/us/app/bowelle-the-ibs-tracker/id1436064640

Bowen, D. J., Balsam, K. F., & Ender, S. R. (2008). A review of obesity issues in sexual minority women. *Obesity, 16*(2), 221–228. https://doi.org/10.1038/oby.2007.34

Braddock, A., Browne, N. T., Houser, M., Blair, G., & Williams, D. R. (2023). Weight stigma and bias: A guide for pediatric clinicians. *Obesity Pillars, 6*, 100058. https://doi.org/10.1016/j.obpill.2023.100058

Brady, T. J., Murphy, L., Beauchesne, D., Bhalakia, A., Chervin, D., Daniels, B., Greenberg, M., House, M., & O'Colmain. (2011). *Sorting through the evidence for the arthritis self management program and the chronic disease self management program: Executive summary of ASMP/CDSMP meta-analyses.* https://stacks.cdc.gov/view/cdc/23175

Bryant, R. V., van Langenberg, D. R., Holtmann, G. J., & Andrews, J. M. (2011). Functional gastrointestinal disorders in inflammatory bowel disease: Impact on quality of life and psychological status. *Journal of Gastroenterology and Hepatology, 26*(5), 916–923. https://doi.org/10.1111/j.1440-1746.2011.06624.x

Buttorff, C., Ruder, T., & Bauman, M. (2017). *Multiple chronic conditions in the United States.* RAND Corporation. https://www.rand.org/pubs/tools/TL221.html

Cahill, A., Martin, M., Beachy, B., Bauman, D., & Howard-Young, J. (2024). The contextual interview: A cross-cutting patient-interviewing approach for social context. *Medical Education Online, 29*(1), 2295049. https://doi.org/10.1080/10872981.2023.2295049

Calzo, J. P., Blashill, A. J., Brown, T. A., & Argenal, R. L. (2017). Eating disorders and disordered weight and shape control behaviors in sexual minority populations. *Current Psychiatry Reports, 19*(8), 49. https://doi.org/10.1007/s11920-017-0801-y

Cardel, M. I., Newsome, F. A., Pearl, R. L., Ross, K. M., Dillard, J. R., Miller, D. R., Hayes, J. F., Wilfley, D., Keel, P. K., Dhurandhar, E. J., & Balantekin, K. N. (2022). Patient-centered care for obesity: How health care providers can treat obesity while actively addressing weight stigma and eating disorder risk. *Journal of the Academy of Nutrition and Dietetics, 122*(6), 1089–1098. https://doi.org/10.1016/j.jand.2022.01.004

Carroll, J. K., Flocke, S. A., Sanders, M. R., Lowenstein, L., Fiscella, K., & Epstein, R. M. (2016). Effectiveness of a clinician intervention to improve physical activity discussions in underserved adults. *Family Practice, 33*(5), 488–491. https://doi.org/10.1093/fampra/cmw036

Centers for Disease Control (CDC). (2024). *State fact sheets | Smoking & tobacco use.* CDC. https://www.cdc.gov/tobacco/stateandcommunity/state-fact-sheets/index.htm

Centers for Disease Control and Prevention (CDC). (2023). *Youth Risk Behavior Surveillance System (YRBSS) results.* https://www.cdc.gov/yrbs/%3FCDC_AAref_Val=, https://www.cdc.gov/healthyyouth/data/yrbs/results.html

Centers for Disease Control and Prevention (CDC). (2024). *The behavioral risk factor surveillance system (BRFSS).* Centers for Disease Control and Prevention. https://www.cdc.gov/brfss/index.html#:~:text=The%20Behavioral%20Risk%20Factor%20Surveillanceand%20use%20of%20preventive%20services

Centers for Disease Control and Prevention (CDC). (2024a). *Childhood obesity facts.* https://www.cdc.gov/obesity/php/data-research/childhood-obesity-facts.html#:~:text=From%202017%20to%20March%202020percentile%20for%20age%20and%20sex

Centers for Disease Control and Prevention (CDC). (2024b). *Discussing sexual health with your patients.* HIV Nexus: CDC Resources for Clinicians. https://www.cdc.gov/hivnexus/hcp/sexual-history/index.html

Centers for Disease Control and Prevention (CDC). (2024c). Adult obesity facts. *Obesity.* https://www.cdc.gov/obesity/php/data-research/adult-obesity-facts.html

Chey, W. D., Keefer, L., Whelan, K., & Gibson, P. R. (2021). Behavioral and diet therapies in integrated care for patients with irritable bowel syndrome. *Gastroenterology, 160*(1), 47–62. https://doi.org/10.1053/j.gastro.2020.06.099

Child and Adolescent Health Measurement Initiative. (2023). *Fast facts: 2021–2022 National Survey of children's health.* Data resource Center for Child and Adolescent Health Supported by the U.S. Department of Health and Human Services, Health Resources and Services Administration (HRSA), Maternal and Child Health Bureau (MCHB). https://www.cdc.gov/sleep/data-research/facts-stats/children-sleep-facts-and-stats.html

Chung, F., Abdullah, H. R., & Liao, P. (2016). STOP-bang questionnaire: A practical approach to screen for obstructive sleep apnea. *Chest, 149*(3), 631–638. https://doi.org/10.1378/chest.15-0903

Claxton, A. J., Cramer, J., & Pierce, C. (2001). A systematic review of the associations between dose regimens and medication compliance. *Clinical Therapeutics, 23*(8), 1296–1310. https://doi.org/10.1016/S0149-2918(01)80109-0

Colten, H. R., Altevogt, B. M., & Institute of Medicine (US) Committee on Sleep Medicine and Research. (2006). Committee on sleep medicine and research. In *Sleep disorders and sleep deprivation: An unmet public health problem.* National Academies Press. https://www.ncbi.nlm.nih.gov/books/NBK19944/

Cooper, A. J., Gupta, S. R., Moustafa, A. F., & Chao, A. M. (2021). Sex/gender differences in obesity prevalence, comorbidities, and treatment. *Current Obesity Reports, 10*(4), 458–466. https://doi.org/10.1007/s13679-021-00453-x

Cortese, S., Wang, F., Angriman, M., Masi, G., & Bruni, O. (2020). Sleep disorders in children and adolescents with autism spectrum disorder: Diagnosis, epidemiology, and management. *CNS Drugs, 34*(4), 415–423. https://doi.org/10.1007/s40263-020-00710-y

Crowe, M. (2012). Couple relationship problems and sexual dysfunctions: Therapeutic guidelines. *Advances in Psychiatric Treatment, 18*(2), 154–159. https://doi.org/10.1192/apt.bp.109.007443

Dao, M. C., Thiron, S., Messer, E., Sergeant, C., Sévigné, A., Huart, C., Rossi, M., Silverman, I., Sakaida, K., Bel Lassen, P., Sarrat, C., Arciniegas, L., Das, S. K., Gaussérès, N., Clément, K., & Roberts, S. B. (2020). Cultural influences on the regulation of energy intake and obesity: A qualitative study comparing food customs and attitudes to eating in adults from France and the United States. *Nutrients, 13*(1), 63. https://doi.org/10.3390/nu13010063

Di Angelantonio, E., Bhupathiraju, S., Wormser, D., Gao, P., Kaptoge, S., Berrington de Gonzalez, A., Cairns, B., Huxley, R., Jackson, C., Joshy, G., Lewington, S., Manson, J., Murphy, N., Patel, A., Samet, J., Woodward, M., Zheng, W., Zhou, M., & Hu, F. (2016). Body-mass index and all-cause mortality: Individual-participant-data meta-analysis of 239 prospective studies in four continents. *Lancet, 388*(10046), 776–786. https://doi.org/10.1016/S0140-6736(16)30175-1

DiClemente, C. C., & Velasquez, M. M. (2002). Motivational interviewing and the stages of change. In W. R. Miller & S. Rollnick (Eds.), *Motivational interviewing: Preparing people for change* (2nd ed., pp. 201–216). Guilford Press.

Doran, G. T. (1981). There's a S.M.A.R.T. way to write managements's goals and objectives. *Management Review, 70*(11), 35.

Edinger, J. D., & Carney, C. E. (2014). *Overcoming insomnia: A cognitive-behavioral therapy approach, therapist guide.* Oxford University Press.

Elnazer, H. Y., & Baldwin, D. S. (2020). Structured review of the use of the Arizona sexual experiences scale in clinical settings. *Human Psychopharmacology: Clinical and Experimental, 35*(3), e2730. https://doi.org/10.1002/hup.2730

Eypasch, E., Williams, J. I., Wood-Dauphinee, S., Ure, B. M., Schmülling, C., Neugebauer, E., & Troidl, H. (1995). Gastrointestinal quality of life index: Development, validation and application of a new instrument. *The British Journal of Surgery, 82*(2), 216–222. https://doi.org/10.1002/bjs.1800820229

Faubion, S. S., & Rullo, J. E. (2015). Sexual dysfunction in women: A practical approach. *American Family Physician, 92*(4), 281–288.

Fehily, C., Hodder, R., Bartlem, K., Wiggers, J., Wolfenden, L., Dray, J., Bailey, J., Wilczynska, M., Stockings, E., Clinton-McHarg, T., Regan, T., & Bowman, J. (2020). The effectiveness of interventions to increase preventive care provision for chronic disease risk behaviours in mental health settings: A systematic review and meta-analysis. *Preventive Medicine Reports, 19*, 101108. https://doi.org/10.1016/j.pmedr.2020.101108

Finan, P. H., Goodin, B. R., & Smith, M. T. (2013). The association of sleep and pain: An update and a path forward. *The Journal of Pain, 14*(12), 1539–1552. https://doi.org/10.1016/j.jpain.2013.08.007

Fink-Miller, E. L., Long, D. M., & Gross, R. T. (2014). Comparing chronic pain treatment seekers in primary care versus tertiary care settings. *Journal of the American Board of Family Medicine, 27*(5), 594–601. https://doi.org/10.3122/jabfm.2014.05.130311

Fischer, V. J., Andersson, G., Billieux, J., & Vögele, C. (2022). The relationship between emotion regulation and sexual function and satisfaction: A scoping review. *Sexual Medicine Reviews, 10*(2), 195–208. https://doi.org/10.1016/j.sxmr.2021.11.004

Fisher, L., Glasgow, R. E., Mullan, J. T., Skaff, M. M., & Polonsky, W. H. (2008). Development of a brief diabetes distress screening instrument. *Annals of Family Medicine, 6*(3), 246–252. https://doi.org/10.1370/afm.842

Flynn, K. E., Lin, L., Bruner, D. W., Cyranowski, J. M., Hahn, E. A., Jeffery, D. D., Reese, J. B., Reeve, B. B., Shelby, R. A., & Weinfurt, K. P. (2016). Sexual satisfaction and the importance of sexual health to quality of life throughout the life course of U.S. adults. *The Journal of Sexual Medicine, 13*(11), 1642–1650. https://doi.org/10.1016/j.jsxm.2016.08.011

Ford, A. C., Quigley, E. M. M., Lacy, B. E., Lembo, A. J., Saito, Y. A., Schiller, L. R., Soffer, E. E., Spiegel, B. M. R., & Moayyedi, P. (2014). Effect of antidepressants and psychological therapies, including hypnotherapy, in irritable bowel syndrome: Systematic review and meta-analysis. *American Journal of Gastroenterology, 109*(9), 1350. https://doi.org/10.1038/ajg.2014.148

Franqueiro, A. R., Yoon, J., Crago, M. A., Curiel, M., & Wilson, J. M. (2023). The interconnection between social support and emotional distress among individuals with chronic pain: A narrative review. *Psychology Research and Behavior Management, 16*, 4389–4399. https://doi.org/10.2147/PRBM.S410606

Gearhardt, A., Roberto, C. A., Seamans, M. J., Corbin, W. R., & Brownell, K. D. (2013). Preliminary validation of the Yale Food addiction scale for children. *Eating Behaviors, 14*(4). https://doi.org/10.1016/j.eatbeh.2013.07.002

Geneen, L. J., Moore, R. A., Clarke, C., Martin, D., Colvin, L. A., & Smith, B. H. (2017). Physical activity and exercise for chronic pain in adults: An overview of Cochrane reviews. *Cochrane Database of Systematic Reviews, 4*. https://doi.org/10.1002/14651858.CD011279.pub3

Gerend, M. A., Zetrenne, S., Sutin, A. R., Naar, S., & Maner, J. K. (2023). Weight discrimination and health risk behavior in racial, ethnic, and sexual minority adults. *Annals of Behavioral Medicine, 57*(7), 571–581. https://doi.org/10.1093/abm/kaad003

Geurts, J. W., Willems, P. C., Lockwood, C., van Kleef, M., Kleijnen, J., & Dirksen, C. (2017). Patient expectations for management of chronic non-cancer pain: A systematic review. *Health Expectations, 20*(6), 1201–1217. https://doi.org/10.1111/hex.12527

Gikas, A., & Triantafillidis, J. K. (2014). The role of primary care physicians in early diagnosis and treatment of chronic gastrointestinal diseases. *International Journal of General Medicine, 7*, 159–173. https://doi.org/10.2147/IJGM.S58888

Glasgow, R. E., Davis, C. L., Funnell, M. M., & Beck, A. (2003). Implementing practical interventions to support chronic illness self-management. *Joint Commission Journal on Quality and Safety, 29*(11), 563–574. https://doi.org/10.1016/s1549-3741(03)29067-5

Goldstein, M. G., Whitlock, E. P., & DePue, J. (2004). Multiple behavioral risk factor interventions in primary care: Summary of research evidence. *American Journal of Preventive Medicine, 27*(2), 61–79. https://doi.org/10.1016/j.amepre.2004.04.023

Goldstein, R. B., Smith, S. M., Chou, S. P., Saha, T. D., Jung, J., Zhang, H., Pickering, R. P., Ruan, W. J., Huang, B., & Grant, B. F. (2016). The epidemiology of DSM-5 posttraumatic stress disorder in the United States: Results from the National Epidemiologic Survey on alcohol and related conditions-III. *Social Psychiatry and Psychiatric Epidemiology, 51*(8), 1137–1148. https://doi.org/10.1007/s00127-016-1208-5

Gordon, A. R., Egan, K. A., Wang, M. L., Ziyadeh, N. J., Kenney, E. L., Rosario, M., & Austin, S. B. (2023). Weight-based discrimination and disordered eating behaviors in a cohort of U.S. sexual minority young adults. *International Journal of Eating Disorders, 56*(10), 1983–1990. https://doi.org/10.1002/eat.24015

Graci, G. (2021). *Sleep disorders: Elements, history, treatments, and research.* Bloomsbury Publishing.

Grider, H. S., Douglas, S. M., & Raynor, H. A. (2021). The influence of mindful eating and/or intuitive eating approaches on dietary intake: A systematic review. *Journal of the Academy of Nutrition and Dietetics, 121*(4), 709–727.e1. https://doi.org/10.1016/j.jand.2020.10.019

Hacker, K. (2024). The burden of chronic disease. *Mayo Clinic Proceedings: Innovations, Quality & Outcomes, 8*(1), 112–119. https://doi.org/10.1016/j.mayocpiqo.2023.08.005

Hall, S. M., & Prochaska, J. J. (2009). Treatment of smokers with co-occurring disorders: Emphasis on integration in mental health and addiction treatment settings. *Annual Review of Clinical Psychology, 5*, 409–431. https://doi.org/10.1146/annurev.clinpsy.032408.153614

Halpert, A., Dalton, C. B., Palsson, O., Morris, C., Hu, Y., Bangdiwala, S., Hankins, J., Norton, N., & Drossman, D. (2007). What patients know about irritable bowel syndrome (IBS) and what they would like to know. National survey on patient educational needs in IBS and development and validation of the patient educational needs questionnaire (PEQ). *American Journal of Gastroenterology, 102*(9), 1972. https://doi.org/10.1111/j.1572-0241.2007.01254.x

Hamilton, W. (2010). Cancer diagnosis in primary care. *British Journal of General Practice, 60*(571), 121–128. https://doi.org/10.3399/bjgp10X483175

HiDoc Technologies GmbH. (2020). *Cara care: IBS, FODMAP tracker* (Version 5.4.5) [Mobile App]. App Store. https://apps.apple.com/us/app/cara-care-ibs-fodmap-tracker/id1133687886

Hunter, C. L., Goodie, J. L., Oordt, M. S., & Dobmeyer, A. C. (2024). *Integrated behavioral health in primary care: Step-by-step guidance for assessment and intervention* (3rd ed.). American Psychological Association. https://doi.org/10.1037/0000380-001

Institute of Medicine (US) Committee on Psychosocial Services to Cancer Patients/Families in a Community Setting. (2008). In N. E. Adler & A. E. Page (Eds.), *Cancer care for the whole patient: Meeting psychosocial health needs.* National Academies Press. http://www.ncbi.nlm.nih.gov/books/NBK4015/

Irvine, E. J., Zhou, Q., & Thompson, A. K. (1996). The short inflammatory bowel Disease questionnaire: A quality of life instrument for community physicians managing inflammatory bowel disease. *The American Journal of Gastroenterology, 91*(8), 1571–1578.

Jehan, S., Zizi, F., Pandi-Perumal, S. R., Myers, A. K., Auguste, E., Jean-Louis, G., & McFarlane, S. I. (2017). Shift work and sleep: Medical implications and management. *Sleep Medicine and Disorders: International Journal, 1*(2), 8.

Jha, P., Ramasundarahettige, C., Landsman, V., Rostron, B., Thun, M., Anderson, R. N., McAfee, T., & Peto, R. (2013). 21st-century hazards of smoking and benefits of cessation in the United States. *New England Journal of Medicine, 368*(4), 341–350. https://doi.org/10.1056/NEJMsa1211128

Johns, M. W. (1991). A new method for measuring daytime sleepiness: The Epworth sleepiness scale. *Sleep, 14*(6), 540–545. https://doi.org/10.1093/sleep/14.6.540

Keefer, L., Palsson, O. S., & Pandolfino, J. E. (2018). Best practice update: Incorporating psychogastroenterology into management of digestive disorders. *Gastroenterology, 154*(5), 1249–1257. https://doi.org/10.1053/j.gastro.2018.01.045

Ketola, E., Sipilä, R., & Mäkelä, M. (2000). Effectiveness of individual lifestyle interventions in reducing cardiovascular disease and risk factors. *Annals of Medicine, 32*(4), 239–251. https://doi.org/10.3109/07853890009011767

Kiernan, G. N., & Frame, P. S. (1996). Cancer occurrence and screening in family practice. A 20-year experience. *The Journal of Family Practice, 43*(1), 49–55.

Kim, L. Y., Rose, D. E., Soban, L. M., Stockdale, S. E., Meredith, L. S., Edwards, S. T., Helfrich, C. D., & Rubenstein, L. V. (2018). Primary care tasks associated with provider burnout: Findings from a veterans health administration survey. *Journal of General Internal Medicine, 33*(1), 50–56. https://doi.org/10.1007/s11606-017-4188-6

Knight, M. G., Anekwe, C., Washington, K., Akam, E. Y., Wang, E., & Stanford, F. C. (2021). Weight regulation in menopause. *Menopause, 28*(8), 960–965. https://doi.org/10.1097/GME.0000000000001792

Knowler, W. C., Barrett-Connor, E., Fowler, S. E., Hamman, R. F., Lachin, J. M., Walker, E. A., Nathan, D. M., & Diabetes Prevention Program Research Group. (2002). Reduction in the incidence of type 2 diabetes with lifestyle intervention or metformin. *The New England Journal of Medicine, 346*(6), 393–403. https://doi.org/10.1056/NEJMoa012512

Kok, G., Peters, G.-J. Y., Kessels, L. T. E., ten Hoor, G. A., & Ruiter, R. A. C. (2018). Ignoring theory and misinterpreting evidence: The false belief in fear appeals. *Health Psychology Review, 12*(2), 111–125. https://doi.org/10.1080/17437199.2017.1415767

Kripalani, S., Yao, X., & Haynes, R. B. (2007). Interventions to enhance medication adherence in chronic medical conditions: A systematic review. *Archives of Internal Medicine, 167*(6), 540–549. https://doi.org/10.1001/archinte.167.6.540

Kroenke, K., Spitzer, R. L., & Williams, J. B. W. (1999). Patient health questionnaire-9. https://doi.org/10.1037/t06165-000

Lackner, J. M., Jaccard, J., Krasner, S. S., Katz, L. A., Gudleski, G. D., & Holroyd, K. (2008). Self-administered cognitive behavior therapy for moderate to severe irritable bowel syndrome: Clinical efficacy, tolerability, feasibility. *Clinical Gastroenterology and Hepatology, 6*(8), 899–906. https://doi.org/10.1016/j.cgh.2008.03.004

Lee, M. (2024). *MyFitnessPal* (version 24.30.0) [Mobile app]. App store. https://www.myfitnesspal.com/

Lenhart, A., Ferch, C., Shaw, M., & Chey, W. D. (2018). Use of dietary management in irritable bowel syndrome: Results of a survey of over 1500 United States gastroenterologists. *Journal of Neurogastroenterology and Motility, 24*(3), 437–446. https://doi.org/10.5056/jnm17116

Li, H., Gao, T., & Wang, R. (2016). The role of the sexual partner in managing erectile dysfunction. *Nature Reviews Urology, 13*(3), 168–177. https://doi.org/10.1038/nrurol.2015.315

Licciardone, J. C., Patel, S., Kandukuri, P., Beeton, G., Nyalakonda, R., & Aryal, S. (2023). Patient satisfaction with medical care for chronic low back pain: A pain research registry study. *The Annals of Family Medicine, 21*(2), 125–131. https://doi.org/10.1370/afm.2949

Lindberg, N. M., Stevens, V. J., Vega-López, S., Kauffman, T., Calderón, M. R., & Cervantes, M. A. (2012). A weight-loss intervention program designed for Mexican-American women: Cultural adaptations and results. *Journal of Immigrant and Minority Health/Center for Minority Public Health, 14*(6), 1030–1039. https://doi.org/10.1007/s10903-012-9616-4

Liu, J., Chey, W. D., Haller, E., & Eswaran, S. (2020). Low-FODMAP diet for irritable bowel syndrome: What we know and what we have yet to learn. *Annual Review of Medicine, 71*, 303–314. https://doi.org/10.1146/annurev-med-050218-013625

Longstreth, G. F. (2007). Avoiding unnecessary surgery in irritable bowel syndrome. *Gut, 56*(5), 608–610. https://doi.org/10.1136/gut.2006.115006

Mahana Therapeutics, Inc. (2024). *Mahana IBS: Treatment and relief* (version 5.14.1) [Mobile app]. App Store. https://apps.apple.com/us/app/mahana-ibs-treatment-relief/id1507233227

Maiorino, M. I., Bellastella, G., & Esposito, K. (2015). Lifestyle modifications and erectile dysfunction: What can be expected? *Asian Journal of Andrology, 17*(1), 5–10. https://doi.org/10.4103/1008-682X.137687

Marchand, E. (2021). Psychological and behavioral treatment of female orgasmic disorder. *Sexual Medicine Reviews, 9*(2), 194–211. https://doi.org/10.1016/j.sxmr.2020.07.007

Masood, B., & Moorthy, M. (2023). Causes of obesity: A review. *Clinical Medicine, 23*(4), 284–291. https://doi.org/10.7861/clinmed.2023-0168

Masters, W., & Johnson, V. E. (1970). *Human sexual inadequacy*. Little, Brown, and Company.

McCuen-Wurst, C., Ruggieri, M., & Allison, K. C. (2018). Disordered eating and obesity: Associations between binge-eating disorder, night-eating syndrome, and weight-related comorbidities. *Annals of the New York Academy of Sciences, 1411*(1), 96–105. https://doi.org/10.1111/nyas.13467

McGahuey, C. A., Gelenberg, A. J., Laukes, C. A., Moreno, F. A., Delgado, P. L., McKnight, K. M., & Manber. (2000). The Arizona sexual experience scale (ASEX): Reliability and validity. *Journal of Sex & Marital Therapy, 26*(1), 25–40. https://doi.org/10.1080/009262300278623

McMullen, S., & Rosen, R. C. (1979). Self-administered masturbation training in the treatment of primary orgasmic dysfunction. *Journal of Consulting and Clinical Psychology, 47*(5), 912–918.

Meg Foundation for Pain. (2024). *Part two: The framework of pain.* Meg Foundation. https://www.megfoundationforpain.org/the-framework-of-pain/

Mehnert, A., Hartung, T. J., Friedrich, M., Vehling, S., Brähler, E., Härter, M., Keller, M., Schulz, H., Wegscheider, K., Weis, J., Koch, U., & Faller, H. (2018). One in two cancer patients is significantly distressed: Prevalence and indicators of distress. *Psycho-Oncology, 27*(1), 75–82. https://doi.org/10.1002/pon.4464

Meltzer, L. J., & Mindell, J. A. (2007). Relationship between child sleep disturbances and maternal sleep, mood, and parenting stress: A pilot study. *Journal of Family Psychology, 21*(1), 67–73. https://doi.org/10.1037/0893-3200.21.1.67

Meston, C. M. (2003). Validation of the female sexual function index (FSFI) in women with female orgasmic disorder and in women with hypoactive sexual desire disorder. *Journal of Sex & Marital Therapy, 29*(1), 39–46. https://doi.org/10.1080/713847100

Metz, M. E., & McCarthy, B. W. (2003). *Coping with premature ejaculation: How to overcome PE, please your partner, and have great sex.* New Harbinger Publications. https://www.newharbinger.com/9781608829293/coping-with-premature-ejaculation

Meyers, D., Wolff, T., Gregory, K., Marion, L., Moyer, V., Nelson, H., Petitti, D., & Sawaya, G. F. (2008). USPSTF recommendations for STI screening. *American Family Physician, 77*(6), 819–824.

Milne, S., Sheeran, P., & Orbell, S. (2000). Prediction and intervention in health-related behavior: A meta-analytic review of protection motivation theory. *Journal of Applied Social Psychology, 30*(1), 106–143. https://doi.org/10.1111/j.1559-1816.2000.tb02308.x

Mindset Health Pty Ltd. (2024). *Nerva: IBS & gut hypnotherapy* (version 33.0) [Mobile app]. App store. https://apps.apple.com/us/app/nerva-ibs-gut-hypnotherapy/id1467398796

Morgan, J. F., Reid, F., & Lacey, J. H. (1999). The SCOFF questionnaire: Assessment of a new screening tool for eating disorders. *BMJ, 319*(7223), 1467–1468. https://doi.org/10.1136/bmj.319.7223.1467

Morin, C. M. (1993). *Insomnia severity index (ISI).* APA PsycTests. https://doi.org/10.1037/t07115-000

Morrissey, E. C., Corbett, T. K., Walsh, J. C., & Molloy, G. J. (2016). Behavior change techniques in apps for medication adherence: A content analysis. *American Journal of Preventive Medicine, 50*(5), e143–e146. https://doi.org/10.1016/j.amepre.2015.09.034

Morton, K., Beauchamp, M., Prothero, A., Joyce, L., Saunders, L., Spencer-Bowdage, S., Dancy, B., & Pedlar, C. (2015). The effectiveness of motivational interviewing for health behaviour change in primary care settings: A systematic review. *Health Psychology Review, 9*(2), 205–223. https://doi.org/10.1080/17437199.2014.882006

mySugr GmbH. (2024). *mySugr—Diabetes tracker log* (version 3.107.0) [mobile app]. App Store. https://apps.apple.com/us/app/mysugr-diabetes-tracker-log/id516509211

Naliboff, B. D., & Mayer, E. A. (2006). Brain imaging in IBS: Drawing the line between cognitive and non-cognitive processes. *Gastroenterology, 130*(1), 267–270. https://doi.org/10.1053/j.gastro.2005.11.034

National Comprehensive Cancer Network. (1999). NCCN practice guidelines for the management of psychosocial distress. *Oncology, 13*(5A), 113–147.

National Institute of Diabetes and Digestive and Kidney Diseases. (2024). *Prescription medications to treat overweight & obesity*. National Institute of Health. https://www.niddk.nih.gov/health-information/weight-management/prescription-medications-treat-overweight-obesity

Nicola, M., Correia, H., Ditchburn, G., & Drummond, P. D. (2022). Defining pain-validation: The importance of validation in reducing the stresses of chronic pain. *Frontiers in Pain Research, 3*. https://doi.org/10.3389/fpain.2022.884335

Nigg, C. R., & Long, C. R. (2012). A systematic review of single health behavior change interventions vs. multiple health behavior change interventions among older adults. *Translational. Behavioral Medicine, 2*(2), 163–179. https://doi.org/10.1007/s13142-012-0130-y

Nijs, J., D'Hondt, E., Clarys, P., Deliens, T., Polli, A., Malfliet, A., Coppieters, I., Willaert, W., Tumkaya Yilmaz, S., Elma, Ö., & Ickmans, K. (2020). Lifestyle and chronic pain across the lifespan: An inconvenient truth? *PM & R: The Journal of Injury, Function, and Rehabilitation, 12*(4), 410–419. https://doi.org/10.1002/pmrj.12244

Nusbaum, M. R. H., Hamilton, C., & Lenahan, P. (2003). Chronic illness and sexual functioning. *American Family Physician, 67*(2), 347–354.

Obesity Action Coalition. (2024). *People-first language for obesity*. https://www.obesityaction.org/wp-content/uploads/1033162_FirstPersonOne-Pager01_041921.pdf

Odorico, M., Le Goff, D., Aerts, N., Bastiaens, H., & Le Reste, J. Y. (2019). How to support smoking cessation in primary care and the community: A systematic review of interventions for the prevention of cardiovascular diseases. *Vascular Health and Risk Management, 15*, 485–502. https://doi.org/10.2147/VHRM.S221744

Ogden, C. L., Carroll, M. D., Kit, B. K., & Flegal, K. M. (2012). Prevalence of obesity in the United States, 2009–2010. *NCHS Data Brief, 82*, 1–8.

Palsson, O. S., & Whitehead, W. E. (2013). Psychological treatments in functional gastrointestinal disorders: A primer for the gastroenterologist. *Clinical Gastroenterology and Hepatology, 11*(3), 208–216. https://doi.org/10.1016/j.cgh.2012.10.031

Patrick, D. L., Drossman, D. A., Frederick, I. O., DiCesare, J., & Puder, K. L. (1998). Quality of life in persons with irritable bowel syndrome: Development and validation of a new measure. *Digestive Diseases and Sciences, 43*(2), 400–411. https://doi.org/10.1023/a:1018831127942

PDQ® Supportive and Palliative Care Editorial Board. (2004). *PDQ grief, bereavement, and coping with loss*. National Cancer Institute. https://www.cancer.gov/about-cancer/advanced-cancer/caregivers/planning/bereavement-hp-pdq

Peery, A. F., Crockett, S. D., Murphy, C. C., Jensen, E. T., Kim, H. P., Egberg, M. D., Lund, J. L., Moon, A. M., Pate, V., Barnes, E. L., Schlusser, C. L., Baron, T. H., Shaheen, N. J., & Sandler, R. S. (2022). Burden and cost of gastrointestinal, liver, and pancreatic diseases in the United States: Update 2021. *Gastroenterology, 162*(2), 621–644. https://doi.org/10.1053/j.gastro.2021.10.017

Perry, L., Morgan, J., Reid, F., Brunton, J., O'Brien, A., Luck, A., & Lacey, H. (2002). Screening for symptoms of eating disorders: Reliability of the SCOFF screening tool with written compared to oral delivery. *International Journal of Eating Disorders, 32*(4), 466–472. https://doi.org/10.1002/eat.10093

Petersen, R., Pan, L., & Blanck, H. M. (2019). Racial and ethnic disparities in adult obesity in the United States: CDC's tracking to inform state and local action. *Preventing Chronic Disease, 16*, E46. https://doi.org/10.5888/pcd16.180579

Polonsky, D. C. (2000). Premature ejaculation. In R. C. Rosen & S. R. Leiblum (Eds.), *Principles and practice of sex therapy* (3rd ed., pp. 305–332).

Prochaska, J. O., & Velicer, W. F. (1997). The transtheoretical model of health behavior change. *American Journal of Health Promotion, 12*(1), 38–48. https://doi.org/10.4278/0890-1171-12.1.38

Puhl, R. M., Peterson, J. L., & Luedicke, J. (2011). Parental perceptions of weight terminology that providers use with youth. *Pediatrics, 128*(4), e786–e793. https://doi.org/10.1542/peds.2010-3841

Qaseem, A., Kansagara, D., Forciea, M. A., Cooke, M., Denberg, T. D., & Clinical Guidelines Committee of the American College of Physicians. (2016). Management of chronic insomnia disorder in adults: A clinical practice guideline from the American College of Physicians. *Annals of Internal Medicine, 165*(2), 125–133. https://doi.org/10.7326/M15-2175

Ramlachan, P., & Naidoo, K. (2024). Enhancing sexual health in primary care: Guidance for practitioners. *South African Family Practice, 66*(1), 5822. https://doi.org/10.4102/safp.v66i1.5822

Recovery Record. (2024). *RR: Eating disorder management* (version 9.5.4) [Mobile app]. App store. https://apps.apple.com/us/app/rr-eating-disorder-management/id457360959

Remington, P. L., Brownson, R. C., & Centers for Disease Control and Prevention (CDC). (2011). Fifty years of progress in chronic disease epidemiology and control. *MMWR Supplements, 60*(4), 70–77.

Riba, M. B., Donovan, K. A., Andersen, B., Braun, I., Breitbart, W. S., Brewer, B. W., Buchmann, L. O., Clark, M. M., Collins, M., Corbett, C., Fleishman, S., Garcia, S., Greenberg, D. B., Handzo, G. F., Hoofring, L., Huang, C.-H., Lally, R., Martin, S., McGuffey, L., & Darlow, S. D. (2019). Distress management, version 3.2019. *Journal of the National Comprehensive Cancer Network, 17*(10), 1229–1249. https://doi.org/10.6004/jnccn.2019.0048

Rikard, S. M. (2023). Chronic pain among adults—United States, 2019–2021. *MMWR. Morbidity and Mortality Weekly Report, 72*. https://doi.org/10.15585/mmwr.mm7215a1

Robinson, P. J., Gould, D. A., & Strosahl, K. D. (2011). *Real behavior change in primary care: Improving patient outcomes & increasing job satisfaction*. New Harbinger Publications. https://www.newharbinger.com/9781626252035/real-behavior-change-in-primary-care

Rollnick, S., Miller, W. R., & Butler, C. C. (2022). *Motivational interviewing in health care: Helping people change behavior* (2nd ed.). Guilford Press. https://www.guilford.com/books/Motivational-Interviewing-in-Health-Care/Rollnick-Miller-Butler/9781462550371

Roohafza, H., Bidaki, E. Z., Hasanzadeh-Keshteli, A., Daghaghzade, H., Afshar, H., & Adibi, P. (2016). Anxiety, depression and distress among irritable bowel syndrome and their subtypes: An epidemiological population based study. *Advanced Biomedical Research, 5*(1), 183. https://doi.org/10.4103/2277-9175.190938

Rossman, J. (2019). Cognitive-behavioral therapy for insomnia: An effective and underutilized treatment for insomnia. *American Journal of Lifestyle Medicine, 13*(6), 544–547. https://doi.org/10.1177/1559827619867677

Ryan, K. L., Arbuckle-Bernstein, V., Smith, G., & Phillips, J. (2018). Let's talk about sex: A survey of patients' preferences when addressing sexual health concerns in a family medicine residency program office. *PRiMER: Peer-Review Reports in Medical Education Research, 2*, 23. https://doi.org/10.22454/PRiMER.2018.728252

Savoy, M., O'Gurek, D., & Brown-James, A. (2020). Sexual health history: Techniques and tips. *American Family Physician, 101*(5), 286–293.

Schaffer, S. D., & Yucha, C. B. (2004). Relaxation & pain management: The relaxation response can play a role in managing chronic and acute pain. *The American Journal of Nursing, 104*(8), 75. https://doi.org/10.1097/00000446-200408000-00044

Schulte, E. M., & Gearhardt, A. N. (2017). Development of the modified Yale Food addiction scale version 2.0. *European Eating Disorders Review: The Journal of the Eating Disorders Association, 25*(4), 302–308. https://doi.org/10.1002/erv.2515

Seamans, M. J., Robinson, W. R., Thorpe, R. J., Cole, S. R., & LaVeist, T. A. (2015). Exploring racial differences in the obesity gender gap. *Annals of Epidemiology, 25*(6), 420–425. https://doi.org/10.1016/j.annepidem.2015.03.010

Senthilvel, E., Auckley, D., & Dasarathy, J. (2011). Evaluation of sleep disorders in the primary care setting: History taking compared to questionnaires. *Journal of Clinical Sleep Medicine, 7*(1), 41–48.

Simmons, V. N., Piñeiro, B., Hooper, M. W., Gray, J. E., & Brandon, T. H. (2016). Tobacco-related health disparities across the cancer care continuum. *Cancer Control, 23*(4), 434–441. https://doi.org/10.1177/107327481602300415

Simpson, C. C., & Mazzeo, S. E. (2017). Calorie counting and fitness tracking technology: Associations with eating disorder symptomatology. *Eating Behaviors, 26*, 89–92. https://doi.org/10.1016/j.eatbeh.2017.02.002

Sirma Medical Systems. (2024). *Diabetes:M* (version 9.0.9) [Mobile app]. App Store. https://apps.apple.com/us/app/diabetes-m/id1196733537

Smith, G. F., & Toonen, T. R. (2007). Primary care of the patient with cancer. *American Family Physician, 75*(8), 1207–1214.

Sturgeon, J. A. (2014). Psychological therapies for the management of chronic pain. *Psychology Research and Behavior Management, 7*, 115–124. https://doi.org/10.2147/PRBM.S44762

Sweetman, A., Zwar, N. A., Grivell, N., Lovato, N., & Lack, L. (2021). A step-by-step model for a brief behavioural treatment for insomnia in Australian general practice. *Australian Journal of General Practice, 50*(5), 287–293. https://doi.org/10.31128/AJGP-04-20-5391

Szigethy, E. (2015). Hypnotherapy for inflammatory bowel disease across the lifespan. *American Journal of Clinical Hypnosis, 58*(1), 81–99. https://doi.org/10.1080/00029157.2015.1040112

Szigethy, E., Kenney, E., Carpenter, J., Hardy, D. M., Fairclough, D., Bousvaros, A., Keljo, D., Weisz, J., Beardslee, W. R., Noll, R., & DeMASO, D. R. (2007). Cognitive-behavioral therapy for adolescents with inflammatory bowel disease and subsyndromal depression. *Journal of the American Academy of Child & Adolescent Psychiatry, 46*(10), 1290–1298. https://doi.org/10.1097/chi.0b013e3180f6341f

Tam, J., Warner, K. E., & Meza, R. (2016). Smoking and the reduced life expectancy of individuals with serious mental illness. *American Journal of Preventive Medicine, 51*(6), 958–966. https://doi.org/10.1016/j.amepre.2016.06.007

Tatineny, P., Shafi, F., Gohar, A., & Bhat, A. (2020). Sleep in the elderly. *Missouri Medicine, 117*(5), 490–495.

Tavares, I. M., Moura, C. V., & Nobre, P. J. (2020). The role of cognitive processing factors in sexual function and dysfunction in women and men: A systematic review. *Sexual Medicine Reviews, 8*(3), 403–430. https://doi.org/10.1016/j.sxmr.2020.03.002

Taylor, B., & Davis, S. (2006). Using the extended PLISSIT model to address sexual healthcare needs. *Nursing Standard, 21*(11), 35.

Telch, M. J., & Pujols, Y. (2013). The erectile performance anxiety index: Scale development and psychometric properties. *The Journal of Sexual Medicine, 10*(12), 3019–3028. https://doi.org/10.1111/jsm.12305

Theodoulou, A., Chepkin, S. C., Ye, W., Fanshawe, T. R., Bullen, C., Hartmann-Boyce, J., Livingstone-Banks, J., Hajizadeh, A., & Lindson, N. (2023). Different doses, durations and modes of delivery of nicotine replacement therapy for smoking cessation. *Cochrane Database of Systematic Reviews, 6*(6). https://doi.org/10.1002/14651858.CD013308.pub2

Thompson, R. D., Craig, A., Crawford, E. A., Fairclough, D., Gonzalez-Heydrich, J., Bousvaros, A., Noll, R. B., DeMaso, D. R., & Szigethy, E. (2012). Longitudinal results of cognitive behavioral treatment for youths with inflammatory bowel disease and depressive symptoms. *Journal of Clinical Psychology in Medical Settings, 19*(3), 329–337. https://doi.org/10.1007/s10880-012-9301-8

Tobacco Use and Dependence Guideline Panel. (2008). A clinical practice guideline for treating tobacco use and dependence: 2008 update. *American Journal of Preventive Medicine, 35*(2), 158–176. https://doi.org/10.1016/j.amepre.2008.04.009

Tran, L., & Mulligan, K. (2019). A systematic review of self-management interventions for children and adolescents with inflammatory bowel disease. *Inflammatory Bowel Diseases, 25*(4), 685–698. https://doi.org/10.1093/ibd/izy299

Tresca, A. (2023). *Phone apps for managing IBS*. Verywell Health. https://www.verywellhealth.com/phone-apps-for-managing-ibs-5090428

Tribole, E., & Huber, H. (2021). *Intuitive eating: A revolutionary anti-diet approach* (4th ed.). https://www.blackstonelibrary.com/intuitive-eating-4th-edition?sp=175017

Tribole, E., & Resch, E. (2017). *The intuitive eating workbook: Ten principles for nourishing a healthy relationship with food*. New Harbinger Publications. https://www.newharbinger.com/9781626256231/the-intuitive-eating-workbook
Troxel, W. M., Germain, A., & Buysse, D. J. (2012). Clinical management of insomnia with brief behavioral treatment (BBTI). *Behavioral Sleep Medicine, 10*(4), 266–279. https://doi.org/10.1080/15402002.2011.607200
U.S. Department of Health and Human Services. (2020). *Smoking cessation: A report of the surgeon general*. US Department of Health and Human Services. https://www.ncbi.nlm.nih.gov/books/NBK555596/table/ch6.tab2/
U.S. Department of Health and Human Services, Centers for Disease Control and Prevention, & National Cancer Institute. (2024). *U.S. cancer statistics data visualizations tool* [Dataset]. https://www.cdc.gov/cancer/dataviz
U.S. Department of Veterans Affairs. (2024a). *Pain coach* [Mobile app]. https://apps.apple.com/us/app/pain-coach-by-va/id6447589030
U.S. Department of Veterans Affairs. (2024b). *CBT-I coach*. (version 3.1.2) [Mobile app]. App Store. https://apps.apple.com/us/app/cbt-i-coach/id655918660
U.S. Food and Drug Administration. (2018). *Smoking—Medicines to help you quit*. Food and Drug Administration Office of Women's Health. https://www.fda.gov/consumers/womens-health-topics/smoking-medicines-help-you-quit
United States Preventative Services Task Force. (2021). *Tobacco smoking cessation in adults, including pregnant persons: Interventions*. United States Preventative Services Task Force.
Van Dyke, N., & Drinkwater, E. J. (2014). Relationships between intuitive eating and health indicators: Literature review. *Public Health Nutrition, 17*(8), 1757–1766. https://doi.org/10.1017/S1368980013002139
Van Frank, B., Malarcher, A., Cornelius, M. E., Schecter, A., Jamal, A., & Tynan, M. (2024). Adult smoking cessation—United States, 2022. *Morbidity and Mortality Weekly Report (MMWR), 73*(29), 633–641. https://doi.org/10.15585/mmwr.mm7329a1
van Tilburg, M. A. L., Palsson, O. S., & Whitehead, W. E. (2013). Which psychological factors exacerbate irritable bowel syndrome? Development of a comprehensive model. *Journal of Psychosomatic Research, 74*(6), 486–492. https://doi.org/10.1016/j.jpsychores.2013.03.004
van't Riet, J., & Ruiter, R. A. C. (2013). Defensive reactions to health-promoting information: An overview and implications for future research. *Health Psychology Review, 7*(sup1), S104–S136. https://doi.org/10.1080/17437199.2011.606782
Velanovich, V. (2007). The development of the GERD-HRQL symptom severity instrument. *Diseases of the Esophagus, 20*(2), 130–134. https://doi.org/10.1111/j.1442-2050.2007.00658.x
Velligan, D. I., Weiden, P. J., Sajatovic, M., Scott, J., Carpenter, D., Ross, R., & Docherty, J. P. (2010). Strategies for addressing adherence problems in patients with serious and persistent mental illness: Recommendations from the expert consensus guidelines. *Journal of Psychiatric Practice, 16*(5), 306–324. https://doi.org/10.1097/01.pra.0000388626.98662.a0
Veteran Affairs National Center for PTSD. (2024). *Mindfulness coach* (version 2.8) [Mobile App]. App Store. https://apps.apple.com/us/app/mindfulness-coach/id804284729
Vlaeyen, J. W. S., & Linton, S. J. (2000). Fear-avoidance and its consequences in chronic musculoskeletal pain: A state of the art. *Pain, 85*(3), 317. https://doi.org/10.1016/S0304-3959(99)00242-0
Walker, J., Muench, A., Perlis, M. L., & Vargas, I. (2022). Cognitive behavioral therapy for insomnia (CBT-I): A primer. *Clinical Psychology and Special Education, 11*(2), 123–137. https://doi.org/10.17759/cpse.2022110208
Warren, J. M., Smith, N., & Ashwell, M. (2017). A structured literature review on the role of mindfulness, mindful eating and intuitive eating in changing eating behaviours: Effectiveness and associated potential mechanisms. *Nutrition Research Reviews, 30*(2), 272–283. https://doi.org/10.1017/S0954422417000154
Weir, K. (2022). Diagnosing and treating sleep disorders. *Monitor on Psychology, 53*(5). https://www.apa.org/monitor/2022/07/ce-sleep-disorders

Wilkinson, A. N. (2021). Cancer diagnosis in primary care. *Canadian Family Physician, 67*(4), 265–268. https://doi.org/10.46747/cfp.6704265

Wolfgang, K. M., Takeshita, J., Fitzsimmons, R., & Guerra, C. E. (2022). The association between sexual orientation, BMI, obesity diagnosis, and provider recommendation for weight management. *BMC Women's Health, 22*(1), 19. https://doi.org/10.1186/s12905-021-01585-x

Yamamoto, M., Lim, C. T., Huang, H., Spottswood, M., & Huang, H. (2023). Insomnia in primary care: Considerations for screening, assessment, and management. *The Journal of Medicine Access, 7*, 27550834231156727. https://doi.org/10.1177/27550834231156727

Zhang, Y., Ren, R., Yang, L., Zhang, H., Shi, Y., Okhravi, H. R., Vitiello, M. V., Sanford, L. D., & Tang, X. (2022). Sleep in Alzheimer's disease: A systematic review and meta-analysis of polysomnographic findings. *Translational Psychiatry, 12*, 136. https://doi.org/10.1038/s41398-022-01897-y

Zimmerman, G. L., Olsen, C. G., & Bosworth, M. F. (2000). A 'stages of change' approach to helping patients change behavior. *American Family Physician, 61*(5), 1409–1416.

Chapter 10
Treatment of Substance Use Disorders in Primary Care

Matthew P. Martin PhD, MS, LMFT, Corina Marshall MD, FAAFP, Michelle Nanda MD, MPH, FAAFP, and Randi Sokol MD, MPH, MMedEd

The Role of Primary Care in Addiction Management

Primary care providers (PCP) are well positioned to identify and treat all substance use disorders (SUD) (Saitz & Daaleman, 2017). Like treating other chronic conditions (e.g., diabetes or heart disease), PCPs should utilize a comprehensive approach that includes both pharmacological options and behavioral support. Ideally, PCPs should be part of an integrated, multidisciplinary team of healthcare professionals who provide comprehensive, continuous, accessible, and coordinated SUD management over a patients' lifetime, supporting them during the "ups" and "downs" of their recovery journey. While this is not always the case, there are still many ways in which the PCP is integral to providing care for patients who struggle with substance use disorders.

Becoming More Involved in Addiction Management PCPs may hesitate to provide or expand SUD treatment for several reasons. Some might feel inadequately equipped to manage complex cases or unfamiliar with current treatment protocols. Others may be affected by unconscious bias toward patients with SUDs. Commonly used terms in medical documentation such as "drug-seeking" and "addict" can

M. P. Martin PhD, MS, LMFT (✉)
Arizona State University College of Health Solutions, Phoenix, AZ, USA
e-mail: matthew.perry.martin@asu.edu

C. Marshall MD, FAAFP · M. Nanda MD, MPH, FAAFP
Guthrie Medical Group, Sayre, PA, USA
e-mail: corina.marshall@guthrie.org

M. Nanda MD, MPH, FAAFP
e-mail: michelle.nanda@guthrie.org

R. Sokol MD, MPH, MMedEd
Tufts Department of Family Medicine, Somerville, MA, USA
e-mail: rsokol@challiance.org

M. L. C. Williamson and D. L. Terry (eds.), *Essentials for Treating Behavioral Health in Primary Care*, https://doi.org/10.1007/978-3-032-09558-9_10

perpetuate such bias. Mentorship, training, and consultation with addiction treatment specialists can increase PCP comfort with providing care for SUDs. We have provided a list of resources at the end of this chapter for further training and support.

Limited exposure to patients with SUD can skew PCP perspective. For example, some clinicians may primarily see hospitalized patients who are actively using substances and are at "rock bottom," suffering the consequences of recent use. Seeing patients in successful recovery in the outpatient setting can broaden a PCPs perspective and generate positive feelings as patients transform their lives (i.e., gaining employment, caring for children, saving money, developing consistent healthy habits). Another solution is for PCPs to spend time with peer recovery support specialists who are lay individuals trained to use their addiction and recovery experiences to teach and support others.

There are logistical and resource challenges. Addiction treatment often requires frequent visits and close monitoring, which can be difficult to squeeze into busy clinic schedules. Many practices lack the necessary support staff, such as addiction counselors or social workers, to effectively manage addiction and its psychosocial comorbidities. In communities with limited healthcare services, PCPs may need to develop additional skills, integrate with other health professionals, and/or identify additional resources to meet patients' behavioral health (BH) and SDOH (social determinants of health) needs. However, lack of resources should not preclude care: Any treatment offered to patients is better than no treatment at all, including expressions of emotional support and empathy. The goal for PCPs managing addiction in primary care should be to view addiction as a chronic condition with medical and psychosocial components and seek to provide continuous, team-based, patient-centered, and holistic care to the fullest extent that matches available resources.

Understanding Addiction Addiction is a chronic brain disorder characterized by compulsive drug seeking and use, despite negative consequences. Over time, the brain adjusts to the substance and requires that substance just to achieve a normal level of contentment or pleasure. Meanwhile, the brain's response to typical stimuli is diminished, meaning a hug from a family member or a favorite food no longer produces a positive response. Addiction knows no boundaries—affecting people of all sociodemographic, ethnic, gender, and age groups. Additionally, each addiction origin and journey is different. There are many factors that can play a role:

(a) *Genetics* can predispose a patient to addiction; those with a family history are much more likely to be susceptible to developing addiction.
(b) *Starting young:* Adolescent brains are especially vulnerable due to ongoing development in both reward and decision-making areas.
(c) *Behavioral Health*: Patients with BH struggles like anxiety or depression may use drugs to self-medicate negative emotions. Personality traits like impulsivity, a desire for new experiences, or low self-esteem can make someone more susceptible. Certain cognitive biases can distort thinking, leading to underestimating risks or overestimating control over drug use.

(d) *Environment ("people, places, and things")*: Surrounding oneself with people who use drugs can normalize and encourage such behavior. Factors like poverty, lack of opportunity, and exposure to violence within one's socioeconomic environment can increase vulnerability. By understanding the complex interplay of biopsychosocial factors that contribute to addiction, PCPs can offer effective and evidence-based treatment strategies to promote long-term recovery.

Diagnosing Addiction PCPs can leverage BH screening methods to effectively diagnose SUDs. Substance use screening should be brief, simple, and easy to integrate into routine visits. Examples of tools include AUDIT-C, DAST-10, ASSIST, and the NIDA SISQ (see Table 10.1). Ideally, support staff should administer the screening while the PCP reviews and interprets the score to the patient. When available, SUD assessment might include an in-depth exploration of a patient's substance use history and its impact on their life. The DSM-5-TR (*Diagnostic and Statistical Manual of Mental Disorders, Fifth Edition*) lists diagnostic criteria for substance use disorders. A shortened way of identifying addiction is that, in addition to having physiological symptoms (tolerance and withdrawal), patients also meet the 4 C's (Jovey, 2012; see Table 10.2).

Substance Use Disorders and Behavioral Health SUDs and BH disorders frequently co-occur, creating a complex dynamic that can each worsen symptoms of the other (see Box 10.1; National Institute on Drug Abuse (NIDA), 2023). Conditions like anxiety disorders (panic disorder, generalized anxiety disorder, and PTSD) are commonly diagnosed alongside SUDs. Conversely, individuals with BH disorders such as depression, bipolar disorder, psychotic disorders, personality disorders, and schizophrenia are also at a significantly higher risk of developing SUDs. A particularly strong association exists between post-traumatic stress disorder (PTSD) and SUDs (see Box 10.2). The trauma associated with PTSD can significantly increase a person's vulnerability to developing an SUD at some point in their life. Individuals with trauma history are more likely to have a SUD compared to those without one.

Box 10.1 Behavioral Health or Substance Use: Which Patient Need Should I Address?

Providers often ask: Can I treat a BH problem if a patient has an SUD, or should I treat the SUD first?
Sometimes it's unclear whether a patient has a primary BH condition, or the BH condition is the result of the SUD. A careful assessment can determine which condition is primary and which is secondary.
PCPs should treat both conditions at the same time. After patients are stable in recovery, the patient and PCP may decide together to taper off and stop any medication for BH conditions.

Table 10.1 Common substance use screening tools

Name	Substance (time)	Description
AUDIT-C (alcohol use disorders identification test—concise)	Alcohol (1–2 min)	This 3-question tool is a quick and easy way to identify risky alcohol use in adults. It asks about frequency of drinking, typical amount consumed on a single occasion, and the frequency of exceeding recommended drinking limits
DAST-10 (drug Abuse screening test)	Drugs and alcohol (2–3 minutes)	This 10-question tool screens for various substance use disorders, including alcohol, illicit drugs, and prescription medications. It asks about frequency of use, cravings, and negative consequences related to substance use
S2BI (short screening for Behavioral interventions)	Drugs and alcohol (2–3 min)	This web-based 6-question tool for adolescents and young adults screens for both alcohol and drug use, as well as depression and risky sexual behavior. It asks about frequency of use, cravings, and risky behaviors associated with substance use
ASSIST (alcohol, smoking and substance involvement screening test)	Multiple (5–10 minutes)	This 8-item core module with optional additional questions screens for alcohol, tobacco, and illicit drug use. It asks about frequency and amount of use, as well as related problems
CRAFFT 2.0 (car, relax, alone, forget, friends, and trouble)	Drug and alcohol (5–10 min)	This 6-item tool screens adolescents for high-risk alcohol and drug use behaviors. A total score of 2 or higher suggests the need for a more comprehensive assessment

Table 10.2 4 C's of addiction and patient interview questions

Craving	"In the past month, how often did you experience strong urges or cravings to use [substance]?" (e.g., alcohol, cigarettes, etc.)
Compulsivity	"Do you feel like you sometimes can't resist using [substance], even if you want to stop?"
Loss of control	"How confident are you in your ability to control your use of [substance] right now?" (use a scale of 1–10, with 1 being not confident and 10 being very confident)
Consequences	"Has your use of [substance] caused any problems in your life, such as health issues, work difficulties, or relationship problems?"

Note: While these screening tools are a helpful reference, PCPs can also make a diagnosis without administering a formalized tool. If you recognize that a patient is using substances illicitly (from the street) and/or substances are consuming their lives (interfering in their daily function), you can make a diagnosis of SUD

Box 10.2 How Do I Ask About Trauma History?

Primary care providers should routinely ask patients with a SUD about trauma.
"I want to understand your health and wellbeing as best as possible. Have you ever experienced trauma, including physical, emotional, or sexual abuse? How have these experiences affected your life, if at all"
Maintain a non-judgmental and supportive environment. Validate the patient's experience, even if they don't disclose specific details. Provide resources or referrals for mental health professionals specializing in trauma

Non-pharmacological Substance Use Disorder Treatment, Patient Engagement, Harm Reduction

For all substance use disorders (SUDs), non-pharmacological treatments are considered the cornerstone of care (see Table 10.3). These interventions address the underlying behavioral and psychological aspects of addiction.

Community Resource Inventory Develop a comprehensive list of non-pharmacological treatment options available in your community. This could include resources like:

- Individual and group therapy.
- Behavioral therapies (CBT, DBT, etc.).

Table 10.3 Non-pharmacological treatment

Psychological and support services
• Individual or group psychotherapy (CBT, mindfulness) • 12 step meetings (AA/NA) + smart recovery (based on CBT rather than spiritual focus) • Other community-based groups (ex: Local community centers, church/mosque/temple) • Sponsor or recovery coach • Community reinforcement approach: Help support job training, education, relationship counseling • Exercise/hobbies/volunteering • Residential living: Halfway house, sober house
Higher levels of care
• Detox (medically managed withdrawal): Usually a 3–5 day stay coupled with 1–3 month inpatient stay (CSS/TSS) • Intensive outpatient program/IOP or partial hospitalization program/PHP: Usually meets 3–5 days/week, last ~1 month

- Support groups (12-step programs, SMART Recovery, etc.)—There are numerous virtual groups that are free and easily accessible to patients, regardless of where they live. You can do a "google search" to find available programs.
- Recovery coaching.
- Vocational rehabilitation programs.

Warm Handoffs and Care Coordination If recovery coaches or BH providers are available onsite, facilitate warm handoffs to these professionals. This smooth transition ensures continuity of care and connects patients with additional support.

Navigating Higher Levels of Care Moving to a more intensive level of care (inpatient or outpatient programs) often requires navigating insurance and healthcare systems. Here's how to support your patients:

- Partner with recovery coaches, social workers, and case managers to assist patients with insurance and healthcare system complexities.
- Help patients understand their treatment options and guide them through the referral process.

Meeting Patient Needs Remember, the goal is to offer patients the highest level of care they are willing to accept and can realistically participate in. Effective communication and collaboration can help patients access the non-pharmacological interventions that form the foundation of successful SUD treatment.

Patient Engagement and Relapse Prevention PCPs can play a vital role in engaging patients with SUDs in treatment using the following approaches.

1. Building rapport and empathy
   (a) *Create a safe and welcoming environment.* A judgment-free atmosphere encourages patients to feel comfortable opening up about their struggles.
   (b) *Active listening.* Pay close attention to what patients say and what they don't say. Validate their experiences and concerns.
   (c) *Focus on the person, not the addiction.* Remember, the patient is not defined by their SUD. Treat them with respect and compassion.
2. Motivational Interviewing
   (a) *Use open-ended questions.* Help patients explore their ambivalence about change and build intrinsic motivation to seek treatment.
   (b) *Affirm their strengths.* Acknowledge their efforts and past successes, no matter how small.
   (c) *Focus on collaboration.* Work together with the patient to develop a treatment plan that aligns with their goals and preferences.
3. Matching patients with the right treatment
   (a) *Assess individual needs.* Consider the specific substance involved, severity of SUD, co-occurring BH conditions, and patient preferences.

(b) *Offer a range of treatment options.* This might include medication-assisted treatment (MAT), behavioral therapy, support groups, or a combination approach.
(c) *Connect patients with appropriate resources.* Provide referrals to specialists, support groups, or treatment centers based on their needs.

4. Using non-stigmatizing language
   (a) *Avoid judgmental terms.* Instead of "addict" or "alcoholic," use terms like "person with a substance use disorder."
   (b) *Focus on behavior, not labels.* Talk about "substance use" or "misuse" rather than attaching labels to the patient.
   (c) *Emphasize recovery potential.* Frame treatment as a path toward improvement and a healthier life.

Supporting Patients in Relapse Prevention Relapse is a common occurrence in the recovery journey from SUDs. PCPs can play a vital role in supporting patients by understanding and preventing relapse triggers and developing personalized relapse prevention strategies and contingency plans. Celebrate small wins, be patient with setbacks, and encourage continued effort. Reassure patients the relapse is part of the recovery journey.

Harm Reduction in Primary Care: A Practical Approach

Harm reduction is a philosophy and set of strategies that aim to minimize the negative consequences associated with drug use, focusing on safety and well-being rather than abstinence as the sole goal (Bartlett et al., 2013). This approach can be effective in primary care settings.

Core Principles of Harm Reduction:

- *Meeting people where they are*: Acknowledges that not everyone is ready or able to stop using substances completely.
- *Emphasis on safety:* Prioritizes strategies to reduce risks associated with drug use, like overdose prevention.
- *Respect for autonomy:* Empowers individuals to make informed choices about their health and drug use.
- *Connection to care:* Provides a bridge to connect people with healthcare services and potential treatment pathways when they are ready.

Harm Reduction Strategies:

- *Screening and assessment:* Identify individuals at risk for substance use complications and tailor interventions accordingly.

- *Naloxone distribution*: Equipping patients, friends and family with naloxone, a medication that reverses opioid overdose and save lives.
- *Safe injection practices*: Use a safe injection site where available or only use with a companion who can contact emergency services and/or administer naloxone.
- *Syringe service programs (SSPs)*: Providing sterile syringes and safe disposal options prevents the spread of bloodborne diseases associated with injection drug use.
- *Vaccination*: Offering vaccinations against Hepatitis A and B, common among people who use drugs, protects their health.
- *Wound care and infection prevention*: Addressing skin and injection-related infections can prevent serious health complications.
- *Motivational interviewing*: Encouraging patients to explore their goals and ambivalence about behavior change can motivate them to consider reducing drug use or seeking treatment.
- *Referral to addiction specialists*: Connecting patients with appropriate treatment resources when they are interested in reducing use or quitting altogether.

Benefits of Harm Reduction in Primary Care:

- Reduces overdose deaths and associated healthcare costs.
- Improves public health outcomes by preventing infectious diseases.
- Builds trust with patients who may be hesitant to seek traditional treatment.
- Opens the door for future conversations about reducing use or quitting.

Harm reduction is not condoning drug use, but rather a pragmatic approach to minimizing risks and promoting overall well-being for people who use substances. By incorporating these strategies, PCPs can expand their toolkit for addressing SUDs and improve patient outcomes.

Pharmacological Management of Specific Substance use Disorders

For all SUDs, effective treatment includes both pharmacological and non-pharmacological approaches, though the evidence for each varies and is ever-evolving, as discussed in more detail below.

Opioid Use Disorder

Medications are the gold standard for treating opioid use disorder (OUD). These medications, known as medication-assisted treatment (MAT) or medication for opioid use disorder (MOUD), include methadone, buprenorphine-naloxone

(Suboxone), and Naltrexone (Substance Abuse and Mental Health Services Administration (SAMHSA), 2019, 2021). Highly effective, MOUD significantly reduces mortality rates by more than threefold. Relapse rates are high without MOUD. Studies show that 90% of patients who start MOUD and then taper off relapse within 3 months (Tuten et al., 2012). However, with long-term MOUD maintenance, roughly 50% of patients are still in recovery after a year. Psychotherapy, while valuable, is not mandatory for MOUD. Some research suggests that buprenorphine-naloxone alone can be sufficient treatment, with minimal additional benefit from psychotherapy. Reflecting this evidence, recent federal guidelines no longer require methadone clinics to provide psychotherapy alongside methadone treatment.

Choosing the Right Medication While various algorithms can help determine the best medication for OUD, a patient's preference should also be a key factor (Lee et al., 2018; Potter et al., 2013). Often, patients have knowledge about treatment options (from personal experience or through friends and family) and may have a strong preference for a specific medication, so simply asking them what medication they prefer can help identify where to start. You should also help them identify non-pharmacological strategies that can support their recovery (see Box 10.3).

Box 10.3 How Can I Better Engage Patients?

Recovery is a journey with setbacks. By revisiting past periods of sobriety, we remind patients of their inner strength and capacity for change. These reminders strengthen self-efficacy, the belief in their ability to achieve their goals. A strong sense of self-efficacy is crucial for staying engaged in treatment. Discussing past victories reminds patients that recovery is possible. This renewed sense of hope fuels their commitment to stay on track

Clinician: "What was your longest period of sobriety? What treatment were you using then (e.g., MOUD, meetings, sponsor, counseling)? What else helped you succeed in the past?"

Similar Effectiveness, Different Initiation All three medications—methadone, buprenorphine-naloxone (B/N; brand name: Suboxone), and Naltrexone—offer similar effectiveness in treating OUD once a patient is stabilized on the medication (Fiellin et al., 2014; Weiss & Rao, 2017). However, Naltrexone can be trickier to initiate because it requires the patient to be opioid-free for at least 7 days beforehand.

Goal of Medication The goal of all three medications is to help patients achieve a sense of normalcy, allowing them to manage daily activities, work, and home life responsibilities without feeling high or sedated (Martin et al., 2018; Mintzer et al., 2007; National Institute on Drug Abuse (NIDA), 2019; RxList, 2019). The medications achieve this by normalizing the body's response to opioids (see Table 10.4).

Table 10.4 Overview of different medications for opioid use, misuse

	Buprenorphine-naloxone (B/N)	Methadone	Naltrexone
Action on mu receptor	Partial agonist	Full agonist	Antagonist
Typical maintenance dose, route	Tablet or film (brand names: Suboxone, Zubsolv): 16–24 mg daily SL (of the buprenorphine component) or Monthly injection (Sublocade or Brixadi)	80–120 mg daily PO (liquid)	50–100 mg daily PO 380 mg IM/monthly
Safety profile	Ceiling effect which limits resp. depression Few drug-drug interactions	Resp depression QT prolongation Multiple drug-drug interactions	7-day minimum opioid washout period before starting
Availability	Any prescriber with a DEA license (no longer need X waiver)	OTP ('methadone clinic') only Daily observed administration Can earn take-homes	No restrictions on prescribing
Who is it best for?	Anyone Convenience of primary care Does well with weekly-monthly rx	Anyone People who need structure, accountability NB: Associated with stigma	Anyone High accountability jobs (e.g., doctors, pilots) Coming from opioid-naive setting (e.g., prison, long hospital stay)

Starting MOUD (Inductions)

- *Methadone*: Methadone can only be started at a federally licensed opioid treatment programs (OTP; methadone clinic) or in the hospital. After starting, the OTP will gradually titrate up the medication until the patient no-longer experiences cravings and is not sedated. While methadone can be prescribed for pain, it cannot be used in primary care for OUD. To find a local OTP by geographic region, visit SAMHSA's website "opioid treatment program directory."
- *Buprenorphine-naloxone (B/N)*: Usually, the patient needs to be in withdrawal as measured by the Clinical Opiate Withdrawal Scale (Wesson & Ling, 2003; COWS >8) before starting B/N or the patient could experience precipitated withdrawal (if they cannot tolerate this, see micro-induction protocol below). A patient who experiences precipitated withdrawals should be given additional doses of B/N to overcome the withdrawals. Below are three B/N induction protocols.

Buprenorphine/Naloxone (B/N) Standard Induction

- *Best suited for*: Patients who ONLY have short-acting opioids in their system (including oxycodone, hydrocodone, morphine, or tramadol). If they are using street drugs, it likely is contaminated with fentanyl, so this induction strategy might not work.
- *How it works*: The patient is started on a medium dose of B/N and ramped up to a therapeutic dose within 1–2 days.

Example protocol: Once a patient scores >8 on COWS, administer 8 mg of B/N. If symptoms of withdrawal persist after 2–4 h, administer additional 4 mg dose. Day 2 administer total dose from previous day in single dose. If symptoms persist after 2–4 h, administer additional 4 mg dose. Continue until patient no longer experiences symptoms or cravings. Each day thereafter, give a therapeutic maintenance dose up to 32 mg q AM.

Buprenorphine/Naloxone (B/N) Micro-Induction:

- *Best suited for*: Patients who do not want to experience ANY withdrawal symptoms (e.g., previous experience of precipitated withdrawal) and can follow a long protocol that takes up to 2 weeks to complete and often requires provider support. This protocol is also recommended for patients who are switching from methadone to B/N.
- *How it works*: The patient is cross tapered from a full opioid agonist while being given small doses of Buprenorphine that increase over time (see Table 10.5).

Buprenorphine/Naloxone (B/N) Macro-Induction:

- *Best suited for*: Patients who have fentanyl in their system (whether using fentanyl directly or other products—even cannabis—laced with fentanyl; check UDS). While fentanyl is short-acting, its lipophilic nature makes it stick around in the

Table 10.5 Example of buprenorphine micro-induction

Day	Bup/nx (only list bup dose)	Other opioid
1	0.5 mg qd	Usual (methadone/fentanyl/oxycodone)
2	0.5 mg bid	Usual (methadone/fentanyl/oxycodone)
3	0.5 mg bid	Usual (methadone/fentanyl/oxycodone)
4	1 mg bid	LESS than usual, if possible
5	1 mg tid	None
6	2 mg tid	None
7	4 mg tid	None
8	8 mg bid	None
9	16 mg qd	None

body for a long time. Hence, patients attempting to use standard B/N induction protocols can precipitate withdrawal because they still have fentanyl in their system.

- *How it works*: Patients receive large amounts of B/N at once; any precipitated withdrawal that occurs is "rescued" by more B/N 1 h later. Because of B/N's ceiling effect for respiratory depression and sedation, this method is considered safe. It also allows the patient to reach a therapeutic dose of B/N within 1 h.
- *Example of a protocol*: Once the patient is feeling uncomfortable (are already in some withdrawal; and for fentanyl, they last used ~24–48 h ago), give 16 mg B/N. If they are still feeling uncomfortable 1 h later, give another 8–16 mg (for a total of 32 mg on induction day); each day thereafter, give a therapeutic maintenance dose of 16–24 mg q AM.

B/N Therapeutic Dose Withdrawal suppression occurs when >50% opioid receptors are occupied (>4 mg B/N/day). Blockade of subjective opioid effects (cravings) requires >80% occupancy (16 mg/ B/N day) and may require >90% occupancy (up to 32 mg/day) in the fentanyl era. Patients should be maintained on 16–32 mg/day to minimize cravings (unless they tell you they feel sedated on that dose). These higher doses likely increase retention in treatment and decrease illicit drug use. Remember: we are not trying to limit B/N dosing: If a patient reports they have cravings at their current dose, increase the dose.

Patient Instructions or "Rule of 15"

- Encourage patients to avoid eating, drinking, and smoking 15 min before taking.
- Let B/N dissolve under the tongue for 15 min (do not swallow).
- Avoid eating, drinking, and smoking 15 min after taking.

Alcohol Use Disorder

While medication plays a vital role in treating OUD, the evidence supporting its use for alcohol use disorder (AUD) is less conclusive (Jonas et al., 2014; Myrick et al., 2009; National Institute on Alcohol Abuse and Alcoholism (NIAAA), 2005). Non-pharmacological (behavioral) therapies remain the cornerstone of AUD treatment (Anton et al., 2006). The choice of medication depends on a patient's goal (i.e., reducing alcohol consumption or complete abstinence). The FDA has approved three medications specifically for AUD.

Naltrexone This medication has the strongest evidence base and can help people drink less overall (Springer & Bisaga, 2018; Substance Abuse and Mental Health Services Administration (SAMHSA), 2009). It's important to note that Naltrexone doesn't prevent drinking entirely. Start the dose at 25 or 50 mg/day. Can take up to 100 mg qd if needed. Check a urine drug screen (UDS) and ensure no opioids before prescribing. Naltrexone is also available in a long-acting depot formulation (brand name Vivitrol). Once you confirm a patient can tolerate Naltrexone orally, they can be transitioned to this injectable formulation. Dosing is 380 mg once monthly by IM injection and can be administered by a nurse or provider. The patient will continue to take the oral formulation until the day of administration. Vivitrol coverage is variable with different insurances, and cost/lack of insurance coverage is the biggest barrier to use. Vivitrol has a program to help with copays and submitting to insurance.

Acamprosate This medication helps people who have already quit drinking to stay abstinent; it minimizes the prolonged withdrawal after cessation. However, it must be taken three times a day (TID). The dosing is 666 mg TID, or 333 mg TID for patients with moderate CKD (eGFR <60; do not prescribe if GFR is less than 30).

Disulfiram (Antabuse) This medication deters impulsive drinking by causing unpleasant side effects if alcohol is consumed. It requires strict adherence and avoiding all products containing alcohol, even some medications, mouthwashes, or hand sanitizers. For optimal effectiveness, some patients benefit from having a trusted friend or family member oversee the medication administration. Because it causes such unpleasant side effects, it is less commonly being utilized.

Two medications, not FDA approved for AUD, but increasingly being utilized “off-label” include:

Topiramate. While the United States Department of Veterans Affairs (VA) recommends it as a first-line option, topiramate can have significant side effects that may prevent patients from reaching an effective dose for reducing alcohol use. The dosing is gradually titrated up from 25–50 mg/day (weekly by 25–50 mg increments) to 300 mg/day.

Gabapentin. This medication can help manage cravings and withdrawal symptoms and can potentially be continued after detoxification if needed. However, due to its high potential for abuse, it’s not considered a first-line treatment for AUD. This is dosed 600 mg BID to TID, titrated up over days to weeks.

The best medication for a patient depends on their individual goals and circumstances. Open communication with the patient is essential to determine the most appropriate treatment approach.

Stimulant Use Disorder

Stimulant use disorders, specifically involving methamphetamine and cocaine, can manifest in various patterns, ranging from daily use to intermittent episodes or binges. Initially, these stimulants can improve mood, concentration, and focus. However, with continued use, they can lead to a range of negative health consequences, including:

- Elevated blood pressure (hypertension).
- Rapid heart rate (tachycardia).

- Seizures.
- Chest pain.
- Paranoia.
- Psychosis.

Treatment of Stimulant Withdrawal Symptoms Discontinuing stimulant use can trigger withdrawal symptoms like depression, anxiety, insomnia, and paranoia. These symptoms can persist for weeks or even months. Early identification and management of withdrawal symptoms can reduce the risk of relapse (returning to stimulant use) and promote long-term recovery (Substance Abuse and Mental Health Services Administration (SAMHSA), 2018).

Acute Management of Stimulant Intoxication Stimulant intoxication, also known as "overamping," typically occurs after extended periods with little to no eating, drinking, or sleeping. This can lead to a state of paranoia and delusions. The primary focus of managing acute stimulant intoxication involves creating a calm and low-stimulation environment. This allows the patient to rest, rehydrate, and receive nourishment. Physical restraints are not recommended in this situation. In some cases, medication might be necessary to manage agitation or psychotic symptoms.

- *For agitation/discomfort.* Benzodiazepines, such as Lorazepam (2–4 mg IV/IM every 10–15 min, up to a total of 8 mg) or Midazolam (2–5 mg IV/IM/IN every 5–15 min, up to a total of 10 mg), can be used to promote calmness.
- *For psychosis.* If the patient becomes psychotic, antipsychotics like Haloperidol (5 mg IV/IM, repeated in 10 minutes, up to a total of 10 mg) or Olanzapine (5–10 mg IM, repeated every 120 min, up to a total of 20 mg) might be administered.

Chronic Stimulant Use The cornerstone of long-term management for chronic stimulant use disorder is psychosocial treatment, using various approaches such as cognitive behavioral therapy, motivational interviewing and enhancement treatment, and community reinforcement approach. There is substantial evidence for the benefits of contingency management for stimulant use disorders.

Box 10.4 What Is Contingency Management?

Contingency Management, an evidence-based intervention, uses principles of operant conditioning (Carroll et al., 2012; Litt et al., 2013). Patients receive rewards (positive reinforcement) for achieving desired behaviors (e.g., negative urine drug screens) and may face consequences (negative reinforcement) for undesired behaviors (e.g., positive urine drug screens). A common example is a "fishbowl" system, where patients can earn entries for negative tests, with the chance to win prizes. While some view this as "bribing" patients, it has strong evidence for promoting long-term abstinence.

While psychosocial interventions are the mainstay of treatment for stimulant use disorder, there are a few medications that hold promise though they lack strong scientific support, and none are FDA approved.

For methamphetamine use disorder:

(a) *Mirtazepine.* 15 mg qd × 1 week, increase to 30 mg qd; cannot be stopped abruptly/need to taper; avoid if concurrent MAOi, renal failure (eGFR <40), severe liver disease; check baseline LFTs and renal function; risk for serotonin syndrome, QTc prolongation.
(b) *Injectable Naltrexone + Bupropion.* 380 mg IM Naltrexone q 3 weeks +450 mg PO bupropion; avoid if concurrent OUD or need for opioid medications, severe liver disease.

For cocaine use disorder:

(a) *Topiramate.* 50 mg PO BID titrating weekly by 50 mg to reach a max tolerated dose or up to 150 mg BID cannot be stopped abruptly, need to taper. Avoid if renal impairment, glaucoma, pregnancy, TBI/memory impairment. Check drug interactions. Can cause dizziness, weight loss, depression, mental slowing.
(b) *Extended release mixed amphetamine salts (like brand names Adderall XR and Vyvanse).* 60–80 mg qd. Best for patients with attention-deficit/hyperactivity disorder (ADHD) and cocaine use disorder; do NOT use in patients with methamphetamine use disorder (could cause psychosis), uncontrolled HTN, cardiovascular disease, or hyperthyroidism. Avoid with serotonergic meds, TCAs. SE include weight loss, dry mouth, h/a, jitteriness/anxiety, cardiac overstimulation. Monitor HR and BP.

You can also combine topiramate and XR mixed amphetamine salts. For patients using cocaine or meth (who do not yet have fentanyl in their UDS), you can provide them daily oral Naltrexone to prevent opioid overdose, since cocaine and meth are often laced with fentanyl.

Patients often complain of concentration problems and may report using cocaine to self-medicate ADHD. They may request prescribed stimulants, and providers may thus find themselves in a challenging situation (see Box 10.3).

Box 10.5 How Do I Help Patients Who Use Stimulants and Request ADHD Treatment?

"Do I potentially treat a patient's ADHD properly, so they are not self-medicating with illicit substances? Or do I avoid prescribing medications with abuse potential when they are actively using cocaine?"

There is no ONE right approach to this situation. PCPs will need to balance patient safety and harm reduction. Some things to consider:

(a) First, assess and treat the patient for other common conditions such as MDD, anxiety, and PTSD
(b) Know that the diagnosis of ADHD cannot be made until the patient is off substances. Consider using a validated tool to assess for ADHD once the patient is off substances
(c) If you suspect ADHD, the first-line treatment is psychotherapy (that helps the patient with executive and organizational skills). Next, you can try non stimulant medications (like atomoxetine or bupropion)
(d) If you decide to use XR mixed amphetamine salts, monitor the patient and provide short prescriptions: Does this prescribing increase their function? Does it cut back/eliminate their illicit substance use?
(e) Explore with the patient their relationship with the cocaine. Are they taking it to get high/escape/numb emotions or to concentrate? If the former, providing them with XR mixed amphetamine salts may support a use disorder; if the latter, providing them with XR mixed amphetamine salts may reduce their illicit substance use

Remember whatever you decide, you can always modify the plan as you continue to assess the patient and weigh the risk vs benefits of the current plan

Naltrexone and Liver Concerns

You may worry about starting Naltrexone in a patient with liver disease or abnormal liver function tests (LFTs; Vannier et al., 2022). The good news is that Naltrexone is generally safe, and in fact, it can often improve LFTs in patients with alcohol-related liver disease.

Here are some key things to remember when starting Naltrexone:

- *Monitor liver function.* Check LFTs after starting Naltrexone and monitor for any signs of worsening liver problems, such as jaundice or confusion.
- *Baseline tests not required.* You do not need LFT testing before starting Naltrexone; the absence of labs should not prevent you from starting Naltrexone.

Combining Naltrexone with Gabapentin Some studies suggest that combining Naltrexone with gabapentin might offer additional benefits in treating AUD.

Outpatient Alcohol Detoxification

For most patients, outpatient management of alcohol withdrawal is considered safe, effective, and allows for a more patient-centered approach to recovery (Kranzler et al., 2019). While healthcare professionals traditionally receive more training in managing alcohol withdrawal in an inpatient setting, research shows that outpatient treatment can be just as safe and effective, resulting in shorter stays and lower costs compared to inpatient detox.

A patient who is drinking ~4–6 standard drinks daily for at least a month likely needs some form of detox (outpatient or inpatient). A patient recently discharged from the hospital after detox might experience some discomfort but since they have not been drinking for 30 days consistently, they do not need another detox.

Who Is Not a Candidate for Outpatient Detoxification? Absolute Contraindications

There are some situations where outpatient detox (managed withdrawal at home) is not recommended, and inpatient detox is advised:

- *Severe past withdrawal.* If a patient experienced severe withdrawal symptoms in the past, such as seizures or hallucinations (DTs), inpatient detox is the safer option.
- *Moderate-severe withdrawal symptoms.* Currently experiencing moderate-to-severe withdrawal symptoms demonstrated by a CIWA-Ar (Clinical Institute Withdrawal Assessment of Alcohol Scale, Revised) >10 indicates a need for inpatient detox.

Alcohol Withdrawal: How Long?

Alcohol withdrawal starts 24 h after the last drink, begins with stimulation symptoms (anxiety, sweats, h/a, n/v/d, tremors), and progresses to hallucinations. At days 3–4, the patient can experience withdrawal seizures and/or delirium tremens (DTs), hence it is important to keep medications on board for at least 3 days after the patient's last drink.

Assessing Alcohol Withdrawal Severity

Short Alcohol Withdrawal Scale (SAWS). The SAWS is a simple tool that patients can use to self-report their symptoms daily. Scores >12 indicate moderate-severe withdrawal, and may warrant either increase in medication or referral for inpatient management.

Medically Managed Alcohol Withdrawal Treatment Protocol

When medically managing alcohol withdrawal, medications can help ease discomfort and prevent complications. Here's a breakdown of common choices:

- *Long-acting benzodiazepine (diazepam).* This should be the first choice for most patients experiencing alcohol withdrawal, even those with severe liver disease or cirrhosis. It works by calming the nervous system and reducing withdrawal symptoms. A short course of long-acting benzodiazepine (diazepam) can be given even in the setting of liver disease. Long-acting benzodiazepines are more stabilizing for withdrawal management than short-acting benzodiazepines (like lorazepam).
- *Gabapentin.* For people with very mild withdrawal symptoms, gabapentin might be a suitable option. This medication can also be used for long-term treatment of AUD and may potentially help prevent more severe withdrawal symptoms in the future.
- *Starting the protocol.* Have the patient start the protocol the morning after their appointment. If the patient consumes >10 drinks per day, double the dose on the first day only (diazepam 20 mg q 6 h or gabapentin 600 mg q 6 h). If the patient consumes <10 drinks/day, keep the first day as is (i.e., Valium 10 q 6 or Gabapentin 300 q6). The other 3 days stay the same, regardless of previous alcohol use. Because we are using long-acting medications, these stay in the system for a while, so it is equivalent to giving 7–10 days of medications. Also, provide 5 extra PRN Tables (1 per day) to be used over the course of the 4 days (see Table 10.6).

Table 10.6 Four day alcohol taper protocol

	Diazepam[a]	Gabapentin
Day 1	10 mg q 6 h	300 mg q 6 h
Day 2	10 mg TID	300 mg TID
Day 3	10 mg BID	300 mg BID
Day 4	10 mg qd	300 mg qd
Additional PRNs (pt can use 1 extra pill/day PRN)	5 × 10 mg tablets	5 × 300 mg tablets

[a] Can substitute chlordiazepoxide 50 mg for diazepam 10 mg

Medically Managed Alcohol Withdrawal Treatment Follow Up

Frequency. Frequent check-ins are crucial for monitoring patient progress and adjusting the treatment plan as needed. This may involve in-person visits, telehealth consultations, or daily phone calls with a healthcare professional (physician, nurse practitioner, or physician assistant). For this reason, it is best to start the protocol early to mid-week so appropriate follow up can occur.
Symptom evaluation. Assess withdrawal symptoms such as tremors, headaches, nausea, vomiting, anxiety, sleep disturbances, and skin crawling. Tracking the improvement or worsening of these symptoms is essential.
Safety Measures. If severe withdrawal symptoms develop, like confusion or seizures, providers should refer the patient to inpatient management. *Patients should be counseled on severe withdrawals and reasons to go to the emergency department.*
Monitoring. Monitor for excessive sleepiness, sedation, or slurred speech. Dosage adjustments might be necessary to address these side effects.

Relative Contraindications for Outpatient Detox

While outpatient detox can be an option for some, there are situations where inpatient detox is strongly encouraged, but the ultimate decision should be patient centered. Here are factors to consider when deciding on outpatient detox:

- *Serious health conditions.* Having four or more of these health conditions—congestive heart failure (CHF), severe chronic obstructive pulmonary disease (COPD) requiring oxygen, advanced liver disease (decompensated cirrhosis), or advanced kidney disease (stage 3 or higher)—increases the risks for complications associated with outpatient detox.
- *Pregnancy.* Outpatient detox is not recommended during pregnancy.
- *Limited support system.* If a patient is homeless, lacks a phone, or has limited social support, outpatient detox might be challenging due to the need for frequent check-ins.
- *Multiple addictions.* Having multiple active substance use disorders is generally a reason to recommend inpatient detox. A patient who is stable in recovery on B/N for OUD is not considered part of this category.
- *Other sedating medications.* Taking high doses of other sedating medications, such as methadone.

Cannabis Use Disorder

Cannabis use disorder (CUD) refers to a problematic pattern of cannabis use leading to significant impairment or distress. While cannabis use is common, not everyone who uses it develops CUD. Cannabis contains a complex mix of thousands of chemicals. The two most relevant are CBD (cannabidiol), a non-psychoactive compound that offers anti-inflammatory properties, and THC (tetrahydrocannabinol), the psychoactive compound responsible for the "high" associated with cannabis. The potency of cannabis depends on the percentage of THC, which has increased significantly over time. "Street" cannabis now averages around 16% THC, while medical dispensaries may offer products with much higher concentrations (up to 88%). Synthetic Cannabinoids are artificial substances that mimic the effects of THC and are often sold under names like "K2," "Spice," or "Synthetic marijuana." They can be dangerous and unpredictable.

Cannabis Use: Weighing the Evidence The evidence for both benefits and harms associated with cannabis use is complex and ongoing. It is crucial to discuss the potential risks and rewards with a patient who is using cannabis (Agrawal et al., 2012).

Potential Benefits:

- *Moderate to substantial evidence.* Cannabis may be helpful in managing chronic pain, chemotherapy-induced nausea, and spasticity associated with multiple sclerosis.

Potential Harms:

- *Substantial evidence.* Cannabis use can lead to respiratory problems, increase the risk of motor vehicle crashes (due to impaired judgment, coordination, and reaction time), and lower birth weight (cannabis use during pregnancy is discouraged). For adolescents, there is substantial evidence that cannabis can increase the risk for schizophrenia, suicidality, and depression (especially with rising THC levels, which has been associated with negative mood).
- *Moderate evidence.* Cannabis use may increase the risk of injuries in children, impair learning, memory, and attention, and even dependence on other substances.
- *Breastfeeding.* Cannabis use is not recommended during breastfeeding as THC can pass through breast milk and potentially cause long-term neurobehavioral effects in the infant.

Treating Cannabis Use Disorder In the primary care setting, between 7–22% of patients using cannabis will develop a cannabis use disorder. Generally, if someone is using cannabis daily, they likely have CUD (Flórez-Salamanca et al., 2013). It will be important to explore their relationship with cannabis and think about the 4 C's described above.

Asking About Cannabis Use It is important to understand your patient's relationship with cannabis. Consider why they are using (what purpose is it serving them) and how they are using to identify if they have a CUD and/or offer harm reduction strategies (Budney et al., 2000; Calomarde-Gómez et al., 2021). You can ask other questions, such as what they like and don't like about using, to help them identify reason to quit or cut back (Flórez-Salamanca et al., 2013). Some useful questions:

- *How often do you use?*
- *How are you using?* (encourage using safer routes: edible/tincture > vaping > smoking).
- *Where do you get cannabis*? (encourage purchasing from a dispensary rather than using off the street, which is often laced with contaminants like fentanyl).
- *How does it make you feel? What do you like about it?*
- *What do you not like about it?*
- *How do you feel about your use overall?*
- *Have you tried to cut down before? Why?*
- *Have you had withdrawal symptoms or cravings?*
- *Have you ever experienced hallucinations or paranoia while using it?*
- *How is it affecting your social life? Work? Health?*

CUD Treatment: Effective Strategies Once you have identified underlying reasons for cannabis use, you can target them. For example, you learn that a patient is using cannabis to self-medicate anxiety or insomnia, you can focus on addressing these concerns through pharmacological and/or non-pharmacological approaches that do not involve cannabis (Chazal et al., 2022; Durbin et al., 2021; Gates et al., 2016; Halladay et al., 2019; Imtiaz et al., 2020).

Goal Setting and Management:

- *Collaboration is Key.* Working collaboratively with the patient, treatment plans establish goals for either:
  - Reduction: Decreasing cannabis use (frequency or potency).
  - Complete Cessation: Abstaining from cannabis entirely.
- *Managing Expectations.* It's important to manage expectations about withdrawal. Complete cessation may take a month or longer for symptoms (e.g., anxiety) to subside and for the patient to feel better.
- *Withdrawal Management.* During the first 2 weeks, anxiety and other withdrawal symptoms might worsen. These can be very uncomfortable for the patient, so it is important to help them to succeed by providing comfort medications (see Table 10.7).

For adolescents and young adults (patients <25 years old), there is moderate quality evidence that N-acetyl cysteine (NAC) can help reduce cravings. Since NAC is considered safe with minimal side effects, it is recommended to prescribe this for your adolescent patients.

Table 10.7 Cannabis withdrawal management

• Nausea: Zofran PO 4 mg TID (if refractory: Haldol 0.5 mg TID (don't give >3 days/24 h or give >7 days) • Insomnia: Melatonin, hydroxyzine • Headaches: Acetaminophen, ibuprofen • Anxiety: Hydroxyzine, buspirone, propranolol, clonidine. AVOID benzodiazepines and gabapentin due to high addiction potential. • Anorexia: Cyproheptadine, megestrol acetate • Abdominal pain: Topical capsaicin cream

Harm Reduction for CUD It is important to meet the patient where they are at. While some patients might not want to stop using cannabis entirely, we can still help support safe use, including encouraging them to:

- Buy from a dispensary
- Avoid adding tobacco (bulking, rolling with cigar paper)
- Use safer routes (edible/tincture> vaping > smoking)
- Avoid driving
- Limit quantity (due to its potency) or down-titrate the amount of THC
- Safe storage, especially with edibles and kids
- Avoid high-THC formulations (e.g., "shatter," "dab")

Urine Drug Screening in Addiction Treatment: A Supportive Tool

Urine Drug Screening (UDS) can be a valuable tool in addiction medicine, providing objective evidence of recent substance use. UDS is most helpful when PCPs use it in intentional ways rather than mandating it as part of treatment. Here's how UDS can be used effectively:

Promoting Accountability

- *Patient-driven.* Some patients in recovery choose to have regular UDS to hold themselves accountable.
- *Provider-driven.* PCPs may have concerns about a patient and ask them to submit a UDS to promote a conversation that offers the patient additional support if they need it. Studies also show that random UDS (with short notice) can be more effective in deterring relapse compared to scheduled UDS.
- *Collaborative approach.* The PCP and patient can work together to determine the appropriate UDS frequency.

Verifying Relapse Concerns:

- *Open communication.* Discussing positive UDS results in a non-judgmental way is crucial. Keep in mind that UDS are subject to false positives and false negatives. The provider should thus discuss results with curiosity (e.g., "*The urine drug test showed something I was not expecting [shares results]. When I see this, I get concerned and you have not brought this up. So, I wanted to check in with you about your recovery and what might be going on and how I can support you*").
- *Exploration and support.* By exploring the reasons behind the relapse, the provider offers support and discusses options for getting back on track. This may include:
  - Community resources like support groups, sponsors, sober living facilities.
  - Higher levels of care like intensive outpatient programs (IOP) or inpatient treatment.
  - Additional psychological support.
  - Activities like work or volunteering that promote recovery.

Box 10.6 Is UDS a Punishment for Patients?

You can help patients understand that urine drug screening (UDS) is not a punishment. Do not use UDS results to dismiss a patient from treatment or a practice. Be transparent about the purpose of urine drug screening. Explain that it's a tool to monitor progress, identify potential relapses early, and adjust treatment accordingly. Emphasize that the goal is to support recovery, not to catch patients in a mistake. A positive UDS signifies an opportunity to intervene with additional support and prevent further relapse. UDS is a valuable tool in addiction treatment, but it is most effective when used in conjunction with other strategies and a focus on patient support. By using UDS judiciously and approaching positive results with openness and empathy, healthcare providers can empower patients in their recovery journey

Key Points

- PCPs are well positioned to identify and treat SUDs like chronic conditions, using both pharmacological and behavioral support. Whenever possible, an integrated, multidisciplinary team for comprehensive SUD management should be used, however lack of these services should not preclude treatment particularly in resource-limited communities. Providing ANY SUD treatment is better than providing NO SUD treatment.
- Addiction is a chronic brain disorder with factors like genetics, BH struggles, personality traits, and social environment playing roles. PCPs can use brief screening tools (e.g., AUDIT-C, DAST-10, ASSIST), and the DSM-5-TR criteria for effective diagnosis.

- SUDs often co-occur with mental health disorders, worsening each other's symptoms. Conditions like anxiety, depression, bipolar disorder, ADHD, and PTSD are commonly associated with SUDs, with PTSD significantly increasing the risk of developing an SUD.
- Effective substance use treatment includes both pharmacological and non-pharmacological approaches. For medications, there is substantial evidence that these are the gold standard of treatment for OUD. For other SUDs, medications can play a role, but have limited evidence. For ALL SUDs, psychosocial approaches are considered cornerstone treatment.
- Primary care doctors should approach patients in a non-judgmental way, use open-ended questions and motivational interviewing to explore the rationale for their drug use, their interest in quitting, and then meet them where they are at. This might include complete cessation, cutting back, or finding safer ways of using. PCPs should offer patients a menu of treatment options (both pharmacological and psychosocial) and encourage the patient to embrace the highest level of care they are willing to accept.

References

Agrawal, A., Budney, A. J., & Lynskey, M. T. (2012). The co-occurring use and misuse of cannabis and tobacco: A review. *Addiction, 107*(7), 1221–1233. https://doi.org/10.1111/j.1360-0443.2012.03837.x

Anton, R. F., O'Malley, S. S., Ciraulo, D. A., Cisler, R. A., Couper, D., Donovan, D. M., Gastfriend, D. R., Hosking, J. D., Johnson, B. A., LoCastro, J. S., Longabaugh, R., Mason, B. J., Mattson, M. E., Miller, W. R., Pettinati, H. M., Randall, C. L., Swift, R., Weiss, R. D., Williams, L. D., Zweben, A., & COMBINE Study Research Group. (2006). Combined pharmacotherapies and behavioral interventions for alcohol dependence. The COMBINE study: A randomized controlled trial. *JAMA, 295*(17), 2003–2017. https://doi.org/10.1001/jama.295.17.2003

Bartlett, R., Brown, L., Shattell, M., Wright, T., & Lewallen, L. (2013). Harm reduction: Compassionate care of persons with addictions. *Medsurg Nursing: Official Journal of the Academy of Medical-Surgical Nurses, 22*(6), 349.

Budney, A. J., Higgins, S. T., Radonovich, K. J., & Novy, P. L. (2000). Adding voucher-based incentives to coping skills and motivational enhancement improves outcomes during treatment for marijuana dependence. *Journal of Consulting and Clinical Psychology, 68*(6), 1051–1061. https://doi.org/10.1037/0022-006X.68.6.1051

Calomarde-Gómez, C., Jiménez-Fernández, B., Balcells-Oliveró, M., Gual, A., & López-Pelayo, H. (2021). Motivational interviewing for cannabis use disorders: A systematic review and meta-analysis. *European Addiction Research, 27*(6), 413–427. https://doi.org/10.1159/000515667

Carroll, K. M., Nich, C., LaPaglia, D. M., Peters, E. N., Easton, C. J., & Petry, N. M. (2012). Combining cognitive behavioral therapy and contingency management to enhance their effects in treating cannabis dependence: Less can be more, more or less. *Addiction, 107*(9), 1650–1659. https://doi.org/10.1111/j.1360-0443.2012.03877.x

Chazal, C., Roux, C., Kinouani, S., Schuers, M., Fortin, F., Pereira, B., Blanc, O., Piñol-Domenech, N., Brousse, G., Vorilhon, P., & Laporte, C. (2022). Effectiveness of brief interventions in primary care for cannabis users aged from 12 to 25 years old: A systematic review. *Family Practice, 39*(6), 1156–1168. https://doi.org/10.1093/fampra/cmac050

Durbin, S., Ayers, C., Harrod, C., Paynter, R., & Kansagara, D. (2021). *Pharmacotherapy for the treatment of cannabis use disorder (the systematically testing the evidence on marijuana project).* Oregon Health & Science University.

Fiellin, D. A., Schottenfeld, R. S., Cutter, C. J., Moore, B. A., Barry, D. T., & O'Connor, P. G. (2014). Primary care–based buprenorphine taper vs maintenance therapy for prescription opioid dependence: A randomized clinical trial. *JAMA Internal Medicine, 174*(12), 1947–1954. https://doi.org/10.1001/jamainternmed.2014.5302

Flórez-Salamanca, L., Secades-Villa, R., Budney, A. J., García-Rodríguez, O., Wang, S., & Blanco, C. (2013). Probability and predictors of cannabis use disorders relapse: Results of the National Epidemiologic Survey on alcohol and related conditions (NESARC). *Drug and Alcohol Dependence, 132*(1), 127–133. https://doi.org/10.1016/j.drugalcdep.2013.01.013

Gates, P. J., Sabioni, P., Copeland, J., Foll, B. L., & Gowing, L. (2016). Psychosocial interventions for cannabis use disorder. *Cochrane Database of Systematic Reviews, 5*. https://doi.org/10.1002/14651858.CD005336.pub4

Halladay, J., Scherer, J., MacKillop, J., Woock, R., Petker, T., Linton, V., & Munn, C. (2019). Brief interventions for cannabis use in emerging adults: A systematic review, meta-analysis, and evidence map. *Drug and Alcohol Dependence, 204*, 107565. https://doi.org/10.1016/j.drugalcdep.2019.107565

Imtiaz, S., Roerecke, M., Kurdyak, P., Samokhvalov, A. V., Hasan, O. S. M., & Rehm, J. (2020). Brief interventions for cannabis use in healthcare settings: Systematic review and meta-analyses of randomized trial. *Journal of Addiction Medicine, 14*(1), 78–88. https://doi.org/10.1097/ADM.0000000000000527

Jonas, D. E., Amick, H. R., Feltner, C., Bobashev, G., Thomas, K., Wines, R., Kim, M. M., Shanahan, E., Gass, C. E., Rowe, C. J., & Garbutt, J. C. (2014). Pharmacotherapy for adults with alcohol use disorders in outpatient settings: A systematic review and meta-analysis. *JAMA, 311*(18), 1889–1900. https://doi.org/10.1001/jama.2014.3628

Jovey, R. D. (2012). Opioids, pain and addiction—Practical strategies. *British Journal of Pain, 6*(1), 36–42. https://doi.org/10.1177/2049463712439132

Kranzler, H. R., Feinn, R., Morris, P., & Hartwell, E. E. (2019). A meta-analysis of the efficacy of gabapentin for treating alcohol use disorder. *Addiction, 114*(9), 1547–1555. https://doi.org/10.1111/add.14655

Lee, J. D., Nunes, E. V., Novo, P., Bachrach, K., Bailey, G. L., Bhatt, S., Farkas, S., Fishman, M., Gauthier, P., Hodgkins, C. C., King, J., Lindblad, R., Liu, D., Matthews, A. G., May, J., Peavy, K. M., Ross, S., Salazar, D., Schkolnik, P., Shmueli-Blumberg, D., Stablein, D., Subramaniam, G., & Rotrosen, J. (2018). Comparative effectiveness of extended-release naltrexone versus buprenorphine-naloxone for opioid relapse prevention (X:BOT): A multicentre, open-label, randomised controlled trial. *The Lancet, 391*(10118), 309–318. https://doi.org/10.1016/S0140-6736(17)32812-X

Litt, M. D., Kadden, R. M., & Petry, N. M. (2013). Behavioral treatment for marijuana dependence: Randomized trial of contingency management and self-efficacy enhancement. *Addictive behaviors, 38*(3), 1764–1775. https://doi.org/10.1016/j.addbeh.2012.08.011

Martin, S. A., Chiodo, L. M., Bosse, J. D., & Wilson, A. (2018). The next stage of buprenorphine care for opioid use disorder. *Annals of Internal Medicine, 169*(9), 628–635. https://doi.org/10.7326/M18-1652

Mintzer, I. L., Eisenberg, M., Terra, M., MacVane, C., Himmelstein, D. U., & Woolhandler, S. (2007). Treating opioid addiction with buprenorphine-naloxone in community-based primary care settings. *Annals of Family Medicine, 5*(2), 146–150. https://doi.org/10.1370/afm.665

Myrick, H., Malcolm, R., Randall, P. K., Boyle, E., Anton, R. F., Becker, H. C., & Randall, C. L. (2009). A double-blind trial of gabapentin versus lorazepam in the treatment of alcohol withdrawal. *Alcoholism: Clinical and Experimental Research, 33*(9), 1582–1588. https://doi.org/10.1111/j.1530-0277.2009.00986.x

National Institute on Alcohol Abuse and Alcoholism (NIAAA). (2005). *Helping patients who drink too much: A clinician's guide (NIH publication no. 05–3769)*. National Institutes of Health. https://www.samhsa.gov/resource/ebp/helping-patients-who-drink-too-much-clinicians-guide

National Institute on Drug Abuse (NIDA). (2019). *How much does opioid treatment cost?* https://www.drugabuse.gov/publications/research-reports/medications-to-treat-opioid-addiction/how-much-does-opioid-treatment-cost

National Institute on Drug Abuse (NIDA). (2023). *Treatment and recovery*. https://nida.nih.gov/publications/drugs-brains-behavior-science-addiction/treatment-recovery

Potter, J. S., Marino, E. N., Hillhouse, M. P., Nielsen, S., Wiest, K., Canamar, C. P., Martin, J. A., Ang, A., Baker, R., Saxon, A. J., & Ling, W. (2013). Buprenorphine/naloxone and methadone maintenance treatment outcomes for opioid analgesic, heroin, and combined users: Findings from starting treatment with agonist replacement therapies (START). *Journal of Studies on Alcohol and Drugs, 74*(4), 605–613. https://doi.org/10.15288/jsad.2013.74.605

RxList. (2019). *Sublocade (buprenorphine injection for subcutaneous use): Side effects, interactions, warning, dosage & uses*. https://www.rxlist.com/sublocade-drug.htm.

Saitz, R., & Daaleman, T. P. (2017). Now is the time to address substance use disorders in primary care. *The Annals of Family Medicine, 15*(4), 306–308. https://doi.org/10.1370/afm.2111

Springer, S. A., & Bisaga, A. (2018). *Monitoring of liver function tests in patients receiving naltrexone or extended-release naltrexone*. PCSS Providers' Clinical Support System: MAT Training. http://pcssmat.org/wp-content/uploads/2014/10/PCSS-MAT-NTX-Liver-Safety-Guideline1.pdf

Substance Abuse and Mental Health Services Administration (SAMHSA). (2009). Chapter 4: Oral naltrexone. In *Incorporating alcohol pharmacotherapies into medical practice*. Substance Abuse and Mental Health Services Administration (US). https://www.ncbi.nlm.nih.gov/books/NBK64042/

Substance Abuse and Mental Health Services Administration (SAMHSA). (2018). *Treatment for stimulant use disorders*. Substance Abuse and Mental Health Services Administration (US).

Substance Abuse and Mental Health Services Administration (SAMHSA). (2019). *Medication-assisted treatment (MAT)*. https://www.samhsa.gov/medications-substance-use-disorders

Substance Abuse and Mental Health Services Administration (SAMHSA). (2021). Medications for opioid use disorder. https://store.samhsa.gov/product/tip-63-medications-opioid-use-disorder/pep21-02-01-002

Tuten, M., DeFulio, A., Jones, H. E., & Stitzer, M. (2012). Abstinence-contingent recovery housing and reinforcement-based treatment following opioid detoxification. *Addiction, 107*(5), 973–982. https://doi.org/10.1111/j.1360-0443.2011.03750.x

Vannier, A. G. L., Shay, J. E. S., Fomin, V., Patel, S. J., Schaefer, E., Goodman, R. P., & Luther, J. (2022). Incidence and progression of alcohol-associated liver disease after medical therapy for alcohol use disorder. *JAMA Network Open, 5*(5), e2213014. https://doi.org/10.1001/jamanetworkopen.2022.13014

Weiss, R. D., & Rao, V. (2017). The prescription opioid addiction treatment study: What have we learned. *Drug and Alcohol Dependence, 173*(Suppl 1), S48–S54. https://doi.org/10.1016/j.drugalcdep.2016.12.001

Wesson, D. R., & Ling, W. (2003). The clinical opiate withdrawal scale (COWS). *Journal of Psychoactive Drugs, 35*(2), 253–259. https://doi.org/10.1080/02791072.2003.10400007

Additional Resources

Providers Clinical Support System (PCSS). (2024). *Comprehensive curriculum and mentorship on substance use treatment*. https://pcssnow.org/courses

Society of Teachers of Family Medicine (STFM). (2024). *National addiction medicine curriculum*. https://www.stfm.org/addictionmodules

Substance Abuse and Mental Health Services Administration (SAMHSA). (2024). *Core curriculum elements on substance use disorder for early academic career medical and health professions education programs.* https://www.samhsa.gov/sites/default/files/core-curriculum-report-final.pdf

The Curbsiders. (2004). Addiction medicine podcast. *The Curbsiders Addiction Medicine Podcast.* https://thecurbsiders.com/addiction

Chapter 11
Peripartum, Pediatric, and Adolescent Considerations

Lisa Ramirez PhD, ABPP, Amy Lacroix MD, and Rachel Herbst PhD

The Peripartum Period

The peripartum period is a critical time for development and regulation. This stage builds the foundation for social emotional health. Specifically, attunement from the caregivers is critical for the development of attachment. Secure attachment has been associated with higher self-esteem, improved stress management, better impulse control, academic success, and a high overall level of social emotional well-being (Miller & Commons, 2010). Therefore, cultivating attunement and attachment represent a social emotional health promotion strategy across the lifespan, starting in the peripartum period.

From a practical standpoint, PCPs are uniquely positioned to identify risk factors and protective factors associated with secure attachment (see Table 11.1). This requires a two-generation approach, given that maternal and caregiver well-being is strongly associated with child well-being (Deave et al., 2008). Various caregiver and child risk factors have been associated with poorer child outcomes. Social determinants of health, or life-enhancing resources such as access to quality food, housing, social relationships, transportation, education, and health care, impact the developmental, mental, and physical health of both the caregiver and the child (Brennan Ramirez et al., 2008). Additionally, adverse childhood experiences (ACES), toxic

L. Ramirez PhD, ABPP (✉)
The MetroHealth System, Cleveland, OH, USA
e-mail: lramirez@metrohealth.org

A. Lacroix MD
Children's Physicians University of Nebraska Medical Center, Omaha, NE, USA
e-mail: aelacroi@unmc.edu

R. Herbst PhD
Cincinatti Children's Hospital Medical Center, Cincinnati, OH, USA
e-mail: Rachel.Herbst@cchmc.org

M. L. C. Williamson and D. L. Terry (eds.), *Essentials for Treating Behavioral Health in Primary Care*, https://doi.org/10.1007/978-3-032-09558-9_11

stress, discrimination, and oppression can impact parenting. These lived experiences of caregivers can unintentionally perpetuate cycles of parenting with limited warmth and responsiveness; however, they also provide opportunities for caregivers' reflections on how they want to parent differently (Rowell & Neal-Barnett, 2022). Conversely, protective factors from the caregiver's history can buffer adverse childhood experiences and toxic stress, supporting their use of positive parenting practices. These factors include benevolent childhood experiences (BCES; including strong relationships with family, teachers). Other protective factors include current social support and faith or spiritual practices (Doom et al., 2021).

Peripartum Screening During the peripartum period, PCPs can inquire about caregivers' goals for their children then link these goals to an acknowledgment that all caregivers want a better life for their child, seeking to decrease their child's ACES and increase their BCES. A natural port of entry for this conversation is during maternal depression screening. Given that the American Academy of Pediatrics recommends this screening occurring during the first 6 months of the infant's life, the screening process provides multiple opportunities to partner with families and begin to understand social drivers of health, both historically (e.g., caregiver mental health history) and currently, that can impact the caregiver-child relationship (Earls et al., 2019).

Identification of depressive symptomatology is a powerful port of entry to impact child social emotional health. Attunement to infant cues can be more challenging for caregivers with depression, which can create difficulties in bonding and infant regulation (Goodman et al., 2011). Children of depressed mothers are at risk for a wide variety of health concerns, including sleep disturbances, developmental delays, externalizing problems (e.g., aggression, conduct problems, and ADHD), internalizing problems (e.g., separation anxiety, social withdrawal, and depression), and increased risk of self-harm (Hammerton et al., 2015). Although most research focuses on maternal depression, depression in any primary caregiver poses similar risks to the child's mental and BH (Marçal, 2021). Therefore, identifying and treating caregiver depression is a key strategy to both promote social emotional well-being in children

Table 11.1 Adverse childhood experiences and benevolent childhood experiences

<table>
<tr><th>Adverse Childhood Experiences</th><th>Benevolent Childhood Experiences</th></tr>
<tr><td>Types of adversity experienced in childhood that increase the risk of various negative mental and physical health outcomes, including shorter life expectancy</td><td>Positive experiences in childhood (independent of socioeconomic status) associated with positive mental and physical health outcomes</td></tr>
<tr><td>Originally included various forms of physical and emotional abuse, neglect, and household dysfunction</td><td rowspan="2">Include perceived internal and external safety and security (e.g., holding beliefs that provided comfort); positive and predictive quality of life (e.g., predictable home routine); and relational support (e.g., having a supportive adult who was not a parent/caregiver)</td></tr>
<tr><td>Have been expanded to include exposure to bullying, community violence, neighborhood safety, racism, and living in foster care</td></tr>
</table>

and mitigate the child's risk of developing a future BH concern. Evidence-based treatment for perinatal mood disorders includes both evidenced-based psychotherapy and pharmacology (Earls et al., 2019).

Various resources can support PCPs and families in promoting social emotional health. During visits, PCPs can support caregivers' attunement to their infant's cues, reinforcing caregivers' responsiveness to their infant's signals of needs such as hunger, sleep, and comfort. Caregivers who experienced ACES or toxic stress in their childhood may benefit from additional guidance, as they seek to provide a different life for their child than what they experienced (HealthySteps, 2021; Mount Sinai Parenting Center, 2024). As the infant grows, PCPs can build upon the attunement of these basic cues to new needs that will remain present across the pediatric lifespan, specifically the need for exploration and comfort (Circle of Security, 2019).

The perinatal period also provides opportunities to intervene early on subclinical or clinical BH concerns. In infants, this can present as increased fussiness, sleep, or feeding problems without a medical cause (Zero to Three, 2024a). PCPs can support the family by reinforcing a focus on caregiver well-being, attunement, and strategies to comfort the infant when distressed.

These key strategies presented in the perinatal period are applicable across the entire pediatric lifespan. Throughout the remainder of the chapter, we will continue to reference cross-cutting themes and demonstrate applicability to all pediatric developmental phases (see Table 11.2).

Infancy and Early Childhood

The foundation of social emotional health that emerges in the perinatal period is further solidified during infancy and early childhood (see Table 11.3). This developmental phase provides PCPs with an opportunity to guide families toward positive parenting practices that align with their cultural and familial values. Anticipatory guidance to promote social emotional health includes:

- Attunement: continuing to support caregivers in recognizing their child's cues (including the need for comfort and support in co-regulation).
- Positive reinforcement: starting to use labeled praise with their child during infancy, describing what they like that their child is doing (which also supports language development, which has linkages to social emotional health).
- Structure: establishing routines, especially around transitions (e.g., giving a warning and saying goodbye before leaving the playground).
- Attachment: spending 5–10 min of special time with their child; quality time without screens where the focus is on letting the child lead play/activities; the caregiver refrains from trying to teach or correct and delights in the interaction with their child.

Table 11.2 Cross cutting themes for promoting social emotional health and addressing mental health concerns

Promoting caregiver Well-being (inclusive of extended family and other support figures)	• Formal screening for caregiver ACES, BCES, and depression • Inquiring during the visit about the caregiver's adjustment to this developmental phase • Identifying the caregiver's protective factors (e.g., social support) • Providing additional support to support caregiver Well-being (e.g., handouts, parenting resources, therapy referrals)
Promoting attunement and attachment	• Identifying the emotional relational environment between the caregiver and the child (e.g., stressors that may impact their emotional health) • Promotion of meaningful nurturing relationships • Explicit anticipatory guidance on the development of emotional regulation
Positive parenting practices	• Regular, brief, special one-on-one time occurs between the caregiver and the child • Positive reinforcement, such as labeled praise, is used to recognize the child's strengths, efforts, and abilities • Differential attention (praising desired behavior and ignoring non-desired behaviors that are not dangerous or destructive) • Boundaries and structure are used in a developmentally-appropriate way to communicate expectations, commands, and consequences (that are appropriately responsive to the negative behavior)

- Limit setting: providing brief, clear explanations of limits, with the emphasis on the caregiver to ensure the boundary is held (e.g., "I know you are angry but I will not let you hit me." [said while putting down the child so they cannot physically hit the caregiver]).
- Emotional regulation: labeling emotions and supporting co-regulation, given that young children need a high level of adult support to regulate. Caregivers can help toddlers and preschoolers practice regulation skills when they are calm. For example, they might teach belly breathing by blowing bubbles or singing the Daniel Tiger "When You Feel So Mad that You Want to Roar" song.

The most common behavior concern during this phase is tantrums. Tantrums are a normal part of development, typically peaking between 18 months and 36 months to occur once a day for an average of 3 minutes (Potegal et al., 2003). However, they are distressing to caregivers, can cause significant challenges, and tantrums that exceed the average duration and frequency can signal emerging BH concerns (Wakschlag

Table 11.3 Takeaways from peripartum through infancy developmental period

• Screening: maternal and caregiver depression; social determinants (e.g., ACES) disruptive behaviors; developmental concerns
• Strategies: positive and effective parenting practices to promote attunement and attachment; evidence-based approaches to managing disruptive behaviors

et al., 2019). Several evidence-based strategies can help with **tantrum management**, including:

- **Attunement and attachment**: Use caregiver's attunement to the child to help identify antecedents to tantrums (i.e., what was happening prior to the onset of the tantrum), which frequently include being tired, hungry, and frustrated. If caregivers can increase their awareness of these antecedents and address the root cause of the behavior, tantrums will be less frequent and less intense.
- **Structure and limit setting**: Engage in differential attention, ignoring the tantrum then praising the child as soon as they start to calm. Note that for some families, ignoring is not a strategy that aligns with their values or their own regulatory capacity (because of the effort required to remain calm and neutral while ignoring).
- **Emotional regulation**: Help with co-regulation. The caregiver empathetically labels the child's emotions, holds the boundary, and helps the child to calm down with support from the adult. For example, "*You're so mad that we have to stop playing and get ready for bed. I know how hard it is to stop doing something fun.*" [Caregiver does not allow the child to keep playing but offers a hug or to listen to a favorite or calming song.]

One of the most common BH diagnoses in this period is a disruptive behavior disorder, such as oppositional defiant disorder, with a prevalence ranging from 1 to 16% (Coto et al., 2018). The pattern of symptoms associated with these disorders, including aggression, defiance of authority, and impulsivity (American Psychiatric Association (APA), 2022). Evidence-based intervention strategies for **disruptive behavior** can be started in primary care while the family is connected to BH resources. These include:

- *Effective commands*: ensuring you have the patient's attention, then clearly stating what the child can do (instead of telling them what they cannot do). For example, if the child is running, the caregiver can tell the child "*Walk slowly while holding my hand.*"
- *Natural and logical consequences*: in place of threatening punishments or trying to convince the child why they should comply, the caregiver uses if/then or when/then statements, indicating what the child has to do to earn a privilege or indicating what the consequence is that will occur if they do not comply. The consequence should match the behavior. For example, "*If you color on the walls, I will take away the crayons and you cannot color until tomorrow.*"
- *Attunement and attachment*: continue praise and special time-Children with disruptive behavior get a disproportionate amount of negative feedback. This

can negatively impact their self-esteem and relationship with caregivers and they may get stuck in cycles where the big reactions and attention from caregivers for negative behaviors becomes reinforcing. Therefore, it is important to continue to praise the child for positive behaviors and have brief, routine special 1:1 time with the child to promote a strong dyadic relationship.

Caregivers' early adoption and understanding of commands, consequences, and attunement lay an important foundation for future child and caregiver interactions. For additional information about navigating common child behavior problems in this developmental phase, Zero to Three (2024b) offers additional guidance.

School-Age Children

As children move into the middle childhood stage, the previous rapid pace of development slows and they enter a relatively calm developmental period (compared to the dramatic nature of toddlerhood and adolescence; see Table 11.4). Even though the vast leaps in motor and language are not explicitly obvious as with the infant through preschool stages, there are still crucial developmental processes occurring under the surface, especially related to physical and cognitive development, executive function, emotion regulation and socialization (Zelazo et al., 2008). The early childhood considerations of ***attunement and attachment, structure and limit setting and emotion regulation*** are equally important in middle childhood, but the expression of these concepts naturally shifts as children begin to explore increased independence around school, friendships, and daily tasks. Additionally, much of the "intervention" in this developmental stage is based upon setting healthy habits in the domains of sleep, socialization, nutrition, physical activity, and academic engagement.

In elementary-age children, there is robust evidence ***that consistent routines and special time*** with caregivers has a multitude of benefits, including family dinners (Eisenberg et al., 2004) and bedtime routines (Mindell & Williamson, 2018). Processing and co-regulating with a parent or meaningful adult following a distressing situation can set the groundwork for appropriate coping strategies for children as they continue to develop. Positive experiences in childhood can provide lifelong protection across physical and mental health conditions (La Charite et al., 2023; Maunder & Monks, 2018). PCPs can incorporate regular screening for family routines

Table 11.4 Takeaways from middle childhood

• Screening: ADHD; autism and developmental delays; school attendance and learning; social connectedness; anxiety and mood disorders; positive parenting practices/routines and structure
• Strategies: Management of medication and behavior related to ADHD; referral to further assessment for concerns about autism or learning disruption; education around anxiety and the reinforcing nature of avoidance (e.g., chronic absence from school)

and quality time with caregivers and include conversations about the importance of positive and predictable routines with adults in their lives.

Friendships and Self-Esteem During the elementary school years, children also begin to cultivate meaningful friendships. Research shows that 1–2 deep friendships are protective over time and promote ***attunement and attachment*** (La Charite et al., 2023; Maunder & Monks, 2018; Nangle et al., 2003), while large groups of friends may lead to a sacrifice in the quality of friendships. PCPs have an opportunity to check in about whether or not a child has at least one close friend and can help a family explore possible reasons for lack of friendships. Research has shown that children with attention-deficit/hyperactivity disorder (ADHD), autism spectrum disorder (ASD), and some anxiety disorders may have difficulty initiating and maintaining friendships over time (Geannopoulos et al., 2024), which could place them at higher risk for depression and anxiety (Gordon-Lipkin et al., 2018). As children enter preteen years, positive peer support can be especially protective against a variety of health outcomes (La Charite et al., 2023; Maunder & Monks, 2018).

Parents appear to value more open conversations with their children about feelings and ***emotional regulation*** than previous generations, but this can sometimes lead to active avoidance of feelings of discomfort in their children. Anxiety can manifest strongly in this age as independence is increasingly introduced, and avoidance of what is feared can make the worry even worse. One of the most prevalent problems related to anxiety and escape, school avoidance, illustrates this example.

School Avoidance School can be a major demand for children, as many children leave their families for the first time and have to adjust to being in a classroom with peers for up to 6 hours a day. Children who feel stress and/or worry related to their school environment may exhibit signs of anxiety that can be troubling to parents: somatic symptoms like headaches or gastrointestinal discomfort; behavioral symptoms like refusing to get out of bed, getting dressed, eating or getting out of the car; and emotional displays of crying or sharing their fears of what may happen at school. Parents are understandably dialed in to their children's emotions and may feel that they are supporting their child's well-being when they allow their child to come home from the school nurse's office when called about somatic symptoms, or even stay home entirely, as parents may believe this will help allay their child's fears and improve the overall situation. However, anxiety is fueled by the ability to avoid the situations we fear, and children do not have the opportunity to develop skills to overcome their worries. It is rarely indicated that a child would benefit from home instruction or online schooling given the impact on socialization and general academic engagement, yet many PCPs will get the inevitable request for a school excuse. Encouraging the parents to work with the school to understand the root of the avoidance (e.g., peer difficulties, academic challenges/learning delays or disorders, separation anxiety, boredom at school) develop a ***structured*** plan for supporting ***emotional regulation and coping*** or re-entry following a prolonged absence can be very effective. See Williamson et al. (2023) for additional information related to addressing school avoidance, including the importance of **limit setting** and **positive reinforcement** for facing their fears.

Bullying Bullying is another common concern raised by parents, and is important to screen for in pediatric practices given the long-term implication. Bullying in childhood has been associated with increased anxiety, depression, and behavioral problems into adulthood (Armitage, 2021). While conflict in childhood, especially middle school, is common, bullying is aggressive, systematic, and targeted and can undermine a child's self-esteem, sense of safety, and overall view of self if not addressed in a timely manner (Mills & Carwile, 2009). If a parent is concerned about bullying, they can submit written concerns and documentation of the bullying and should expect the school to respond with a written plan of action in a timely manner. The U.S. Department of Health and Human Services provides extensive resources related to advocacy around bullying at StopBullying.gov, state policies and laws related to bullying concerns (StopBullying.gov, 2019). Additional ***structure*** and support with ***emotional regulation*** can support emotional health during and after bullying.

Screening and Brief Intervention Middle childhood is a common time for children to begin to exhibit signs and symptoms of BH disruptions or disorders. Common disorders that manifest symptoms during this time period are ADHD, ASD, and anxiety and mood disorders. The benefit of pediatric populations is that the emphasis on prevention and early identification, and of course intervention when warranted. By establishing meaningful connections, talking with children and families, and using validated screeners, PCPs can gain valuable information and make recommendations based on level of symptomatology and severity of disruptions on activities of daily living and developmental milestones and tasks. Evidence-based clinical interventions have been successfully implemented in primary care settings. The American Academy of Pediatrics has comprehensive toolkits available for clinicians providing care for children. These toolkits provide resources related to screening and, when appropriate, treatment in clinical settings around ADHD, ASD, Bright Futures, BH, and Trauma and Resilience (American Academy of Pediatrics (AAP), 2024a). See Chap. 4 for further discussion regarding screening tools for children and adolescents.

Two critical considerations when considering BH presentations in children are sleep and trauma. Chronic sleep deprivation and trauma histories (acute, but especially chronic or complex) can mimic symptoms of other BH disorders including ADHD and disruptive behavior disorders (Siegfried & Blackshear, 2016). However, it is critical to understand that the mechanism behind the symptoms is inherently different. As the National Childhood Traumatic Stress Network (Siegfried & Blackshear, 2016) emphasizes, the core ADHD symptoms of inattention, hyperactivity, and impulsivity due to an understimulated brain would actually be attributed to an overstimulated brain in the case of a child with trauma, despite similar profiles on symptom checklists. Asking for clarification around sleep quality and quantity as well as trauma history of a child is necessary to avoid clinical errors, such using the front-line ADHD psychopharmacological intervention of a stimulant medication on an already overstimulated brain or on a child with chronic insomnia.

The Adolescent Patient

When considering the care of the adolescent and young adult patient, providers must consider the primary goals of the adolescent: (1) becoming an adult capable of separating from their guardians and functioning independently, (2) having their own social support network, and (3) being financially solvent. To this end, the adolescent must learn to care for themselves, build their own friendships, identify both innate talents and their ability to learn new skills, and interact within complex social structures of the educational and/or working world (see Table 11.5).

Behavioral health in adolescents and young adults can be impacted by past experiences and relationships. Knowing patient history is essential to informing care. "Don't ask what is wrong with your patient, ask what has happened to them" is a mantra taught to health care providers. Adolescents are a mix of their own temperament and lived experiences. Lived trauma and ACES compete with protective factors (BCES), learned skills, and relationships to shape a developing adult. These are further affected by factors such as sleep, parenting styles, social media influences, sense of belonging, and self-image. Managing and identifying co-occurring morbidities such as (ADHD), anxiety, depression, obsessive-compulsive disorder (OCD), and other mood disorders can best be done by providers whose patients and their families trust them with this holistic conceptualization.

Authoritative parenting, that is, parenting by setting known limits, consequences, and earned privileges, is more likely to result in adolescent and young adults who can make decisions independently and appreciate their own influence on natural outcomes. Adolescents who are raised in an atmosphere with modeled respect and voiced input learn the importance of respect and collaboration (Ginsburg & Jablow, 2011). Patients who come from unstable environments with inconsistent parenting or abuse may have problems with their own ability to feel in control of their own outcomes. They may also be more inclined to reject suggestions from authority figures, including their health care providers. They especially need to be involved in formulating their own care plan. And though early adolescents may be guided into counseling by a trusted adult, they need to come to any therapeutic alliance of their own will for it to be effective. Buy-in from the older adolescent and young adult patient is essential.

Parents, Adolescents, and Confidentiality As children move from preteen years to adolescence, caring for them should change in step with their evolving independence and needs. They should be allowed "me time" with their provider (Chung et al., 2024).

Table 11.5 Takeaways from adolescence

• Screening: Mood and other mental health disorders; suicide and risk; appropriate use of technology/social media; sleep quality and quantity; substance use
• Strategies: Empowerment around appropriate independence and identity formation; education around healthy social, sexual, digital and physical functioning; referral for mental and BH concerns; sleep hygiene

This should be previewed with parents in late childhood, so that it is no surprise when you ask a parent for time alone with their child or ask them to wait in the waiting room until the visit's end. Anyone who works with adolescents and young adults will tell you that they glean more complete information from patients in private than when parents are sitting next to them. And when meeting with your adolescent and young adult patient in private, it is also essential to let them know the limits of their privacy. Especially as this relates to BH. It is essential that patients know that they are the owners of their information and are not required to share it. But information that identifies abuse or threat to life moves outside of what can be kept confidential.

Sleep The importance of good sleep habits with consistent routines in adolescent and young adults cannot be over-emphasized. All the new emotions that the midbrain juggles are amplified by lack of sleep. Depression, anxiety, OCD, and other BH issues are harder to manage and symptoms can manifest more severely in patients with poor sleep. Sleep disorders such as sleep apnea, restless leg syndrome, and posttraumatic stress disorder (PTSD) have a strong impact on attention, learning, and emotional regulation (Kansagra, 2020).

Working with parents of early adolescents to set regular sleep routines, encourage limits to evening screen time, avoid late night caffeine and other stimuli, and reward good sleep hygiene can go a long way in maintaining adolescent and young adults' health. Having consistent wake times throughout the week and limited naps can allow for development of established sleep routines that decrease the risk of developing insomnia. Using natural relaxants like warm milk, chamomile tea, and lavender as well as white (or brown, green, etc.) noise can all help. Teaching relaxation exercises or meditation, or using soothing music are also tools that can aid in healthy sleep. Regular daily physical activity helps to create a physically tired body to prepare for a good night's sleep. Melatonin is often used by parents and can be helpful, however much still needs to be learned about long-term effects of melatonin in children and adolescents and it is more useful as a short-term sleep aid (Edemann-Callesen et al., 2023). Many adolescents with poor sleep related to BH issues resort to illicit drugs, such as alcohol, marijuana, opiates, and anxiolytics. Making sure to identify these sleep issues and offer care options that are neither disabling nor addictive is crucial to maintaining mental health.

Social Media We are just beginning to get a better idea of the enormous impact of social media on the BH of adolescent and young adult patients. Resources available to today's teens are vast and at their fingertips. Encouraging parents to control access for early adolescents and monitor vigilantly is paramount to avoid their victimization and check their perception of reality. Balancing screen time with school and other in-person activities should be a priority. PCPs can empower parents and caregivers to educate their children and adolescents about benefits and risks of the internet and social media, with emphasis on recognizing predators and protecting personal information (especially given the dangerous rise in sextortion rates), recognizing trusted sources, and maintaining relationships. Early adolescents should be educated about the role of social media in bullying and how to protect themselves. PCPs can encourage direct and simple ground rules for posting on the internet and social media:

(1) no posting anything you wouldn't want your grandmother to see; (2) no digital messaging of content that you wouldn't feel comfortable saying directly to someone in person; (3) no personal identifiers to someone you don't know in real life.

Gaming, while great fun, should also have limits. Recognizing problematic internet usage (Pluhar et al., 2019) can prompt important discussions about how media can promote or harm physical and BH. Encouraging schools to adopt curricula on social media education is a public health matter of significant importance. With a world of information in their pockets adolescents have access to the best and worst of the whole planet, and while that is an amazing resource, it can also be an anxiety-producing burden. Discussing sextortion and internet porn should be a part of sexual health education, as well as information on what constitutes addiction for older adolescents and young adults.

Special Populations

Youth with disabilities may come from families where they have been carefully protected, and rightfully so. Parents sometimes forget that their disabled adolescents and young adults may have doubts, anxiety, or depression. Adolescents with disabilities and young adults also experience issues with relationships and are developing sexual beings. Adolescents all need to be treated with the highest level of respect and confidentiality that is possible (Chung et al., 2024). Guaranteeing time alone with a provider and offering developmentally appropriate medical guidance and treatment is essential. Providers can help parents to know when that is indicated. Identifying mood disorders and treating them appropriately may make a great difference in these patients' day to day lives.

Youth who speak different languages or come from diverse cultures should have accommodations whenever possible to assure that they can communicate their stories effectively. Immigrant and refugee youth have often experienced significant mental, physical, and emotional traumas that need to be addressed.

System-involved youth deserve special attention and care. Whether involved in social services for abuse, in the legal system due to school related issues like truancy or fighting, or detained for substance use or other crimes, these youth have been traumatized and need extra support. Many have both BH and substance use issues and should be cared for by providers who are well versed in management of both. Some also have cognitive disabilities and may not have had the support that they need to function to the top of their ability. Educational evaluations for learning disabilities may also be indicated.

Another group at high risk for BH care needs is LQBTQIA++ youth. Many adolescents who are gender non-conforming or have sexual preferences outside of societal norms have suffered rejection, exclusion, abuse, depression, anxiety, and serious issues with self-image. They also are more likely to suffer from substance use, abuse and eating disorders (The Trevor Project, 2024). Asking about patients' preferred pronouns, gender identity, sexual preferences and preferred names is paramount to providing an environment where they feel acknowledged, respected, and cared about. All office staff should be comfortable with asking these questions respectfully and supportively while being careful not to "out" patients if they are not yet ready. Having a list of resources for LGBTQIA++ youth, for example a QR code with a link to community support groups, is just one way to provide support. Knowing state laws related to LGBTQIA++ health care and who the experts in the community are for providing the care that is legal is another important piece of essential health care for this group (Dawson et al., 2022).

In summary, adolescent and young adult patients are a diverse group who are interested in their own health care and becoming independent. As providers, it is our duty to support them and their parents in identifying their strengths and needs, being their resource and linking them to supports in the community that fit them best. It is also important to advocate for adolescent and young adult needs at all levels.

Conclusion

Comprehensive and developmentally-appropriate approaches to identifying and addressing BH concerns in children, adolescents, and young adults is an area in which PCPs are uniquely positioned. PCPs can partner with and support families around the common threads of attending to caregiver well-being, positive child-caregiver relationships and ***attunement***, focusing on protective factors (e.g., meaningful relationships, ***quality time***, appropriate ***structure and routines*** for sleep, physical activity and nutrition, ***limit setting*** around technology use, and appropriate friendships) and promoting ***emotional regulation*** through positive coping strategies are important throughout all stages of childhood and adolescence.

The majority of children and families will benefit from support and education around positive parenting practices and promoting self-efficacy through the increasing independence of successive developmental stages. Screening, brief intervention and referrals are incredibly impactful during this critical period. Finally, primary care visits offer valuable opportunities to apply proactive and preventative frameworks to avert future BH crises. With this whole-child and systemic lens, PCPs can be an ongoing catalyst for healthy emotional functioning across the lifespan.

Key Points

- Primary care is an ideal setting to promote social emotional health, identify and address early signs of BH concerns, and provide evidence-based interventions for BH conditions.
- Experiences in infancy and early childhood establish the foundation for future health. The relationship between the child and caregiver(s) is a powerful vehicle for promoting wellness and mitigating the impact of stressors.

- Understanding prior and current adverse and benevolent childhood experiences provide an opportunity to understand symptoms and protective factors in a trauma-informed, culturally responsive manner.
- Key strategies (i.e., promoting caregiver well-being, attunement and attachment, and positive parenting practices) apply to the prevention, early intervention, and management of social emotional health across the pediatric lifespan.
- Many resources exist for ongoing learning. The American Academy of Pediatrics offers free parenting resources (www.healthychildren.org) and Mount Sinai Keystones of Development (https://parenting.mountsinai.org/providers/) to discuss with parents during primary care visits. Some states have a multitude of BH and consultation resources. One example is The Massachusetts Child Psychiatry Access Program (MCPAP, 2014). Additionally, the American Academy of Pediatrics provides free, virtual, BH-related Extension for Community Healthcare Outcomes (ECHO) programming to members (American Academy of Pediatrics (AAP), 2024b).

References

American Academy of Pediatrics (AAP). (2024a). *AAP toolkits*. American Academy of Pediatrics. https://publications.aap.org/toolkits

American Academy of Pediatrics (AAP). (2024b). *Project ECHO*. https://www.aap.org/en/practice-management/project-echo/

American Psychiatric Association (APA). (2022). *Diagnostic and statistical manual of mental disorders* (5th ed.). American Psychiatric Publishing. https://psychiatryonline.org/doi/book/10.1176/appi.books.9780890425787

Armitage, R. (2021). Bullying in children: Impact on child health. *BMJ Paediatrics Open, 5*(1), e000939. https://doi.org/10.1136/bmjpo-2020-000939

Brennan Ramirez, L. K., Baker, E. A., & Metzler, M. (2008). *Promoting health equity; A resource to help communities address social determinants of health.* United States Centers for Disease Control and Prevention. https://stacks.cdc.gov/view/cdc/11130

Chung, R. J., Lee, J. B., Hackell, J. M., Alderman, E. M., & Committee on Adolescence, & Committee on Practice & Ambulatory Medicine. (2024). Confidentiality in the care of adolescents: Technical report. *Pediatrics, 153*(5), e2024066327. https://doi.org/10.1542/peds.2024-066327

Circle of Security. (2019). *What is the circle of security.* Circle of Security International. https://www.circleofsecurityinternational.com/circle-of-security-model/what-is-the-circle-of-security/

Coto, J., Garcia, A., Hart, K. C., & Graziano, P. A. (2018). Associations between disruptive behavior problems, parenting factors, and sleep problems among young children. *Journal of Developmental & Behavioral Pediatrics, 39*(8), 610–620. https://doi.org/10.1097/DBP.0000000000000595

Dawson, L., Kates, J., & Musumeci, M. (2022). *Youth access to gender affirming care: The federal and state policy landscape.* Kaiser Family Foundation. https://www.kff.org/other/issue-brief/youth-access-to-gender-affirming-care-the-federal-and-state-policy-landscape/

Deave, T., Heron, J., Evans, J., & Emond, A. (2008). The impact of maternal depression in pregnancy on early child development. *BJOG: An International Journal of Obstetrics and Gynaecology, 115*(8), 1043–1051. https://doi.org/10.1111/j.1471-0528.2008.01752.x

Doom, J. R., Seok, D., Narayan, A. J., & Fox, K. R. (2021). Adverse and benevolent childhood experiences predict mental health during the COVID-19 pandemic. *Adversity and Resilience Science, 2*, 193–204. https://doi.org/10.1007/s42844-021-00038-6

Earls, M. F., Yogman, M. W., Mattson, G., Rafferty, J., Baum, R., Gambon, T., Lavin, A., & Wissow, L. (2019). Incorporating recognition and management of perinatal depression into pediatric practice. *Pediatrics, 143*(1), e20183259. https://doi.org/10.1542/peds.2018-3259

Edemann-Callesen, H., Andersen, H. K., Ussing, A., Virring, A., Jennum, P., Debes, N. M., Laursen, T., Baandrup, L., Gade, C., Dettmann, J., Holm, J., Krogh, C., Birkefoss, K., Tarp, S., & Händel, M. N. (2023). Use of melatonin for children and adolescents with chronic insomnia attributable to disorders beyond indication: A systematic review, meta-analysis and clinical recommendation. *EClinicalMedicine, 61*. https://doi.org/10.1016/j.eclinm.2023.102049

Eisenberg, M. E., Olson, R. E., Neumark-Sztainer, D., Story, M., & Bearinger, L. H. (2004). Correlations between family meals and psychosocial well-being among adolescents. *Archives of Pediatrics & Adolescent Medicine, 158*(8), 792–796. https://doi.org/10.1001/archpedi.158.8.792

Geannopoulos, Z. F., Moody, C. T., McGregor, H. A., Baertschi, D., Bates, S., & Laugeson, E. A. (2024). Outcomes in PEERS® for adolescents across neurodevelopmental disorders: ADHD, autism, and their co-occurrence. *Advances in Neurodevelopmental Disorders*. https://doi.org/10.1007/s41252-023-00380-z

Ginsburg, K. R., & Jablow, M. M. (2011). *Building resilience in children and teens: Giving kids roots and wings*. American Academy of Pediatrics. https://doi.org/10.1542/9781581106190

Goodman, S. H., Rouse, M. H., Connell, A. M., Broth, M. R., Hall, C. M., & Heyward, D. (2011). Maternal depression and child psychopathology: A meta-analytic review. *Clinical Child and Family Psychology Review, 14*(1), 1–27. https://doi.org/10.1007/s10567-010-0080-1

Gordon-Lipkin, E., Marvin, A. R., Law, J. K., & Lipkin, P. H. (2018). Anxiety and mood disorders in children with autism spectrum disorder and ADHD. *Pediatrics, 141*(4), e20171377. https://doi.org/10.1542/peds.2017-1377

Hammerton, G., Mahedy, L., Mars, B., Harold, G. T., Thapar, A., Zammit, S., & Collishaw, S. (2015). Association between maternal depression symptoms across the first eleven years of their child's life and subsequent offspring suicidal ideation. *PLoS One, 10*(7), e0131885. https://doi.org/10.1371/journal.pone.0131885

HealthySteps. (2021). *ACEs, toxic stress, and resilience: Parent handouts (English)*. Healthy Steps. https://www.healthysteps.org/resource/aces-toxic-stress-resilience-parent-handouts-english/

Kansagra, S. (2020). Sleep disorders in adolescents. *Pediatrics, 145*(Supplement_2), S204–S209. https://doi.org/10.1542/peds.2019-2056I

La Charite, J., Khan, M., Dudovitz, R., Nuckols, T., Sastry, N., Huang, C., Lei, Y., & Schickedanz, A. (2023). Specific domains of positive childhood experiences (PCEs) associated with improved adult health: A nationally representative study. *SSM - Population Health, 24*, 101558. https://doi.org/10.1016/j.ssmph.2023.101558

Marçal, K. (2021). Caregiver depression and child behaviour problems: A longitudinal mixed effects approach. *Child & Family Social Work, 26*(1), 26–37. https://doi.org/10.1111/cfs.12786

Massachusetts Child Psychiatry Access Program (MCPAP). (2014). *MCPAP: Massachusetts child psychiatry access project*. Retrieved November 4, 2024, from https://www.mcpap.com/Default.aspx

Maunder, R., & Monks, C. (2018). Children's friendships in middle childhood: How number of friends, reciprocity and friendship quality relate to peer and school identification, and general self-worth. *British Journal of Developmental Psychology, 37*(2), 211–229. https://doi.org/10.1111/bjdp.12268

Miller, P. M., & Commons, M. L. (2010). The benefits of attachment parenting for infants and children: A behavioral developmental view. *Behavioral Development Bulletin, 16*(1), 1–14. https://doi.org/10.1037/h0100514

Mills, C. B., & Carwile, A. M. (2009). The good, the bad, and the borderline: Separating teasing from bullying. *Communication Education, 58*(2), 276–301. https://doi.org/10.1080/03634520902783666

Mindell, J. A., & Williamson, A. A. (2018). Benefits of a bedtime routine in young children: Sleep, development, and beyond. *Sleep Medicine Reviews, 40*, 93–108. https://doi.org/10.1016/j.smrv.2017.10.007

Mount Sinai Parenting Center. (2024). Mount Sinai parenting Center—Keystone curriculum. https://parenting.mountsinai.org/providers/

Nangle, D. W., Erdley, C. A., Newman, J. E., Mason, C. A., & Carpenter, E. M. (2003). Popularity, friendship quantity, and friendship quality: Interactive influences on children's loneliness and depression. *Journal of Clinical Child & Adolescent Psychology, 32*(4), 546–555. https://doi.org/10.1207/S15374424JCCP3204_7

Pluhar, E., Kavanaugh, J. R., Levinson, J. A., & Rich, M. (2019). Problematic interactive media use in teens: Comorbidities, assessment, and treatment. *Psychology Research and Behavior Management, 12*, 447. https://doi.org/10.2147/PRBM.S208968

Potegal, M., Kosorok, M., & Davidson, R. (2003). Temper tantrums in young children: 2. Tantrum duration and temporal organization. *Journal of Developmental & Behavioral Pediatrics, 24*(3), 148–154. https://doi.org/10.1097/00004703-200306000-00003

Rowell, T., & Neal-Barnett, A. (2022). A systematic review of the effect of parental adverse childhood experiences on parenting and child psychopathology. *Journal of Child & Adolescent Trauma, 15*(1), 167–180. https://doi.org/10.1007/s40653-021-00400-x

Siegfried, C. B., & Blackshear, K. (2016). *Is it ADHD or child traumatic stress? A guide for clinicians.* National Center for Child Traumatic Stress.

StopBullying.gov. (2019). *Laws, policies & regulations.* https://www.stopbullying.gov/resources/laws

The Trevor Project. (2024). *Support homepage.* The Trevor Project. Retrieved November 4, 2024, from https://www.thetrevorproject.org/

Wakschlag, L. S., Roberts, M. Y., Flynn, R. M., Smith, J. D., Krogh-Jespersen, S., Kaat, A. J., Gray, L., Walkup, J., Marino, B. S., Norton, E. S., & Davis, M. M. (2019). Future directions for early childhood prevention of mental disorders: A road map to mental health, earlier. *Journal of Clinical Child & Adolescent Psychology, 48*(3), 539–554. https://doi.org/10.1080/15374416.2018.1561296

Williamson, M. L. C., Roberman, S., Sopchak, K., & Mosley, T. M. (2023). School avoidance: How to help when a child refuses to go. *Journal of Family Practice, 72*(7), 304–319. https://doi.org/10.12788/jfp.0653

Zeanah, C. H. (2018). *Handbook of infant mental health.* Guilford Publications. https://www.guilford.com/books/Handbook of Infant Mental-Health/Charles-Zeanah/9781462537105?srsltid=AfmBOopiEKCWNOGUt319VmiwuoBF2bd4K_imQ-bUrBxiKYktTzIzaxJZ

Zelazo, P. D., Carlson, S. M., & Kesek, A. (2008). The development of executive function in childhood. In *Handbook of developmental cognitive neuroscience* (p. 553). Boston Review.

Zero to Three. (2024a). *DC: 0–5 manual and training.* An essential guide to infant and early childhood mental health diagnostic formulation with infants, young children, and their families, in a wide range of settings. https://www.zerotothree.org/our-work/learn-professional-development/dc0-5-manual-and-training/

Zero to Three. (2024b). *For families.* Resources for families: Supporting your child's growth. https://www.zerotothree.org/resources/for-families/

Chapter 12
Models of Behavioral Health Assessment and Treatment in Primary Care

Christina L. Lee MD, MPH, Deepu George PhD, LMFT, and Yajaira Johnson-Esparza PhD

An Overview of the Collaborative Care Model (CoCM)

The Collaborative Care Model (CoCM) was initially developed and piloted by Dr. Wayne Katon and colleagues at the University of Washington in the 1990s as a systematic strategy for treating BH conditions in the primary care setting (Raney, 2015). Its overall goal is to increase access and quality of BH care through a team-based approach within the primary care setting. The PCP remains the primary treatment manager of the patient, with the assistance of a BH care manager who offers brief psychotherapeutic intervention, and a psychiatric consultant who provides psychopharmacologic recommendations.

Since its conception in the 1990s, the CoCM has evolved into a model with a robust evidence base. The Improving Mood-Promoting Access to Collaborative Treatment (IMPACT) trial published in 1995 represents the first large scale study of collaborative care in the treatment of depression in older adults (Katon et al., 1995). Over the last two decades, there have since been over 90 randomized controlled trials in the United States and abroad that have been conducted utilizing the CoCM model and demonstrate its effectiveness across numerous treatment settings, patient populations, diagnoses, and payor groups (Archer et al., 2012; Ell et al., 2009; Fortney et al., 2007; Panagioti et al., 2016). This evidence supports the use of CoCM in the

C. L. Lee MD, MPH (✉)
University of California Davis School of Medicine, Sacramento, CA, USA
e-mail: cnalee@health.ucdavis.edu

D. George PhD, LMFT
University of Texas Rio Grande Valley School of Medicine, Edinburg, TX, USA
e-mail: deepu.george@utrgv.edu

Y. Johnson-Esparza PhD
University of Texas San Antonio, San Antonio, TX, USA
e-mail: johnsonespar@uthscsa.edu

M. L. C. Williamson and D. L. Terry (eds.), *Essentials for Treating Behavioral Health in Primary Care*, https://doi.org/10.1007/978-3-032-09558-9_12

treatment of depression, depression and chronic medical conditions, anxiety, post-traumatic stress disorder, chronic pain, and dementia. There is also growing literature to support its effectiveness in the treatment of substance use disorder, attention deficit hyperactivity disorder, bipolar disorder, and other conditions within child and adolescent populations (Gerrity, 2016; Melek et al., 2018). A meta-analysis of collaborative care treatment of depression and chronic medical conditions also found significant improvements in physical and mental quality of life and social role functioning of patients (Woltmann et al., 2012). Furthermore, studies have demonstrated that CoCM is both cost-effective, with an estimated healthcare savings of $3363 per patient over a 4-year period, and garners high satisfaction rates among a large majority of patients and providers (Levine et al., 2005; Unützer et al., 2002, 2008).

Core Principles of Collaborative Care

In 2011, a panel of national experts in integrated BH convened by the Advancing Integrated Mental Health Solutions (AIMS) Center identified five core principles that define effective collaborative care programs (University of Washington, 2023).

1. Patient-centered care team: primary care and BH providers collaborate effectively as a team in the care of both the physical and mental health of patients using shared care plans.
2. Population-based care: the care team shares a defined group of patients tracked in a registry to ensure no one falls through the cracks. The patient registry is used to track and outreach patients who are not improving, and the psychiatric consultant provides caseload-focused consultation to help adjust treatment if needed.
3. Measurement-based care: each patient's treatment plan articulates personal goals and clinical outcomes are routinely measured by evidence-based screening tools.
4. Evidence-based care: patients are offered evidence-based treatment that supports their efficacy in treating the target condition. This includes a variety of psychotherapies proven to work in primary care and medications.
5. Accountable care: providers are accountable and reimbursed for the quality of care and clinical outcomes, not just the volume of care provided.

Collaborative Care Team

CoCM is often combined with a Stepped Care Approach, which is based on the principle that different patients may need different levels of care for the same problem (Von Korff & Tiemens, 2000). Providers are tasked with continually monitoring symptoms to determine where on the continuum of care the patient should be treated, including moving patients from lower or higher and more specialized levels of care depending on severity of symptoms and response to treatment. This approach can improve outcomes and assist with cost savings.

In the outpatient setting, stepped care starts with self-care management techniques, watchful waiting, and follow up for subthreshold symptoms. Care can be escalated from interventions implemented by the primary care physician to enrollment in collaborative care with psychiatric consultation or brief BH interventions in the primary care setting. A referral can also be made to a psychiatrist for ongoing care for more complex or intensive interventions (see Fig. 12.1).

The implementation of collaborative care requires the PCP to work with a team of providers to support the treatment of the patient (see Fig. 12.2). The members of this team and their roles and responsibilities include the following:

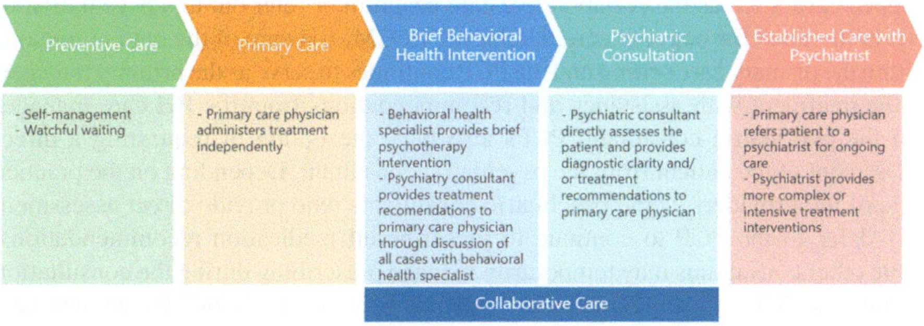

Fig. 12.1 Stepped care approach

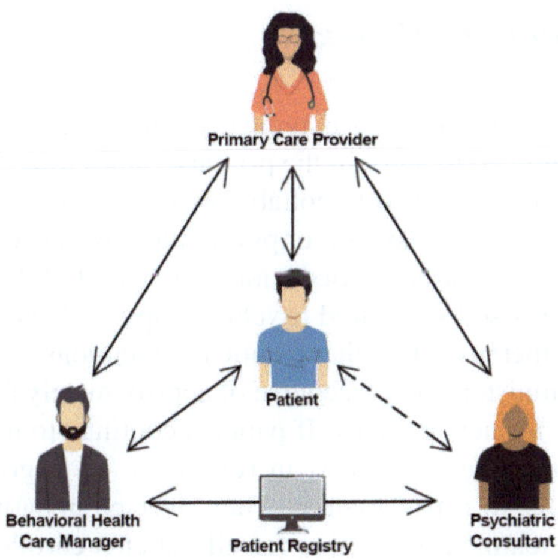

Fig. 12.2 Collaborative care model

Primary Care Provider

The PCP screens for BH symptoms, makes the initial psychiatric diagnosis, and initiates psychopharmacologic treatment. Evidence-based screening tools, such as the Patient Health Questionnaire (PHQ-9) for depression and the Generalized Anxiety Disorder Scale (GAD-7), should be used to identify the presence of a diagnosis, measure the severity of symptoms, detect potential suicidal ideation, and track response to treatment. See Chap. 4 for a complete discussion of screening measures.

If the PCP feels they need assistance with diagnostic clarification or the patient is not improving under their management, they can refer the patient to a higher stepped care, such as the collaborative care program or refer out to a psychiatrist or psychotherapist for ongoing care. Under the CoCM, BH care of the patient remains within the primary care setting and the PCP continues to serve as the primary manager of the treatment with assistance and recommendations from the BH care manager and the psychiatric consultant. PCPs also have the option of requesting a direct assessment of the patient from the psychiatric consultant. Depending on the practice style of the providers, some psychiatric consultants who provide direct assessment may defer to the PCP to continue to prescribe all medication recommendations, while other consultants may temporarily manage prescribing during the consultation period. The PCP typically remains in frequent contact with all CoCM team members regarding the development and implementation of the care plan.

Behavioral Health Care Manager

The behavioral health care manager is typically a nurse, clinical social worker, or psychologist who is trained to work in the primary care setting. They provide initial BH screenings of patients referred to collaborative care, and are trained to provide diagnostic assessment, brief behavioral or psychotherapy interventions, care coordination, and support the initiation of medications by the PCP. They are often trained in providing evidence-based structured psychotherapy such as cognitive behavioral and problem-solving therapy. Their therapeutic interventions are intended to be time limited, typically administered over a course of approximately four months, to allow for ongoing capacity for new patients. If patients continue to need specialized care afterward, the care manager can assist in referral to an ongoing psychotherapist or recommend transfer to a psychiatrist. They oversee updating and maintaining a registry, in which treatment responses for all patients enrolled in the CoCM are systematically tracked with evidence-based measurement tools (e.g., PHQ-9 and GAD-7). This registry helps the CoCM team identify patients who are not reaching treatment goals and need treatment adjustment. They discuss all CoCM patients with the psychiatric consultant through frequent, typically weekly, case review meetings. Cases prioritized for review often include new patients enrolled in CoCM, patients who are not responding to treatment, and patients who are "graduating" from the

CoCM program. Diagnostic and treatment recommendations discussed during these case review meetings are shared with the PCP. Though there is no specific consensus on caseload size, it is common for care managers to have between 50 and 100 patients when they are at full capacity.

Psychiatric Consultant

The psychiatric consultant is usually a psychiatrist, though can alternatively be a nurse practitioner or physician assistant certified in psychiatry, who advises the CoCM team in the treatment of the patient. They help to refine diagnoses and make treatment recommendations to the PCP through discussion of patients with the BH care manager during the CoCM case review meetings and do not typically assess the patient directly. These recommendations can include medication adjustment. If the patient would benefit from a more specialized assessment, the PCP can refer the patient for direct assessment with the psychiatric consultant, typically provided over a course of one to three visits. The psychiatric consultant is often located offsite, but colocation of the psychiatric consultant within the primary care office often helps to improve collaboration with PCPs and allow for curbside consultation.

The patient is responsible for attending and remaining an active participant in their care. They work with the PCP and BH care manager in achieving care goals and track response to treatment. Some patients may also work directly with the psychiatric consultant.

CoCM: Practical Considerations for the Primary Care Provider

Establishing Value

A critical step in starting a CoCM program is establishing value (American Medical Association (AMA), 2024). Key stakeholders who need to be included and considered in the planning stages include providers, support staff, payers, organizational management, and patients. Sharing evidence-based outcomes and patient case studies with leadership can help to convince them of the potential positive impact of CoCM. It can be important to frame that CoCM can help to reduce workload and burnout of PCPs through the creation of more accessible and effective BH treatment resources.

Reimbursement for CoCM

There are various strategies that an organization can adopt to help fund collaborative care (American Psychiatric Association (APA), 2024; Centers for Medicare and Medicaid Services, 2023). Medicare, commercial payers, and many Medicaid plans now provide reimbursement for these services. In a healthcare organization (HCO) that is fully capitated, such as in a managed care organization, the cost of CoCM will need to be covered by the organization. In a partially capitated program, in which care is funded through a combination of capitated premiums and fee-for-service, clinics may be able to obtain a case rate payment for the BH care management services. Some payers may reimburse through case rate payment, in which the organization is reimbursed a flat rate per episode of care, or value-based payments, which reimburse according to quality of service or patient outcomes. Most commonly, organizations are utilizing strategies of direct billing through a combination of traditional fee-for-service and collaborative care billing codes. Additionally, there are also specific billing codes that Federally Qualified Health Centers and Rural Health Clinics can use to bill for services.

Incorporating Psychiatric Screening into the Workflow

Diagnosing psychiatric disorders and utilizing evidence-based screening tools may seem challenging in the primary care setting, where providers often have limited time with patients. Consider having support staff send self-administered screeners to the patient prior to their appointment, via the electronic medical record and online patient portal. For patients who do not have access to a patient portal, they can be prompted to fill out the screeners in the waiting room upon check-in, so as not to take up time during the appointment. Medical assistants, if present, may be able to assist with inputting responses into the medical record, where the PCP can review the responses and scores and determine if further exploration or discussion is needed during the appointment. See Chap. 13 for additional tips on how to maximize use of the medical team.

Deciding Where to Refer Patients

A difficult task for PCPs can include deciding what level of care would be most appropriate to refer a patient to if they are not improving under initial treatment management. Ideal patients for the CoCM include patients with more straightforward diagnosis who may stabilize with brief intervention and recommendations from the BH specialists. The PCP should feel comfortable maintaining management of the patient with the help of additional consultation. In contrast, patients with multiple psychiatric or complex diagnoses, a history of multiple failed medication trials, significant safety concerns, or serious mental illness like Schizophrenia or Bipolar 1 Disorder may benefit from a referral to a psychiatrist for ongoing care when available.

Building Relationships with the Behavioral Health Team

One of the key features to successful collaborative care is effective communication and teamwork. Co-locating the BH care manager and psychiatric consultant within the primary care clinic and situating their clinical space centrally within the office space can help to foster more in-person interaction between team members. Increased opportunity to pass each other in the hallway can lead to informal relationship building. Communication is also a two-way street. PCPs can help the team further optimize the care plan by sharing any clinical updates while the patient is enrolled in CoCM. They can also consider inviting the psychiatric consultant and care manager to provide educational lectures to all the PCPs in the office on high yield topics, which can help to build knowledge base and comfort level with managing psychiatric conditions for the entire practice at once.

Implementing in a Small Clinical Practice

Only 25 percent of primary care practices in the United States have an on-site BH specialist (Fortney et al., 2007). The CoCM can be adapted to help expand BH care in smaller or rural clinics. In the early 2000s, the Veterans Administration (VA) conducted a randomized control trial that demonstrated the successful implementation of telemedicine-based CoCM for depression in their VA community-based outpatient clinics. Telemedicine technologies (e.g., telephone, interactive video, electronic medical records, and the internet) were used to facilitate communication between patients and primary care physicians at smaller satellite community clinics and telepsychiatrists located at a more centrally located VA medical center. Telemedicine partnerships with larger medical centers or urban centers may be a feasible way to implement collaborative care in small clinical practice.

Bringing It Home: A Case Study

Patient A.S. is a 45-year-old woman with a history of depression, anxiety, fibromyalgia, and hypertension who presents for an appointment with her PCP. Her PHQ-9 score is 13 and GAD-7 score is 12. Her PCP interprets these scores to be indicative of worsening depressive and anxiety symptoms and discusses further with the patient. A.S. has a several year history of depression and anxiety that was previously well managed on maximum dose escitalopram. However, she now reports her symptoms have steadily worsened over the last 6 months after recently losing her job, facing increasing financial stress, and ongoing pain related to her fibromyalgia. Her PCP decides to switch her medication to Sertraline and places a collaborative care referral.

Two weeks later, A.S. has an intake with the BH care manager, who repeats the screeners and finds her PHQ-9 score has increased to 15 and GAD-7 score remains at 12. Her diagnosis is further clarified to be recurrent Major Depressive Disorder and Generalized Anxiety Disorder. Her BH care manager begins cognitive behavioral therapy with A.S. every 2 weeks. After 3 sessions, PHQ-9 and GAD-7 scores have still not significantly improved.

Her care manager discusses A.S. with the psychiatric consultant in their weekly case review meeting, and the psychiatrist suggests switching her medication to duloxetine, with the hopes that it may co-treat her mental health and pain symptoms. This recommendation is communicated to A.S.'s PCP in a brief note written in her electronic medical record and includes detailed cross-titration instructions and recommendations to monitor for a potential side effect of increased blood pressure. Her PCP reviews these recommendations and decides to prescribe these changes. Two months later, A.S. describes an improvement in her depression, anxiety, and pain symptoms with a combination of duloxetine and brief psychotherapy. Her PHQ-9 score has improved to 3 and her GAD-7 score is 2. The care manager and psychiatric consultant review A.S.'s positive treatment progress during their case review meeting and decide to "graduate" her from the collaborative care program and remove her from the patient registry.

An Overview of the Primary Care Behavioral Health Model (PCBH)

The Primary Care Behavioral Health (PCBH) has been implemented across a number settings, including the U.S. Veterans health Administration, the U.S. Department of Defense, community health centers, and university health centers (Hunter et al., 2018). Although there is a lack of studies that compare the PCBH model to other models of integration, the existing literature provides substantial evidence in support of PCBH.

The PCBH model is associated with positive patient outcomes, including improvement in functioning and symptomatology across adults (Angantyr et al., 2015; Bridges et al., 2015) and pediatric populations (Bridges et al., 2014). Improvements are observed across clinical presentations, such as depression and anxiety (Angantyr et al., 2015; Cigrang et al., 2011), suicidal ideation (Bryan et al., 2012), posttraumatic stress disorder (Cigrang et al., 2011, 2015), sleep/wake dysfunction (Goodie et al., 2009), and general mental health (Corso et al., 2009). PBCH is also associated with health behavior change (Sadock et al., 2014) and improvements in management of chronic conditions (Cummings et al., 2019). Further, patients receiving care within the PCBH model report satisfaction with the services they have received (Funderburk et al., 2010, 2012; Ogbeide et al., 2018).

Implementation of PCBH is associated with greater provider satisfaction (Aguirre & Carrion, 2013) and the perception that patients benefit from BH services (Funderburk et al., 2012). Importantly, the implementation of the PCBH model has been shown to increase access to BH services. In a system serving over 30,000 patients, the implementation of a PCBH model increased access to BH by almost 400% (Brawer et al., 2010).

Like the CoCM model, the PCBH model is a team-based approach. PCBH differs from CoCM in that PCBH emphasizes same-day accessibility of BH consultation and focused behavioral support around managing BH problems and health conditions influenced by biopsychosocial factors. CoCM, in contrast, is typically disease-specific and offers a more intensive BH intervention over many months with the option of psychiatric consultation.

There is still much research to be conducted to further support the effectiveness and value of the PCBH model. Among the biggest barriers to adequately understanding the effectiveness of PCBH has been the issue with fidelity to the model. Without a standardized definition of the PCBH model, it has been difficult to know to what extent many research studies truly adhered to the PCBH model. Reiter et al. (2018) provide what has become a widely accepted definition of the PCBH model of consultation.

The PCBH model is a team-based primary care approach to managing BH problems and biopsychosocially-influenced health conditions. The model's main goal is to enhance the primary care team's ability to manage and treat such problems/conditions, with resulting improvements in primary care services for the entire clinic population. The model incorporates a BH consultant (BHC) into the primary care team.

Core Principles of PCBH

The PCBH model, similar to primary care, is rooted in population health management. As such, the PBCH model aims to address health at the general population level, as opposed to providing direct high-intensity care to a segment of the patient population as is the case in specialty mental health (Robinson & Reiter, 2016). Importantly, what differentiates the PCBH model from other models of integration is its foundation in a consultant approach (Robinson & Reiter, 2016). BH providers in this model serve as consultants and as such, are referred to as behavioral health consultants (BHCs).

In a consultant approach, the primary consumer is the PCP. As such, the goal of the BHC is to assist the PCP in management of the behavioral needs of the patient population—the BHC is an extension of the PCP. In fact, in the PCBH model, the

PCP maintains ownership of the care of the patient, which differs from specialty mental health models where the BH clinician would have ownership of care. To effectively meet the various needs of the patient population, a team-based approach that includes effective communication and shared treatment planning is essential. Given the primary consumer of the BHC is the PCP, the extent to which the BHC is utilized will depend on how effectively the BHC is able to assist the PCP in caring for their patients.

Consistent with a population health management approach, a BHC must be accessible and available to provide "on-demand" visits, thus increasing the likelihood of engagement in BH services. The "on-demand" visits are facilitated through "warm handoffs" (Tolliver et al., 2022). A consultant approach allows for greater productivity and a higher patient volume, as it does not emphasize higher-intensity care to a segment of the patient population. The scope of practice is wide, which means that patients of all ages and with all presentations are within the scope of the BHC. Finally, care will be provided until a patient progresses toward goals (e.g., improved functioning), as opposed to providing care until a patient's goals have been met (e.g., symptom remission).

The PCBH Team

In the PCBH model (see Fig. 12.3), the role of the Behavioral Health Consultant (BHC) is to serve as an extension of the PCP and to provide support to the treatment team in an effort to meet the health needs of the patient population. To this effect, the BHC must be prepared to meet the needs of patients across the developmental continuum and across health presentations (e.g., BH conditions, lifestyle management, chronic disease management). BHCs must provide evidence-based nonpharmacological services that are accessible, team-based, and routine. The BHC is a BH clinician with a license to practice in a healthcare setting (e.g., PhD/PsyD in psychology, a masters in social work, masters in professional counseling, and masters in marriage and family therapy).

The introduction of the BHC as part of the primary care team offers up new ways of working as a team both for the PCP and the BHC. This new way of working together is designed to amplify principles of population health. This implies that a strong implementation of PCBH will prioritize: (a) a systematic, team-based (BHC + Primary Care Provider + primary care team) approach to improving the health of all in the given population; (b) aim to maximize impact through lower intensity, evidence-based, BH interventions to a large number patients than a high-intensity intervention for a smaller number of patients; and (c) develop clinical pathways and standard procedures for patients with specific conditions or risk factors. The BHC and PCP are working together to address common biological, psychological, relational and spiritual quests of the patient. Like the PCP, the BHC can equally impact the following conditions through evidence-based, nonpharmacological interventions:

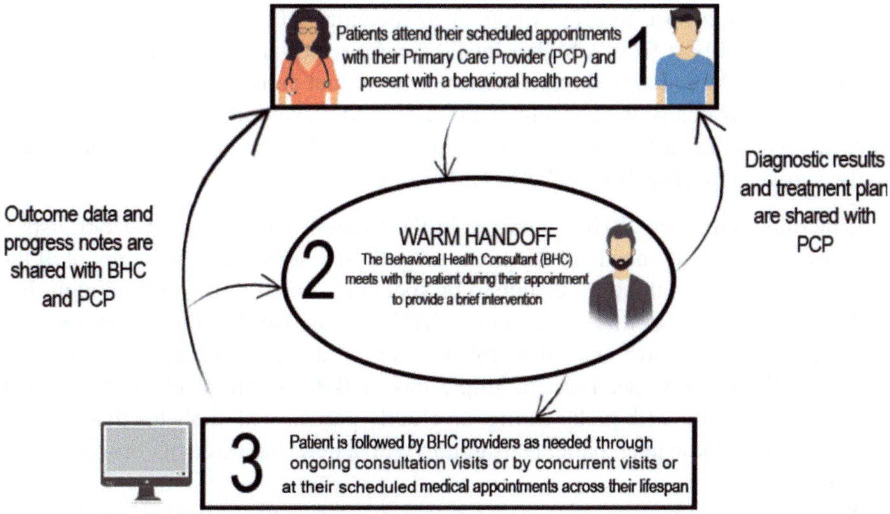

Fig. 12.3 Primary care behavioral health model

1. Preventive care needs (e.g., tobacco cessation, healthy eating, improved fitness).
2. Chronic disease (e.g., diabetes, hypertension, asthma, COPD, chronic pain).
3. Psychiatric comorbidities (e.g., depression, anxiety, PTSD, ADHD, unhealthy alcohol, and illicit substance use).
4. Sub-threshold and social problems (e.g., divorce and separation, child behavior problems, domestic violence).
5. Medically unexplained symptoms (e.g., chronic fatigue, chronic dizziness).
6. Factors impacting standard care (e.g., boundary setting, lack of resources/support, problem solving for social barriers, improving treatment adherence).

In a care episode that presents with any of the above instances, both PCPs and BHCs can work together in a way that comprehensively addresses patient needs (pharmacological and nonpharmacological interventions) and serve as professional support for each other in their clinical work.

The Behavioral Health Consultant

Whereas in specialty BH (i.e., traditional referral for BH from PCP) the customer is typically the client/patient, in the PCBH model, the customer is the PCP. As such, BHC visits typically involve "warm-handoffs" and scheduled appointments. These visits typically take 15–30 min. A treatment episode with a BHC can consist of a single visit or several visits across several months until symptoms and/or functioning improve. Importantly, a BHC can be re-engaged in the care of a patient as needed, whether for a similar issue/problem or a completely different referral reason. BHCs may sometimes choose to refer a patient to specialty BH if it is deemed a patient would be served best from a higher level of care, which might be the case when a patient has not demonstrated improvement after repeat contact with the BHC.

As noted above, a BHC working in a PCBH model exemplifies several characteristics and works toward meeting certain expectations. These can be best remembered by the acronym GATHER (see Table 12.1; Reiter et al., 2018).

- **G**eneralist approach: BHCs working in the PCBH model must be generalists if they are to meet the needs of the patient population versus a small segment of the population. BHCs do not presume to be specialists in all things BH, though they do have expertise in this area. Rather, BHCs recognize that they cannot have a narrow focus and must instead be able to take on various clinical problems across the developmental spectrum. In single day, a BHC might work with a family with a 3-year-old with picky eating, an elderly patient with diabetes that is not at goal, and a middle aged patient struggling with a new diagnosis of chronic kidney disease.
- **A**ccessibility: In PCBH, same-day is key. BHCs strive to see patients on the same day that the PCP has requested assistance in what is commonly referred to as a "warm handoff" versus a scheduled consultation. At times, due to time constraints, a full visit might not be possible. Even then a BHC will strive to have some level of contact with the patient to increase the likelihood of a full visit at a later time, whether at the scheduled consultation with the BHC or at the next PCP visit. Additionally, BHCs are available for curbside consultations when full visit with a patient may not be warranted. Curbside consultations are typically brief and informal discussions to help a PCP or other team members with management of a patient's care. It is also common for BHCs to have their workstations alongside those of PCPs and other team members to increase access.
- **T**eam-based approach: The BHC is an essential member of the team, as is any other team member (e.g., nurse, medical assistant, primary care provider, community health workers). A BHC serves as an extender of the PCP, just as would another team member. Recognizing that a 15-min medical visit does not allow a PCP to address the myriad of issues patients might be experiencing, particularly those with complex presentations, a BHC makes themselves available to assist the PCP in addressing some of these issues. For instance, a BHC can assist with addressing biopsychosocial factors contributing to a patient's poor management of a chronic disease. Serving as an active member of the treatment team contributes to the effectiveness of primary care.
- **H**igh productivity/volume: BHCs strive for high penetration of the patient population. To this goal, BHCs will typically provide care to 10–14 patients a day as compared to 5–7 patients, as might be the case in specialty mental health. Productivity goals typically mirror those of PCPs. If a PCP has a panel of 15-min visits and is expected to average approximately 20 patients a day, a BHC who has 30-minute visits might be expected to care for 20 patients a day on average. To ensure that a high percentage of the patient population is cared for, BHCs make sure that they are not seeing the same group/panel of patients for numerous follow

up visits, but are instead having unique patient visits. Some patients might be seen for a single visit while other patients might receive a series of follow up visits until improvement in functioning is observed.

- **E**ducator: The goal of the BHC is to improve the efficiency of the primary care team, which can happen not only through direct patient care and consultation, but through functioning as an educator. Given expertise in biopsychosocial factors impacting health and wellbeing, among other areas of expertise (e.g., communication skills), BHCs provide education to the PCP and other team members with the goal of improving care provided to patients and other areas, including team dynamics, screening procedures, among others. This education can take place during curbside consultations, if precepting medical learners, during morning huddles, and during staff meetings.
- **R**outine: The BHC is fully integrated into the treatment team. BH services are regarded by the treatment team and introduced to patients as a routine aspect of their care. This is a shift in how BH services might be perceived in other settings in which there is a clear demarcation between primary care services and mental health services. By regarding BH services as routine, one increases the likelihood of routinely using these services when necessary, and importantly, it has the added benefit of reducing stigma. PCPs are encouraged to use language that highlights the routine nature of these services when introducing them to patients. For instance, a PCP might choose to say, "whenever I am working with a patient who could benefit from additional support with management of diabetes, I always bring in a team member who can help me."

The goal of the PCBH model and its core components closely align with the functions of primary care, as described by Starfield (1998) including first contact, continuity, comprehensiveness, and coordinated care.

Table 12.1 Characteristics of an effective BHC in the PCBH model

Generalist	Works with patients across the lifespan for any BH concerns
Accessible	Accessible to assist the PCP at all times, whether for a warm handoff or curbside consultation
Team-based	Essential and active member of the team, collaborates with other team members from the PCP to other staff
High productivity	High volume of patients seen for BH concerns, greater penetration of the patient population
Educator	Educates PCPs and staff in biopsychosocial factors impact health and wellbeing and other areas of expertise (e.g., communication skills)
Routine	Engagement in BH services is recognized as a routine aspect of care

PCBH: Practical Considerations for the Primary Care Provider

While the PCBH definition outlines the expected boundaries of GATHER to guide BHC competencies and behaviors in primary care, we will provide a similar set of behavioral anchors for PCPs. To maximize the impact of the PCBH model, PCPs can monitor key behaviors in six competence domains to improve PCBH integration efforts:

Clinical Practice Skills

The PCP has basic knowledge of best practice guidelines for biopsychosocial interventions for common presenting problems. From a practical point of view, this means that the PCP is skilled at rapidly identifying the problem and the functional impact of the problem. For example, for a patient with uncontrolled diabetes, rather than alternating treatment plans, the PCP should consider barriers or challenges to adherence or other situational factors that have led to low compliance. In addition to recognizing this, the PCP can quickly include the BHC to resolve these challenges. In a follow-up appointment, the PCP will support the BHC interventions by checking-in on progress or making it part of their review.

Practice Management Skills

The PCP can effectively activate the BHC as a treatment extender. Primarily, the PCP can rely on the BHC to improve an encounter in several ways. For example, they can use the BHC to save a visit by scheduling a follow-up visit for a patient who has just started on psychiatric meds. By scheduling with the BHC, the PCP saves a visit and the appointment can be utilized differently.

Consultation Skills

While PCPs are likely to be familiar with working with consultants during their hospital work, there is a tendency to view the BHC like a traditional BH provider. As a consultant to the PCP and the team, a primary goal of the BHC is to complete as many same-day visits as possible. A PCP who understands this consultant role of the BHC is willing to interrupt BHC appointments to request a consult or other assistance. Similarly, the PCP also recognizes the BHC can be consulted for non-clinical aspects of patient care such as feedback on a difficult patient encounter, improving the PCP-patient relationship, or managing the relationship with a patient with biomedical and psychosocial adversities.

Documentation Skills

A benefit of an integrated BHC is the ability to receive immediate feedback on a patient, which may either confirm the plans discussed or provide new directions. A PCP who embraces the full spectrum of possibilities with PCBH will make time to receive feedback from the BHC. Practices may vary in frequency and form of communication, however communication between the PCP and BHC about patients remains critical. The PCP should be mindful of documenting the integration of BHC as part of the treatment plan in the chart note, write down salient points from curbside consultations indicated, and review the BHC plan before a follow-up meeting with a returning patient for a PCP visit.

Team Performance Skills

The central element of the PCBH model is the relationship between the PCP and the BHC. As one of the influential members of the primary care team, the PCP will provide support to the BHC services. These supporting mechanisms can include standing orders for BHC services or collaborating with the BHC in the design and implementation of an effective pathway.

Administrative Skills

PCBH is more than placing a BHC in a primary care setting for mental health needs. A PCP is a powerful partner in helping the BHC actualize its full potential. In addition to understanding multiple ways, the PCBH services can enhance patient care. An ideal PCP champion will also advocate for PCBH with clinic or health system leadership. As front line providers, PCPs have an important voice in the processes of health systems. BHC colleagues need these partnerships to advance the integration mission.

Reimbursement for PCBH

Billing strategies for PCBH are similar with CoCM. As with COCM, there are various strategies to fund PCBH. Medicare, commercial payers and many Medicaid plans now provide reimbursement for these services. In a healthcare organization (HCO) that is fully capitated, such as in a managed care organization, the cost of CoCM will need to be covered by the organization. In a partially capitated program, in which care is funded through a combination of capitated premiums and fee-for-service, clinics may be able to obtain a case rate payment for the BH care management services. Some payers may reimburse through case rate payment, in which the organization is reimbursed a flat rate per episode of care, or value-based payments, which reimburse according to quality of service or patient outcomes. Most commonly, organizations are utilizing strategies of direct billing through a combination of traditional fee-for-service and collaborative care billing codes. Additionally, there are also specific billing codes that Federally Qualified Health Centers and Rural Health Clinics can use to bill for services.

Other Considerations for the PCP and the Practice

All of the competencies discussed above are geared toward a single direction: how to provide contextual and compassionate care as a team. PCPs working within the PCBH model therefore must know how to effectively work with their BHC colleagues. Compared to a refer-out model, in PCBH, a PCP must function with a keen awareness of the interplay between biology, psychological factors, and social factors (e.g., social determinants of health). Oftentimes, this means recognizing that an individual's presentation does not occur within a vacuum, void of context. Recognizing that multiple contextual factors impact a patient's presentation means a PCP might be more apt to seek the involvement of their BHC colleagues.

A PCP might build this competency as they go through their schedule of the day to chart check. For example, if they routinely ask themselves, "How can the BHC help me with this patient?" as they review patient charts for the day, it will naturally lead to more collaborative work with the BHC. Routinely asking themselves this question versus asking themselves, "Can the BHC help me with this patient?" can force a PCP to consider a patient's context and how it impacts the patient's health and wellbeing. Additionally, in doing so, the PCP can involve the BHC earlier on by placing these patients on their radar.

A pitfall to avoid is to see the work of the BHC as limited. For example, there might be a tendency to say "This patient is too complex." Just like a PCP encounter, a BHC encounter is not designed to "resolve" complexity in a single visit. BHC visits are designed to help the patient self-manage some aspects of their life to improve their functioning. In other words, BHCs follow the same principle of having a long-term relationship with the patient and working with the PCP to guide them in their steps toward health. In the same way, BHCs also see patients with PCPs longitudinally and do not have "visit" limits.

Implementing in Rural Clinical Practices

PCBH has been successfully implemented in rural clinical practices (e.g., Gouge et al., 2016) and is associated with increased access and improved patient outcomes and cost. However, there are several considerations when implementing this model in rural practices, including workforce shortages, geographic isolation, and limited resources. Due to BH workforce shortages and geographic isolation, PCPs' options for referral are limited. For this reason, the role of a BHC in primary care is critical, as BHCs can be consulted rather than relying on referrals to specialty mental health clinics. Even in urban settings, patients are more likely to accept BH services in primary care than seek out specialty mental health services (Ogbeide et al., 2018).

The BH workforce shortage can also impact a rural practice specifically, as hiring can be challenging. Practices can consider becoming training sites for psychology, counseling, marriage and family therapy students, social work students and interns; thus, developing a pipeline for BHCs (Selby-Nelson et al., 2018).

Bringing It Home: A Case Study

Dr. Martinez is a family medicine physician in a clinic that has adopted PCBH as a model of integration. Since starting at this clinic, Dr. Martinez has become appreciative of the role of the BHC in helping her more effectively care for her patients, especially those with complex presentations. Today, like every other day, she arrives at the clinic early to chart-check her patients for the day. Throughout her time at this clinic, she has made it a routine practice to consider the many ways in which her BHC colleague, Dr. Wilson, a licensed clinical health psychologist, can support her in caring for her patients. Although she is a firm believer that the BHC could help her with each of her patients, she wants to prioritize those who would especially benefit from a BHC visit today. She checks in with the BHC who is sitting in the same workroom as her and reviews the patients she would like Dr. Wilson to visit during the morning clinic. Dr. Martinez discusses the following patients with Dr. Wilson: a 55-year-old woman with multiple chronic conditions and poor adherence, a 27-year-old male with chronic pain, a 3-year-old with picky eating, and a 63-year-old man with recent myocardial infarction and depression.

Dr. Martinez has also informed her medical assistant of the patients with whom Dr. Wilson plans to have a visit to ensure workflow is not significantly impacted. At the end of her morning clinic, Dr. Martinez cares for a patient who is establishing care. This patient complains of issues with long-standing insomnia. Dr. Martinez introduces BH services, informing her that it is routine for her to request Dr. Wilson's assistance when patients express concern about insomnia. Dr. Martinez sends a chat through the electronic health record to Dr. Wilson asking for assistance with this patient. Dr. Wilson is able to complete a same-day visit (i.e., warm handoff) with this patient and provides an evidence-based intervention to assist with management of insomnia. Given that the warm handoff was completed within 30 min, Dr. Wilson is then available for another PCP requesting assistance with a patient who is reporting forgetfulness.

After the morning clinic, Dr. Martinez realizes that she has not followed up with Dr. Wilson regarding the last patient. Dr. Martinez makes it a point to always follow up with Dr. Wilson to make sure there is a shared treatment plan. Dr. Martinez documents in her note a summary of her discussion with Dr. Wilson so she knows to follow up regarding the intervention provided by Dr. Wilson at the next visit.

Conclusions

PCBH and CoCM are both evidence and population-based models of integrating BH services within primary care. They both offer increased BH support to primary care physicians, making it more accessible to deliver comprehensive mental health care within the primary care setting. Strengths of the PCBH model include same-day BH interventions, particularly helpful in addressing more acute issues, and "warm handoffs" between PCPs and the BH consultant which maximizes collaboration and helps to optimize clinic workflow. However, this model does not typically include a psychiatric consultant on the team or systemically track response to treatment. Strengths of CoCM include a more intensive brief psychotherapeutic interventions delivered over many months and inclusion of psychiatric consultation which can provide psychopharmacologic recommendations. CoCM also utilizes a measurement-based approach and tracks treatment response for all patients enrolled in the program through a registry, which can help to identify patients who are not reaching targeted treatment goals and in need of treatment adjustment. Limitations of this model include that it is typically diagnosis specific (most often focusing on depression and anxiety) and the offers less immediate accessibility of services.

Determining which model will be best for a practice depends on the needs and goals of the practice, among other factors (e.g., billing considerations, financial sustainability, team composition). To help identify an ideal model for a specific clinic, consider examining the psychiatric and BH needs among the population served. A systematic review of patient panels can reveal patterns of need that may be suited for one model over the other or a blend of both. For example, a primary care practice with a higher percentage of patients with physical or chronic disease management and a lower percentage of active BH needs may benefit from a PCBH strategy to help the system integrate more broadly. However, if psychiatric comorbidities are higher compared to physical health needs, the site may consider a CoCM approach—a more focused, vertical integration strategy.

Many health systems, however, are likely to have a high level of physical health needs and BH complications. Several systems have therefore chosen a blended model that combines PCBH and CoCM. In a blended approach, a BH provider would serve as a core member of the primary care team who is available for warm handoffs to meet the acute BH needs and other routine care of the patient population. The BH clinician could also serve as the BH manager consistent with the CoCM model with a clear delineation of roles. As BH care, this team member would track systemic treatment response with a registry for a subscribed group of patients receiving more intensive collaborative care services, with assistance of a psychiatric consultation as needed.

Key Points

- PCBH and CoCM are both evidence and population-based models of integrating BH services within primary care. They both offer increased BH support to primary care physicians, making it more accessible to deliver comprehensive mental health care within the primary care setting.
- The BH workforce shortage can impact a rural practice specifically, as hiring can be challenging. Practices can consider becoming training sites for psychology, counseling, marriage and family therapy students, social work students and interns; thus, developing a pipeline for behavioral health consultants.
- Determining which model will be best for a practice depends on the needs and goals of the practice, among other factors (e.g., billing considerations, financial sustainability, team composition).

References

Aguirre, J., & Carrion, V. G. (2013). Integrated behavioral health services: A collaborative care model for pediatric patients in a low-income setting. *Clinical Pediatrics, 52*(12), 1178–1180. https://doi.org/10.1177/0009922812470744

American Medical Association (AMA). (2024). Behavioral health integration compendium. The BHI Collaborative. https://www.ama-assn.org/system/files/bhi-compendium.pdf

American Psychiatric Association (APA). (2024). *Getting paid in the collaborative care model.* https://www.psychiatry.org:443/psychiatrists/practice/professional-interests/integrated-care/get-paid

Angantyr, K., Rimner, A., Nordén, T., & Norlander, T. (2015). Primary care behavioral health model: Perspectives of outcome, client satisfaction, and gender. *Social Behavior and Personality: An International Journal, 43*(2), 287–301. https://doi.org/10.2224/sbp.2015.43.2.287

Archer, J., Bower, P., Gilbody, S., Lovell, K., Richards, D., Gask, L., Dickens, C., & Coventry, P. (2012). Collaborative care for depression and anxiety problems. *Cochrane Database of Systematic Reviews, 10.* https://doi.org/10.1002/14651858.CD006525.pub2

Brawer, P. A., Martielli, R., Pye, P. L., Manwaring, J., & Tierney, A. (2010). St. Louis initiative for integrated care excellence (SLI^{2}CE): Integrated-collaborative care on a large scale model. *Families, Systems & Health, 28*(2), 175–187. https://doi.org/10.1037/a0020342

Bridges, A. J., Andrews, A. R., III, Villalobos, B. T., Pastrana, F. A., Cavell, T. A., & Gomez, D. (2014). Does integrated behavioral health care reduce mental health disparities for Latinos? Initial findings. *Journal of Latina/o Psychology, 2*(1), 37–53. https://doi.org/10.1037/lat0000009

Bridges, A. J., Gregus, S. J., Rodriguez, J. H., Andrews, A. R., III, Villalobos, B. T., Pastrana, F. A., & Cavell, T. A. (2015). Diagnoses, intervention strategies, and rates of functional improvement in integrated behavioral health care patients. *Journal of Consulting and Clinical Psychology, 83*(3), 590–601. https://doi.org/10.1037/a0038941

Bryan, C. J., Corso, K. A., Corso, M. L., Kanzler, K. E., Ray-Sannerud, B., & Morrow, C. E. (2012). Therapeutic alliance and change in suicidal ideation during treatment in integrated primary care settings. *Archives of Suicide Research, 16*(4), 316–323. https://doi.org/10.1080/13811118.2013.722055

Centers for Medicare and Medicaid Services. (2023). *Behavioral health integration services booklet*. Medicare Learning Network.

Cigrang, J. A., Rauch, S. A. M., Avila, L. L., Bryan, C. J., Goodie, J. L., Hryshko-Mullen, A., & Peterson, A. L. (2011). Treatment of active-duty military with PTSD in primary care: Early findings. *Psychological Services, 8*(2), 104–113. https://doi.org/10.1037/a0022740

Cigrang, J. A., Rauch, S. A. M., Mintz, J., Brundige, A., Avila, L. L., Bryan, C. J., Goodie, J. L., Peterson, A. L., & STRONG STAR Consortium. (2015). Treatment of active duty military with PTSD in primary care: A follow-up report. *Journal of Anxiety Disorders, 36*, 110–114. https://doi.org/10.1016/j.janxdis.2015.10.003

Corso, K., Bryan, C., Morrow, C., Appolonio, K., Dodendorf, D., & Baker, M. (2009). Managing posttraumatic stress disorder symptoms in active-duty military personnel in primary care settings. *Journal of Mental Health Counseling, 31*(2), 119–136. https://doi.org/10.17744/mehc.31.2.1m2238t85rv38041

Cummings, D. M., Lutes, L. D., Littlewood, K., Solar, C., Carraway, M., Kirian, K., Patil, S., Adams, A., Ciszewski, S., Edwards, S., Gatlin, P., & Hambidge, B. (2019). Randomized trial of a tailored cognitive behavioral intervention in type 2 diabetes with comorbid depressive and/or regimen-related distress symptoms: 12-month outcomes from COMRADE. *Diabetes Care, 42*(5), 841–848. https://doi.org/10.2337/dc18-1841

Ell, K., Katon, W., Cabassa, L. J., Xie, B., Lee, P.-J., Kapetanovic, S., & Guterman, J. (2009). Depression and diabetes among low-income Hispanics: Design elements of a socio-culturally adapted collaborative care model randomized controlled trial. *The International Journal of Psychiatry in Medicine, 39*(2), 113–132. https://doi.org/10.2190/PM.39.2.a

Fortney, J. C., Pyne, J. M., Edlund, M. J., Williams, D. K., Robinson, D. E., Mittal, D., & Henderson, K. L. (2007). A randomized trial of telemedicine-based collaborative care for depression. *Journal of General Internal Medicine, 22*(8), 1086–1093. https://doi.org/10.1007/s11606-007-0201-9

Funderburk, J. S., Fielder, R. L., DeMartini, K. S., & Flynn, C. A. (2012). Integrating behavioral health services into a university health center: Patient and provider satisfaction. *Families, Systems & Health, 30*(2), 130–140. https://doi.org/10.1037/a0028378

Funderburk, J. S., Sugarman, D. E., Maisto, S. A., Ouimette, P., Schohn, M., Lantinga, L., Wray, L., Batki, S., Nelson, B., Coolhart, D., & Strutynski, K. (2010). The description and evaluation of the implementation of an integrated healthcare model. *Families, Systems & Health: The Journal of Collaborative Family Healthcare, 28*(2), 146–160. https://doi.org/10.1037/a0020223

Gerrity, M. (2016). *Evolving models of behavioral health integration: Evidence update 2010–2015*. Milbank Memorial Fund.

Goodie, J. L., Isler, W. C., Hunter, C., & Peterson, A. L. (2009). Using behavioral health consultants to treat insomnia in primary care: A clinical case series. *Journal of Clinical Psychology, 65*(3), 294–304. https://doi.org/10.1002/jclp.20548

Gouge, N., Polaha, J., Rogers, R., & Harden, A. (2016). Integrating behavioral health into pediatric primary care: Implications for provider time and cost. *Southern Medical Journal, 109*(12), 774–778.

Hunter, C. L., Funderburk, J. S., Polaha, J., Bauman, D., Goodie, J. L., & Hunter, C. M. (2018). Primary care behavioral health (PCBH) model research: Current state of the science and a call to action. *Journal of Clinical Psychology in Medical Settings, 25*(2), 127–156. https://doi.org/10.1007/s10880-017-9512-0

Katon, W., Von Korff, M., Lin, E., Walker, E., Simon, G. E., Bush, T., Robinson, P., & Russo, J. (1995). Collaborative management to achieve treatment guidelines: Impact on depression in primary care. *JAMA, 273*(13), 1026–1031. https://doi.org/10.1001/jama.1995.03520370068039

Levine, S., Unützer, J., Yip, J. Y., Hoffing, M., Leung, M., Fan, M.-Y., Lin, E. H. B., Grypma, L., Katon, W., Harpole, L. H., & Langston, C. A. (2005). Physicians' satisfaction with a collaborative disease management program for late-life depression in primary care. *General Hospital Psychiatry, 27*(6), 383–391. https://doi.org/10.1016/j.genhosppsych.2005.06.001

Melek, S. P., Norris, D. T., Paulus, J., Matthews, K., Weaver, A., & Davenport, S. (2018). *Potential economic impact of integrated medical-behavioral healthcare.* Milliman. https://www.milliman.com/-/media/milliman/importedfiles/uploadedfiles/insight/2018/potential-economic-impact-integrated-healthcare.ashx

Ogbeide, S. A., Landoll, R. R., Nielsen, M. K., & Kanzler, K. E. (2018). To go or not go: Patient preference in seeking specialty mental health versus behavioral consultation within the primary care behavioral health consultation model. *Families, Systems & Health, 36*(4), 513–517. https://doi.org/10.1037/fsh0000374

Panagioti, M., Bower, P., Kontopantelis, E., Lovell, K., Gilbody, S., Waheed, W., Dickens, C., Archer, J., Simon, G., Ell, K., Huffman, J. C., Richards, D. A., van der Feltz-Cornelis, C., Adler, D. A., Bruce, M., Buszewicz, M., Cole, M. G., Davidson, K. W., de Jonge, P., & Coventry, P. A. (2016). Association between chronic physical conditions and the effectiveness of collaborative care for depression: An individual participant data meta-analysis. *JAMA Psychiatry, 73*(9), 978–989. https://doi.org/10.1001/jamapsychiatry.2016.1794

Raney, L. E. (2015). Integrating primary care and behavioral health: The role of the psychiatrist in the collaborative care model. *American Journal of Psychiatry, 172*(8), 721–728. https://doi.org/10.1176/appi.ajp.2015.15010017

Reiter, J. T., Dobmeyer, A. C., & Hunter, C. L. (2018). The primary care behavioral health (PCBH) model: An overview and operational definition. *Journal of Clinical Psychology in Medical Settings, 25*(2), 109–126. https://doi.org/10.1007/s10880-017-9531-x

Robinson, P. J., & Reiter, J. T. (2016). *Behavioral consultation and primary care: A guide to integrating services.* Springer International Publishing. https://link.springer.com/book/10.1007/978-3-319-13954-8

Sadock, E., Auerbach, S. M., Rybarczyk, B., & Aggarwal, A. (2014). Evaluation of integrated psychological services in a university-based primary care clinic. *Journal of Clinical Psychology in Medical Settings, 21*(1), 19–32. https://doi.org/10.1007/s10880-013-9378-8

Selby-Nelson, E. M., Bradley, J. M., Schiefer, R. A., & Hoover-Thompson, A. (2018). Primary care integration in rural areas: A community-focused approach. *Families, Systems & Health, 36*(4), 528–534. https://doi.org/10.1037/fsh0000352

Starfield, B. (1998). *Primary care: Balancing health needs, services and technology* (Vol. 1). Oxford University Press.

Tolliver, M., Dueweke, A. R., & Polaha, J. (2022). Interprofessional microteaching: An innovation to strengthen the behavioral health competencies of the primary care workforce. *Families, Systems & Health, 40*(4), 484–490. https://doi.org/10.1037/fsh0000735

University of Washington. (2023). Principles of collaborative care—AIMS Center. AIMS Center. https://aims.uw.edu/principles-of-collaborative-care/.

Unützer, J., Katon, W., Callahan, C. M., Williams, J. W., Hunkeler, E., Harpole, L., Hoffing, M., Della Penna, R. D., Noël, P. H., Lin, E. H. B., Areán, P. A., Hegel, M. T., Tang, L., Belin, T. R., Oishi, S., Langston, C., Investigators, I. M. P. A. C. T., Access, I. M.-P., & to Collaborative Treatment. (2002). Collaborative care management of late-life depression in the primary care setting: A randomized controlled trial. *JAMA, 288*(22), 2836–2845. https://doi.org/10.1001/jama.288.22.2836

Unützer, J., Katon, W. J., Fan, M.-Y., Schoenbaum, M. C., Lin, E. H. B., Penna, R. D. D., & Powers, D. (2008). Long-term cost effects of collaborative care for late-life depression. *The American Journal of Managed Care, 14*(2), 95.

Von Korff, M., & Tiemens, B. (2000). Individualized stepped care of chronic illness. *Western Journal of Medicine, 172*(2), 133–137. https://doi.org/10.1136/ewjm.172.2.133

Woltmann, E., Grogan-Kaylor, A., Perron, B., Georges, H., Kilbourne, A. M., & Bauer, M. S. (2012). Comparative effectiveness of collaborative chronic care models for mental health conditions across primary, specialty, and behavioral health care settings: Systematic review and meta-analysis. *American Journal of Psychiatry, 169*(8), 790–804. https://doi.org/10.1176/appi.ajp.2012.11111616

Chapter 13
Maximizing the Use of the Medical Team for Behavioral Health Needs

Danielle L. Terry PhD, ABPP, Ashley Cipriano DO, and Eboni Winford PhD, MPH

The importance of collaboration of teams to provide whole person care cannot be understated. The 2021 National Academy of Sciences, Engineering, and Medicine report, *Implementing high-quality primary care: Rebuilding the foundations of health care,* identifies interprofessional teams as one of the key factors necessary to facilitate high-quality care delivery in primary care (2021). To achieve better health, interprofessional teams should be composed of individuals who meet the needs of the communities served and who work collaboratively and at the top of their skill set. Effective medical teams can improve and facilitate clinical care. Working within a team allows individuals more agency and efficacy in solving problems, generating ideas, and applying knowledge to make decisions compared to those working alone (Larson, 2010). In essence, working effectively within a team allows the primary care provider (PCP) the potential to manage behavioral health (BH) conditions more proficiently, diagnose more accurately, develop care plans, and follow up at appropriate intervals.

Conversely, it is clear that there are harmful consequences when the team is not utilized effectively. Inadequate communication and failure to use available expertise can decrease quality of care and increase the frequency of medical errors (Christian et al., 2006; Institute of Medicine (US) Committee on Quality of Health Care in America, 2001; The Joint Commission, 2024).

D. L. Terry PhD, ABPP (✉) · A. Cipriano DO
Guthrie Medical Group, Sayre, PA, USA
e-mail: danielle.terry@guthrie.org

A. Cipriano DO
e-mail: Ashley.Cipriano@guthrie.org

E. Winford PhD, MPH
Cherokee Health Systems, Knoxville, TN, USA
e-mail: Eboni.Winford@cherokeehealth.com

M. L. C. Williamson and D. L. Terry (eds.), *Essentials for Treating Behavioral Health in Primary Care*, https://doi.org/10.1007/978-3-032-09558-9_13

Despite the growing awareness of the benefits of team-based care for patients, staff, and organizations, one of the biggest barriers organizations face is identifying and utilizing the "best" team members. Furthermore, in areas that may be under-resourced, finding strategies to creatively implement and manage BH care via coordination with other staff is essential. While Chap. 12 highlights the PCBH and CoCM integrated care models, which both actively use a team-based approach, there are many organizations that do not have access to BH providers, care managers, or others with professional expertise in BH. This chapter will provide an overview of strategies to maximize use of the patient's social support, the medical team, and other resources for the PCP if they are the sole provider for BH concerns. When providing BH care, it is often essential to maximize the use of team members in creative ways. These recommendations highlight the need to identify the functions of PCP and to match team members to these functions in ways that maximize each.

Maximizing Your Team: A Tiered Approach

When determining how to maximize use of one's team, the PCP must first determine who is on their team. It is important to remember that the patient and their chosen social support should always be included when considering the PCPs team.

Patient and Their Social Support System Considering the patient and their social support system is critical when determining who is on the team to address BH concerns. The PCP, the patient, and the family system or broader social support system create the foundational team within primary care. It is imperative that PCPs engage in contextual interviewing (See Chap. 2) early on in the patient-provider relationship to understand the patient's cultural background and social support system because these factors will greatly influence the success or failure of BH treatment. McDaniel et al. (2013) provide an in-depth review of treating BH concerns in primary care from a systems perspective.

Clinical Team Clinical team members may include front desk staff, nursing staff, allied health professional including BH providers along with other PCP colleagues. It may also include those they interact with less frequently, including outside providers, agencies, or other resources. PCPs should consider the function and strengths of different members of the office staff within the primary care office and those who may be affiliated with, but also work outside the office. Certain staff have pre-assigned roles and responsibilities in the function of the office. These established niches can be further refined, defined, and creatively utilized to maximize your team's success in caring for your patients more effectively and efficiently. A working understanding of how your office functions, the roles and responsibilities of individual team members or groups of members in your office, as well as the gifts and interests of your staff members will help you create an effective and specific model of care to meet the needs of your patients and community. Each situation and office is unique and will

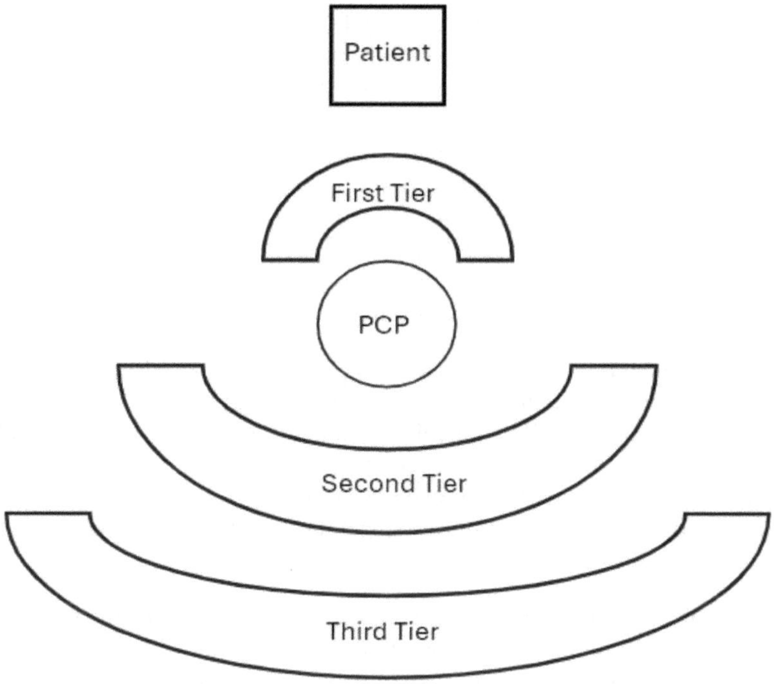

Fig. 13.1 Tiers of support

likely have to adjust to have a seamless workflow that best meets the unique and individual needs of your patient panel and population. Conceptualizing your team in a "tiered" model may be helpful in considering how you might effectively utilize different team members in addressing different BH concerns of patients. This tiered approach considers team members that act directly with the PCP and patient (first tier) to those that have a less direct or more distant role (Second and Third Tiers), and the provider might maximize their team members beginning with the closest to most distant resources. See Fig. 13.1.

The First Tier

Front Desk Staff The first tier is composed of team members that your patient encounters first when they enter the clinic. This typically consists of your front desk staff and nursing staff. The front desk staff may be the first ones to identify a change in the patient's presentation, mood, or concern. They may recognize a certain need or concern that the patient has and can then pass this information on to the nurse and/or provider so that they can be better prepared to help the patient. They can also help facilitate scheduling follow-ups and handling referrals. Front desk staff are often underutilized as they are physically separated from the rest of the staff, constrained to the "front desk" area. There may be limited staff interaction with them during the day due to this physical barrier and their need to stay in that specific area to answer phones, check patients in and out of appointments, etc. Finding an effective way to communicate with them and include them in the team is key. Consider implementing daily huddles either in the morning prior to the start of the day, or even a short huddle before each half day of clinic. There may be an easy way to communicate throughout the day, perhaps through a "chat" function already established in your EHR (Electronic Health Record) or other platform that your facility uses. When all else fails, you can stop by their desk or office space.

Hot Words Offices might establish a list of certain "hot words" that when mentioned by the patient or identified during a patient interaction, trigger the staff to communicate that interaction further down the line to nursing staff and/or other clinical staff. Setting expectations that underscore the important role that they play in the care of the patient can reinforce their involvement, along with reinforcing their use of compassion and effective communication can increase the likelihood that they will do this again.

Nursing Staff The nursing staff are the first line of defense once the patient enters the exam room. If you have the same nurse each time, they have likely formed a relationship and rapport with your patient panel. The patient may confide in them about a struggle, mood concern, or a subject that they would like to discuss with the provider that is different from the "reason for visit" listed on the schedule. Again, touching base with your nurse at the outset of your clinic, or prior to seeing patients can be helpful in streamlining visits that may be complicated by BH concerns.

"Real Reason" for Visits Sometimes it is useful to think about the "real" reason for the visit. Often, the listed "reason for visit" on the schedule prior to entering the room may no longer be pertinent. Support and nursing staff may have clues to other priorities patients may be presenting with when interacting with the patient prior to the PCP entering the room. Most providers work closely with their nurses. They understand that they are an integral part of the team and feel empowered to make recommendations to the PCP when they are finished rooming the patient. For example, a PCP may enter a room planning to discuss blood pressure or a diabetic follow up, and the nurse rooms the patient, and checks in with the PCP to inform them that the patient has confided to them that they are struggling with depression, grief, or anxiety. These interactions aid the PCP in their efficiency and expectations during the encounter. It allows the PCP the opportunity to discuss these critical issues at the start of the visit rather than talking about diabetes for 20 minutes and the patient stating, "by the way..." as the visit comes to a close. Making sure that there is adequate time to discuss these critical issues is vital in forming a safe and appropriate treatment plan and makes the patient feel heard and cared for.

Screening as a Vital Sign At times, the "reason for visit" listed has been identified as a BH concern *prior* to the nursing staff entering the room. In this scenario, nursing staff can complete all behavior health screenings before the provider enters the room to allow for review before the visit starts. Staff should complete the BH screenings as a type of "vital sign" that can immediately be completed following the medical vital signs. Having the same person assessing for medical and BH wellness and changes can help reduce the stigma associated with BH assessments and reinforce the importance of BH. In the same way that one would not obtain medical vital signs (e.g., height, weight, blood pressure, pulse, etc.) in the waiting room, it is best to avoid completing BH screenings/vitals in the waiting room. This should be completed in the exam room to create a seamless workflow. These assessments are sometimes available in certain EHRs and easily accessible during the rooming process. Other facilities or EHRs may not have that function and utilize paper copies of these assessments instead. Whatever the preferred method in your office, ensuring that assessments are easily accessible to the nursing staff during the rooming process and that there is an established process in place is key to ensuring that patients feel comfortable, and that no valuable information goes unnoticed. This is particularly important during a visit where the nursing staff may identify a new BH concern in a patient and need to unexpectantly complete an assessment. Ensuring that staff does not have to leave the room to obtain an assessment form and that it can quickly be completed when other vitals are being obtained helps patients feel comfortable and helps with efficiency in the encounter.

Appropriate Follow Up Care Finally, this important tier of patient care can be utilized for following up with patients to see how they are doing with potential medication changes or completing safety or post-crisis check-ins. For example, if the PCP makes a medication change during a patient visit and their schedule is tight, having the nurse check in with the patient a few weeks after the medication change to assess for side effects, tolerability, and effectiveness of the medication change may be appropriate. Based on the information obtained the PCP may decide to adjust the dose of medication, determine that a sooner appointment is needed, or that a new referral needs to be made. Similarly, using this tier for assistance may also be appropriate if a patient has BH conditions that may increase their suicide risk and/or they may need increased monitoring following a crisis period. However, staff should be well trained on assessment and documentation of these encounters and know when and how to seek additional instruction should the need arise.

The Second Tier

The "second tier" of support refers to people that PCPs may interact with daily, but the patient does not directly interact with until referred. This may include team members such as other PCPs in your office, onsite BH providers, community health workers, care coordinators, or case managers.

Many providers may work in busy clinics with multiple other providers, inpatient care duties, and/or medical learner supervision and teaching. Due to this, the schedule can be challenging, and PCPs may not have the availability or flexibility in their clinics to schedule a patient follow-up in the time frame that they would like. Ensuring that patient follow-up and care is timely and appropriate is critical in the safe care of patients.

Care Teams One way to rectify these problems is by utilizing your second tier of support. Forming "care teams" can be an excellent way of ensuring that patient outreach, follow-up, and care remains seamless. Care teams may consist of other PCPs in the office who work caring for patients within the same patients and can also include nursing staff, allied health professionals, a BH provider in the same clinic, or additional support staff. For example, a PCP may discuss a patient with a fellow physician in the office who will aid in the care of the patient when the PCP is unavailable. This creates an environment of safety and familiarity for the patient. The patient will form a relationship with the other provider who will then be familiar with the patient's current symptoms, problems, and past medical history. While retaining all rights and privileges as PCP of the patient, it provides a familiar and informed alternative to discuss issues or needs should they arise when the assigned PCP is unavailable.

Many providers may hesitate to use an onsite BH provider, due to unfamiliarity, stigma, or concerns of overwhelming that provider. While this luxury is not available everywhere, most BH providers have training or experience in managing and triaging, and even more experience in giving difficult feedback. These individuals are a resource to PCPs, and their job is to assist with managing these concerns. See Chap. 12 regarding models that PCPs might advocate for in their offices.

As the patient centered medical home and team-based care becomes more of an emphasis in modern medicine, many offices now have Care Coordinators or other support staff available to them. Care Coordinators are often invested in the community as well as the office and can be a tremendous asset in facilitating the coordination between a patient's needs and local available resources. They may exist as part of a Collaborative Health Model team, or they may function as a stand-alone resource to an office. They often play an important role in checking in with patients after a medication change, as discussed above, particularly if nursing staff is unavailable. Using a team-based approach or "huddle" and meeting prior to or after a patient encounter can be a strategic way to maximize and involve the Care Coordinator.

The Third Tier

The third tier of support available includes resources outside the office, in the PCP's local and expanded community. This may consist of local psychiatrists, psychologists, community mental health agencies, peer support, hospice care services and counseling, or other providers. While they may not be as readily available to collaborate with as an onsite BH provider, their knowledge and insight are important in the safe and effective care of the patient. Taking the opportunity to engage with local and frequently referred to providers will make communication between PCPs and the provider easier, more frequent, and more effective.

Local and Community Resources It is important that PCPs spend time learning about the local resources available. Having knowledge of local resources and a readily available list of resources will help providers be more effective and efficient in meeting the needs of your patient, whether they be medical, psychological, physical, or social. Gathering this information upfront takes time and effort. Using other vested parties, such as a BH provider or care coordinator, who may have additional knowledge of local resources (or better yet, may have a working relationship with some of these resources) can be incredibly beneficial in directing patients to appropriate care and finding support. Often members in these roles may already have relationships with other organizations' employees as they may have more opportunities to interact with them given their practices' scope. The PCP should be aware of local drug and alcohol programs in their community, grief resources (Hospice may be a good place to start if you are unsure what resources are available), rape and abuse clinics, food banks, and the local Area Agencies on Aging. Many of these organizations have flyers and pamphlets available, provided free of charge. Reaching out to local resources to gather information in regard to their programs and scope of work is also helpful. Often these organizations are eager to help and can be a wealth of information. They are also often willing to come to the office or hospital to meet with your office staff to discuss how they can uniquely meet some of the community's needs. Taking advantage of this benefits PCPs in meeting the needs of patients, but will also result in educating coworkers and staff.

Utilizing the Electronic Medical Record For PCPs that work within a larger electronic system, it may be useful to utilize the electronic health record to create "smart lists" of local resources that can easily and seamlessly be provided to the patient prior to the end of the visit. Devising a point-person or strategy for updating resources is essential, and this can often be completed by the first tier support staff to ensure that numbers, businesses, and other contacts are still in-service and available.

While all of these efforts may sound cumbersome and effortful (and yes, they can be) being proactive and strategically approaching BH concerns by maximizing the use of the team ultimately benefits the patient and the provider.

Reluctance of Team Members

Unfortunately, some team members may not be passionate about addressing the BH concerns of their patients or being part of the PCPs tiered approach. They may feel overwhelmed by the number of local resources available to them and simply not know where to start. They may be uncomfortable addressing certain topics with a patient or feel limited in their ability to address these topics adequately due to the time constraints that often plague providers during a busy clinic day. Or, some staff may not believe this is within their scope of practice and dismiss these topics or try to "pawn them off' on another provider or staff member. If the former, some strategies in this chapter will serve as a starting point and foundation on how to create a tailored approach for your office in effectively addressing BH concerns. Overtime, the workflow of how a specific office runs may evolve from what is discussed in this chapter. All offices and communities have different specific needs and resources.

A more challenging issue exists within the office's mindset when other staff members do not feel that addressing BH concerns with their patients is part of their job. BH concerns affect all aspects of a patient's life, including the management of other chronic diseases. The first tenet of osteopathic medicine states that "the body is a unit; the person is a unit of body, mind, and spirit." This mindset emphasizes the duty and privilege of every health care provider to care for all aspects of their patient to the absolute best of their ability. Changing the mindset and culture of a practice can be challenging but is imperative in providing adequate and effective care. In addition to modeling appropriate behavior, appropriately addressing specific concerns that arise, this may also start with considering who is permitted to be a member of the team.

Qualities of the "Best" Team Members for Behavioral Health Care

In the same way that each healthcare organization and each patient is different, team-based care will vary based upon the needs of your community, your organization, and most importantly, your patients. Thus, there is no magic recipe for identifying the team members who will be best for your team. Team members may include nurses or clinical assistants, front desk staff, or other health providers throughout your organization. Being involved in the hiring process depends on the organization, and may require that the PCP volunteer or offer to assist with weighing in on these decisions. Despite the variability in settings, there are several guiding principles that can inform who PCPs might reach out to within any of the tiers, to assist with BH care.

Flexibility A flexible team member will identify a way to meet the needs of the patient (i.e., labs, BH screening, diabetes education) while they wait for the PCP to enter the room and address their concerns. Often, individuals who present with BH concerns are more complex, presenting with a variety of psychosocial circumstances that impact their punctuality, appointment show rates, adherence to treatment, and ability to provide a clear and concise history of symptoms. This can negatively impact the efficiency of patient encounters and generate distress when providers are already pressed for time.

Team-based care thrives off flexible and compassionate team members—those who will collaborate with the PCP and the patient to get the job done. Flexible team members recognize and appreciate that the schedule will not look the same at the beginning of the day as it will at the end of the day, nor will it look the same from day to day. A flexible team member rolls with it—no matter what "it" is. Finding team members who are willing to go off schedule while still maintaining appropriate boundaries and to prioritize the needs of the patient above their need for rigidity and strict structure are often better suited to assist with BH needs.

Openness to Change A strong team member has an open mindset and is willing to try new things. They are not afraid of failure because they recognize that an idea that does not work out as anticipated represents an opportunity to learn, to reflect, and to try again. Team members who complicate healthcare delivery are those who have fixed mindsets. The very idea of change seems to cause them personal offense. In a world that has increased use of technology, screening and integrated electronic systems, a team member that is willing to maximize the use of incoming tools, strategies, or approaches (e.g., regularly administering screening tools, use of electronic reminders for follow up) can be a great asset to collecting information necessary to address BH needs.

Effective Communication and Psychological Insight While Chap. 2 provides a full discussion on communication skills, working within an interdisciplinary team requires team members to understand the language of the other team members, have a basic working knowledge of BH conditions, and respect for how BH interfaces with medical care. It can be helpful for PCPs to understand the language of case managers, for example, to facilitate the most useful linkages to resources. Similarly, a PCP may need to gently educate specific staff, such as nurses, or front desk staff regarding procedures, screening, or other protocol that might be helpful in assisting the PCP in providing care. Those staff members who have a basic working knowledge of BH conditions, and even signs and symptoms are best equipped to aid in efficient detection and intervention by the PCP.

Recruitment of Behavioral Health Providers

If you are privileged enough to hire a BH provider to work within your primary care team, there are several things to consider. A commonly observed frustration when identifying the "best" team members is that the team member you have in mind when you post the job description is nowhere to be found. This does not mean you do not receive any applications. In fact, you may receive several; however, another component of finding the "best" team members is that the job advertisement accurately reflects the role and functions of the team member you are hoping to hire.

When looking for BH team members to join an interdisciplinary medical team, Human Resource departments often advertise for a specific licensure level or degree. While advertising for team members this way is not inherently flawed, it does add additional barriers to successful identification and selection of the most appropriate team members. Narrow advertising of this type tends to yield a narrow field of prospective candidates—those who meet the licensure and/or degree requirements that are specified within the job description. And nothing else. What is more useful is to outline the functions that the team member would be expected to fulfill and the traits that would help them be most successful at the job.

If the team needs a BH provider who can be flexible in terms of location where services are provided (e.g., in an exam room vs. in a private office), willingness to accommodate patients while they are in the clinic instead of scheduling for follow up only, and scope of practice (e.g., depression and anxiety as well as tobacco cessation and diabetes management), the team would be well served to advertise for a BH member who can fulfill those functions and who has those characteristics. One of the requirements for that position would then be a certain level of training. However, advertising for level of training alone does not often yield the specific skills and personality characteristics that contribute to high-performing interdisciplinary teams. In sum, you should advertise for the team member you *actually* want. Hire for fit and train for skill. And never, ever, EVER hire out of desperation. It is a decision that you will regret every time.

Qualities and Culture of the Team

When maximizing team members in the assessment and treatment of BH conditions, there are several ways in which the PCP might reinforce and maximize the team. Interdisciplinary teams are complex entities that function most optimally when all members recognize not only their roles and skills but also the needs of the entire team and their unique healthcare system. Among other characteristics, interactions between team members reflect communication, coordination, collaboration, comprehensiveness, and continuity (Jimenez et al., 2021; Kroenke, 2004), and when team members are allowed to fulfill any of these functions, regardless of their title or degree, and within the scope of their training, the highest level of functioning can be achieved. Sometimes, individual team members must detach their duties from their titles alone, and if the PCP is the team lead, they can help set this expectation. For example, a PCP that has concerns about a patient with suicidal ideation, may note that the patient works closely with physical therapy, several times a week. The PCP may alert the therapist to these concerns. While it is not the role of the occupational therapist to assess and treat these concerns, they can alert the team. In addition, the front desk staff can be placed on high alert for any calls from the physical therapist and/or the patient, who might later help with communicating and soothing patients (providing bottled water for example) when the provider is off schedule.

This is the hallmark of a high-functioning interdisciplinary team. Within reason, titles alone do not dictate what roles they each play and the ways in which the team members can collaborate in order to meet the patient's needs.

Teams that struggle to fulfill the core functions of primary may hold too tightly to their titles as the sole determinant of the functions they can fulfill. The phrase, "that's not my job" is sometimes necessary to delineate between what legally and ethically can be provided by a specific member. However, when the phrase is used as a way to minimize reciprocal workload, it can be problematic. When identifying team members who can contribute to multidisciplinary medical teams, awareness of the top of each team member's competence is crucial to empowering every team member to fulfill any function that reflects their highest level of performance.

As mentioned in early on, the importance of team collaboration to provide whole person care cannot be understated. Building a team that is capable of identifying and creatively meeting the unique needs of a patient is vital in successfully providing high-quality care to patients. Hiring staff members who are flexible, clear communicators, and able to "roll with the punches" can be of high value in these circumstances. Once your team is built, identifying the different "tiers" and how each tier can be best utilized within the flow of your specific office and community will equip you to quickly identify and address various and complex patient concerns. Having the right people who are able to effectively work together as a team and have a working knowledge of available resources is foundational to the delivery of high-quality patient care.

Key Points

- PCPs should consider the function and strengths of different members of the office staff within the primary care office.
- Addressing BH needs as a sole provider can use direct support staff (Tier 1), others who work within the office (Tier 2) or outside organizations or referrals (Tier 3).
- While there is an upfront time investment with creating resource lists, educating staff, and identifying helpful collaborators, patients with BH needs and the provider will ultimately benefit from this investment.

References

Christian, C. K., Gustafson, M. L., Roth, E. M., Sheridan, T. B., Gandhi, T. K., Dwyer, K., Zinner, M. J., & Dierks, M. M. (2006). A prospective study of patient safety in the operating room. *Surgery, 139*(2), 159–173. https://doi.org/10.1016/j.surg.2005.07.037

Institute of Medicine (US) Committee on Quality of Health Care in America. (2001). *Crossing the quality chasm: A new health system for the 21st century*. National Academies Press. https://doi.org/10.17226/10027

Jimenez, G., Matchar, D., Koh, G. C. H., Tyagi, S., Kleij, R. M. J. J., Chavannes, N. H., & Car, J. (2021). Revisiting the four core functions (4Cs) of primary care: Operational definitions and complexities. *Primary Health Care Research & Development, 22*, e68. https://doi.org/10.1017/S1463423621000669

Kroenke, K. (2004). The many c's of primary care. *Journal of General Internal Medicine, 19*(6), 708–709. https://doi.org/10.1111/j.1525-1497.2004.40401.x

Larson, J. R. (2010). *In search of synergy in small group performance* (1st ed.). Psychology Press. https://www.routledge.com/In-Search-of-Synergy-in-Small-Group-Performance/LarsonJr/p/book/9780805859447

McDaniel, S. H., Doherty, W. J., & Hepworth, J. (2013). *Medical family therapy and integrated care* (2nd ed.). American Psychology Association. https://www.apa.org/pubs/books/4317314

National Academies of Sciences, Engineering, and Medicine. (2021). *Implementing high-quality primary care: Rebuilding the foundation of health care*. The National Academies Press. https://doi.org/10.17226/25983

The Joint Commission. (2024). *Sentinel event data: 2023 annual review*. The Joint Commission. https://www.jointcommission.org/-/media/tjc/documents/resources/patient-safety-topics/sentinel-event/2024/2024_sentinel-event-_annual-review_published-2024.pdf

Chapter 14
Conclusions and Future Directions in Primary Care

Molly Clark PhD, ABPP and Jay Brieler MD

Regier and colleagues described primary care as the de facto behavioral health (BH) care system in their seminal article many years ago (Regier et al., 1978). Much has changed, but much remains the same. Primary care physicians (PCPs) still provide a greater portion of BH care than psychiatrists in the United States (Jetty et al., 2021; Olfson, 2016), and that proportion may be increasing (Rotenstein et al., 2023). BH issues still drive up to 70% of primary care visits (Hunter et al., 2009) and PCPs still prescribe the majority of antidepressant medication (Muench et al., 2022).

What *has* changed in the last 50 years is the recognition that the role of PCPs in the BH arena has shifted due to the natural outgrowth of the relationship between PCPs and their patients. The bio-psycho-social-spiritual context (See Chap. 2) has become embedded in care, and managing BH needs has become an essential part of the role of many PCPs. PCPs are often the first contact for patients for many issues, and continuity of care over time is a foundational principle of the field. Indeed, many organizations are calling for strengthening of the delivery of BH care by PCPs that includes improvements at the practice, community, and policy level (American Academy of Family Physicians (AAFP), 2023; Bipartisan Policy Center, 2023). Primary care provides a stopgap while the United States struggles with access to BH specialty care. Each PCP defines their personal scope of care in all areas of practice—deciding what issues to manage themselves, which issues require consultation, and when to refer out. The call to expand the role of PCPs in BH care requires reconsideration of these choices for many providers. Finding a balance of challenging one's comfort zone and providing responsible care can be difficult. For example, PCPs who are trying to improve BH delivery in their clinics will need to optimize their

M. Clark PhD, ABPP (✉)
University of Mississippi Medical Center, Jackson, MS, USA
e-mail: MClark@umc.edu

J. Brieler MD
Saint Louis University School of Medicine, St. Louis, MO, USA
e-mail: jay.brieler@health.slu.edu

M. L. C. Williamson and D. L. Terry (eds.), *Essentials for Treating Behavioral Health in Primary Care*, https://doi.org/10.1007/978-3-032-09558-9_14

skills in psychopharmacology, behavioral change, and basic psychotherapy skills (see Chaps. 8 and 9). They may need to stay abreast of knowledge and recommendations for those patients who are struggling with trauma or addiction. Providers may also need to learn common language used across BH fields to effectively communicate with BH professionals outside of medicine. This book has sought to provide resources to assist in making these kinds of changes.

Various obstacles affect PCPs' ability to enhance their scope of care to include BH. BH training in medicine is limited and varies widely within and among specialties (Hodges et al., 2001). The breadth of issues that PCPs address often circumvents attention to BH care. Health systems frequently place productivity demands on PCPs that limit time per patient. Since patients with BH diagnoses or psychosocial stressors often require additional time (Miller et al., 2011), caring for them can add additional stress for the PCP. In many geographic areas, access to specialty BH care is quite limited (Negaro et al., 2023), forcing PCPs to care for issues that are more complex than their training.

Different cultures and populations vary in their acceptance of BH care (Jimenez et al., 2013). Practice systems vary widely in terms of available resources and the willingness of administration to deploy those resources. Referral networks outside PCP office walls are very different across geographic location and practice environment. All of these unique practice attributes can serve both as assets and obstacles to the process of enhancing BH care. However, PCPs are unlikely to deliver the best care if they try to tackle it alone.

Integrated BH care has emerged as one of the foremost methods to support PCP delivery of behaviorally minded whole person care. Chapter 12 highlights different types of integrated systems and BH models including strategies for implementing those systems in their own practices. It is essential that providers recognize the unique aspects of their practice environment when attempting to adopt integrated care. Unfortunately, insurance companies also continue to create considerable barriers related to integrating BH coverage and reimbursement for PCPs and BH providers working within integrated BH teams.

Much of the initial development and study of integrated BH care was conducted by leaders associated with academic family medicine departments (Blount, 2015). It is important to recognize that primary care includes other specialties including internal medicine, pediatrics, and obstetrics-gynecology, as well as other training pathways such as advanced practice nurses and physician assistants. Those who have experience in integrated BH care will be tasked with helping others adopt the practice models. Training support staff is an important component of system implementation, especially when working with diverse populations and those who have experienced trauma. Advocacy with peers within the practice and the local communities will be necessary. In spite of the work required, adoption of integrated BH can yield great rewards. It has been associated with increased satisfaction both for providers and patients (Ede et al., 2015).

In summary, integrated BH care has a number of beneficial practice outcomes despite the system challenges faced with its implementation. The integrated BH care values of whole person, patient-centered care resonate with the foundations of primary care creating this wonderful opportunity to raise the bar of health care for all stakeholders (Ede et al., 2015). The PCP plays an important role in providing BH services while advocating for integrated BH implementation in their own work environments. In this rapidly changing healthcare environment, future research and clinical implementation will need to examine the intersection of integrated BH, technology, evolution of the healthcare team, and advocacy for advancing primary care for better health outcomes.

Future Directions: Technology and Artificial Intelligence

With the rise in BH complaints and obstacles that limit access to treatment, there is an opportunity to meet these healthcare needs using technology. However, technologic development moves at a rapid pace and, in fact, the next wave of technology has already been developed and researched. The use and continued development of telehealth, website and mobile applications (apps), and artificial intelligence will have a substantial impact on the delivery of BH care within the primary care setting. Faced with limited access to BH care and treatment, PCPs may be able to expand their reach via strategic use of these resources.

Telehealth has been demonstrated as a mechanism for BH care delivery for many years, and the COVID-19 pandemic forced rapid implementation across settings (McCord et al., 2022; Molfenter et al., 2021). Telehealth can increase access to general and specialty care by allowing patients with physical mobility and transportation barriers to receive care in their own homes. Patients who live in rural areas might especially benefit from the convenience of telehealth through reduction of stigma, increased confidentiality, and reduced travel costs (Hand, 2022).

Despite these benefits, there are continued challenges that should be addressed in the future. There is a lack of infrastructure to support quality and reliable internet connectivity in rural and other resource deprived areas. In addition, rapid hardware and software development leads to significant concerns about access to equipment that will remain viable over time. In addition, digital literacy and proficiency in the use of technology or devices will need to be addressed. In spite of these challenges, telehealth may be a viable option for integrated BH support for PCPs in rural and underserved (Hand, 2022).

Mobile apps and websites are another means for delivering on time and accessible care. For example, software solutions can allow patients to access traditionally manualized CBT content in a "choose your own adventure" style when and where they wish to access it (Milne-Ives et al., 2020). The Veterans Administration and Department of Defense also have open-access applications and resources (U.S. Department of Veterans Affairs, 2024). At the same time, the effectiveness and impact of the modalities are complicated by the overwhelming number of websites and mobile applications offered, the number of health concerns addressed, and the lack of high-quality research. While there is some data to suggest that these platforms may have some level of effectiveness, there continues to be a number of concerns that need to be addressed in order to fully understand the potential impact of these healthcare delivery methods for the PCP (Lattie et al., 2019; Milne-Ives et al., 2020).

For example, technology and websites can be created without quality control and evidence-based interventions. Privacy concerns may not be fully addressed as patients may enter their own personal health information shared through the internet as part of using a website. Furthermore, questions concerning the impact of lack of socialization while interacting with technology have not been addressed. Despite the complications within these modalities, PCPs can still use telehealth resources to increase hope and agency to their patients along with psychoeducation and brief behavioral skills (Lattie et al., 2019; Milne-Ives et al., 2020).

Artificial intelligence (AI) is already being used in clinical practice to assist in clinical decision-making, documentation, and risk prediction (Balasubramanian, 2023; Edavally et al., 2021; Khosravi et al., 2024). The use of text generating AI software is being piloted to generate patient education materials that are customized to specific patient needs (Robinson et al., 2024). In the BH arena, virtual reality paired with AI can provide enhanced exposure therapy in a safe environment for patients with a history of trauma (Knaust et al., 2020). AI can be paired with mobile technology to assist patients who have difficulty remembering medications or attending other treatments (Mikhail, 2022). In addition, AI can analyze natural language patterns, genetic information, and imaging data to assist in the diagnosis of BH conditions (Zhang et al., 2022). These latter applications are still being refined and developed, and their effectiveness remains to be seen. In addition, issues of bias based on patterns in AI training data and the impact of reduced human interaction during mental healthcare delivery have not been fully addressed.

Future Directions: Scope of Care and Evolution of the Healthcare Team

With the development of technology and treatment strategies, primary care delivery must remain flexible and open to new forms of meeting patient care needs. This concept is not new to primary care, and the PCP is a leader that embraces the healthcare team mantra (Iroku-Malize et al., 2013). Communication within and between systems to assist patient care navigation has remained a challenge and is essential for patient care. The core value of timely, compassionate, and effective communication is crucial to quality care delivery. Effective communication requires a patient-centered relationship. Primary care clinicians are well trained within this competency, and it appears to be a core value within the specialty (Kahn, 2021). Therefore, it is critical that primary care leadership continue to incorporate effective communication and emphasize its value in future care models and technology.

Primary care clinicians are on the frontlines of health care and have been providing the necessary care for a variety of healthcare needs. In a culture where "on demand" is more of a norm, primary care as a discipline will need to consider how it will either address this need within our culture, explain the value of comprehensive quality care, or create a model that incorporates both on demand care and comprehensive care (Neves & Burgers, 2022). Patients currently have access to on demand niche market areas via mobile apps that will mail prescriptions. However, these services do not address comprehensive care. The services often do not appreciate the holistic context of each individual patient. Primary care settings will need to continue to be nimble to provide BH services. Research on these models of online consultations in primary care have begun and stress the need for more research and problem solving to meet the on demand need without adding burden (Turner et al., 2022). Furthermore, continued considerations for a variety of integrated care teams within primary care are needed to reduce provider burnout and improve patient care outcomes.

Finally, PCPs should have an awareness and understanding of new modalities for treatment of chronic BH concerns and the models of care under which they are performed. The integration of treatment for opioid use disorders within primary care clinics has been researched along with implementation hurdles (Austin et al., 2023). In addition, research is being conducted for specialized BH interventions including ketamine and psychedelic medications for treatment resistant BH conditions (Evans et al., 2024) along with transcranial magnetic stimulation (TMS) for tobacco cessation and chronic BH conditions (Young et al., 2021). While some of these newer therapies are continuing to be researched, they will likely have implications in primary care, especially in integrated care settings where PCPs are active participants in an expanded scope of BH care delivery.

Future Directions: Advocacy

Engaging in meaningful advocacy in addition to the work of primary care is a daunting task. However, there are many ways in which PCPs can advocate for systems level changes at a manageable scale (Brown et al., 2023). Many of the activities PCPs are already doing lead to system change. The adaptation of practice models to reduce burdens and address patient care needs, making efforts to focus on preventative care, volunteering to educate others, especially marginalized populations, are just a few examples. There are numerous opportunities to financially support organizations who are advocating for changes in reimbursement and patient care models. Any support is vital to moving toward a healthier population and making a meaningful impact.

Conclusions

Despite its challenges, BH care delivery in the primary care office can be one of the most rewarding aspects of practice. Many chose primary care due to an intrinsic desire for human connection, an appreciation for human stories, and the goal of patient empowerment (Scott et al., 2007). These values are symbiotic with the treatment of BH conditions, and the science and art of primary care. In a time when PCPs are feeling increasingly removed from sources of meaning in their careers, focusing on the behavioral aspects of medicine can provide a reconnection to this personal mission.

While developments in technology and care systems can be very helpful in the expansion of BH care delivery, many of the skills described in this book should be useful for PCPs in any healthcare setting. Behavioral change is the cornerstone of prevention of disease and the management of chronic conditions. Prescribing (at least some) psychotropic medication is a core primary care skill. The patient-provider relationship remains a key component of healing. Bolstering skills in these areas allows providers the privilege of helping patients participate more fully in their own health care. In times where access is limited, nurturing and developing skills in treatment of BH conditions in primary care is just another part of the continuum of whole person care.

Key Points

- Primary care provides a stopgap while the United States struggles with access to BH specialty care.
- Engaging in flexible approaches that utilize artificial intelligence and other types of technology are essential for expanding reach and adapting to a technologically driven environment.
- PCPs will need to stay abreast of new modalities for treatment of chronic BH concerns and the models of care under which they are performed.
- PCPs play an important role in advocacy and can engage in this process at varying levels.
- The treatment of BH conditions in primary care is another part of treating patients as a whole and behavioral change is a cornerstone of prevention of disease along with management of chronic conditions.

References

American Academy of Family Physicians (AAFP). (2023). *Mental and behavioral health care services by family physicians (position paper)*. American Academy of Family Physicians. https://www.aafp.org/about/policies/all/mental-health-services.html

Austin, E. J., Chen, J., Briggs, E. S., Ferro, L., Barry, P., Heald, A., Merrill, J. O., Curran, G. M., Saxon, A. J., Fortney, J. C., Ratzliff, A. D., & Williams, E. C. (2023). Integrating opioid use disorder treatment into primary care settings. *JAMA Network Open, 6*(8), e2328627. https://doi.org/10.1001/jamanetworkopen.2023.28627

Balasubramanian, S. (2023). *Is ambient dictation the future of clinical documentation?* Forbes. https://www.forbes.com/sites/saibala/2023/12/26/is-ambient-dictation-the-future-of-clinical-documentation/

Bipartisan Policy Center. (2023). *Strengthening the integrated care workforce*. https://bipartisanpolicy.org/report/strengthening-the-integrated-care-workforce/

Blount, A. (2015). *A brief history of the integration of behavioral health in primary care.* Collaborative Family Healthcare Association (CFHA Blog). https://members.cfha.net/blogpost/689173/213334/A-Brief-History-of-the-Integration-of-Behavioral-Health-in-Primary-Care

Brown, A., Wall, T. N., Pratt, G., Talen, M. R., O'Grady, C., & Reitz, R. (2023). Even one voice: Teaching legislative advocacy as a core competency in family medicine. *The International Journal of Psychiatry in Medicine, 59*(4), 424–431. https://doi.org/10.1177/00912174231190136

Edavally, S., Miller, D. D., & Youssef, N. A. (2021). Artificial intelligence to aid detection and diagnostic accuracy of mood disorders and predict suicide risk: A systematic review. *Annals of Clinical Psychiatry, 33*(4), 270–281. https://doi.org/10.12788/acp.0041

Ede, V., Okafor, M., Kinuthia, R., Belay, Z., Tewolde, T., Alema-Mensah, E., & Satcher, D. (2015). An examination of perceptions in integrated care practice. *Community Mental Health Journal, 51*(8), 949–961. https://doi.org/10.1007/s10597-015-9837-9

Evans, V. D., Arenas, A., Shinozuka, K., Tabaac, B. J., Beutler, B. D., Cherian, K., Fasano, C., & Muir, O. S. (2024). Psychedelic therapy: A primer for primary care clinicians-ketamine. *American Journal of Therapeutics, 31*(2), e155–e177. https://doi.org/10.1097/MJT.0000000000001721

Hand, L. J. (2022). The role of telemedicine in rural mental health care around the globe. *Telemedicine and e-Health, 28*(3), 285–294. https://doi.org/10.1089/tmj.2020.0536

Hodges, B., Inch, C., & Silver, I. (2001). Improving the psychiatric knowledge, skills, and attitudes of primary care physicians, 1950–2000: A review. *American Journal of Psychiatry, 158*(10), 1579–1586. https://doi.org/10.1176/appi.ajp.158.10.1579

Hunter, C. L., Goodie, J. L., Oordt, M. S., & Dobmeyer, A. C. (2009). *Integrated behavioral health in primary care: Step-by-step guidance for assessment and intervention.* American Psychological Association. https://doi.org/10.1037/11871-000

Iroku-Malize, T., Matson, C., Freeman, J., McGrew, M., & David, A. (2013). Interprofessional education. *The Annals of Family Medicine, 11*(2), 188–189. https://doi.org/10.1370/afm.1523

Jetty, A., Petterson, S., Westfall, J. M., & Jabbarpour, Y. (2021). Assessing primary care contributions to behavioral health: A cross-sectional study using the medical expenditure panel survey. *Journal of Primary Care & Community Health, 12.* https://doi.org/10.1177/21501327211023871

Jimenez, D. E., Bartels, S. J., Cardenas, V., & Alegría, M. (2013). Stigmatizing attitudes toward mental illness among racial/ethnic older adults in primary care. *International Journal of Geriatric Psychiatry, 28*(10), 1061–1068. https://doi.org/10.1002/gps.3928

Kahn, N. B. (2021). Redesigning family medicine training to meet the emerging health care needs of patients and communities: Be the change we wish to see. *Family Medicine, 53*(7), 499–505. https://doi.org/10.22454/FamMed.2021.897904

Khosravi, M., Zare, Z., Mojtabaeian, S. M., & Izadi, R. (2024). Artificial intelligence and decision-making in healthcare: A thematic analysis of a systematic review of reviews. *Health Services Research and Managerial Epidemiology, 11.* https://doi.org/10.1177/23333928241234863

Knaust, T., Felnhofer, A., Kothgassner, O. D., Höllmer, H., Gorzka, R.-J., & Schulz, H. (2020). Virtual trauma interventions for the treatment of post-traumatic stress disorders: A scoping review. *Frontiers in Psychology, 11,* 562506. https://doi.org/10.3389/fpsyg.2020.562506

Lattie, E. G., Adkins, E. C., Winquist, N., Stiles-Shields, C., Wafford, Q. E., & Graham, A. K. (2019). Digital mental health interventions for depression, anxiety, and enhancement of psychological Well-being among college students: Systematic review. *Journal of Medical Internet Research, 21*(7), e12869. https://doi.org/10.2196/12869

McCord, C., Ullrich, F., Merchant, K. A. S., Bhagianadh, D., Carter, K. D., Nelson, E., Marcin, J. P., Law, K. B., Neufeld, J., Giovanetti, A., & Ward, M. M. (2022). Comparison of in-person vs. telebehavioral health outcomes from rural populations across America. *BMC Psychiatry, 22*(1), 778. https://doi.org/10.1186/s12888-022-04421-0

Mikhail, A. (2022). *The first AI-driven personal health assistant is here for seniors.* Fortune Well. https://fortune.com/well/2022/10/07/renee-ai-driven-personal-health-assistant

Miller, B. F., Teevan, B., Phillips, R. L., Jr., Petterson, S. M., & Bazemore, A. W. (2011). The importance of time in treating mental health in primary care. *Families, Systems & Health, 29*(2), 144–145. https://doi.org/10.1037/a0023993

Milne-Ives, M., Lam, C., De Cock, C., Van Velthoven, M. H., & Meinert, E. (2020). Mobile apps for health behavior change in physical activity, diet, drug and alcohol use, and mental health: Systematic review. *JMIR mHealth and uHealth, 8*(3), e35479. https://doi.org/10.2196/17046

Molfenter, T., Heitkamp, T., Murphy, A. A., Tapscott, S., Behlman, S., & Cody. (2021). Use of telehealth in mental health (MH) services during and after COVID-19. *Community Mental Health Journal, 57*, 1244–1251. https://doi.org/10.1007/s10597-021-00861-2

Muench, U., Jura, M., Thomas, C. P., Perloff, J., & Spetz, J. (2022). Rural-urban prescribing patterns by primary care and behavioral health providers in older adults with serious mental illness. *BMC Health Services Research, 22*(1), 1440. https://doi.org/10.1186/s12913-022-08813-6

Negaro, S. N. D., Hantman, R. M., Probst, J. C., Crouch, E. L., Odahowski, C. L., Andrews, C. M., & Hung, P. (2023). Geographic variations in driving time to US mental health care, digital access to technology, and household crowdedness. *Health Affairs Scholar, 1*(6), qxad070. https://doi.org/10.1093/haschl/qxad070

Neves, A. L., & Burgers, J. (2022). Digital technologies in primary care: Implications for patient care and future research. *The European Journal of General Practice, 28*(1), 203–208. https://doi.org/10.1080/13814788.2022.2052041

Olfson, M. (2016). The rise of primary care physicians in the provision of US mental health care. *Journal of Health Politics, Policy and Law, 41*(4), 559–583. https://doi.org/10.1215/03616878-3620821

Regier, D. A., Goldberg, I. D., & Taube, C. A. (1978). The de facto US mental health services system: A public health perspective. *Archives of General Psychiatry, 35*(6), 685–693. https://doi.org/10.1001/archpsyc.1978.01770300027002

Robinson, C. L., D'Souza, R. S., Yazdi, C., Diejomaoh, E. M., Schatman, M. E., Emerick, T., & Orhurhu, V. (2024). Reviewing the potential role of artificial intelligence in delivering personalized and interactive pain medicine education for chronic pain patients. *Journal of Pain Research, 17*, 923–929. https://doi.org/10.2147/JPR.S439452

Rotenstein, L. S., Edwards, S. T., & Landon, B. E. (2023). Adult primary care physician visits increasingly address mental health concerns. *Health Affairs, 42*(2), 163–171. https://doi.org/10.1377/hlthaff.2022.00705

Scott, I., Wright, B., Brenneis, F., Brett-MacLean, P., & McCaffrey, L. (2007). Why would I choose a career in family medicine? Reflections of medical students at 3 universities. *Canadian Family Physician, 53*(11), 1956–1957.

Turner, A., Morris, R., Rakhra, D., Stevenson, F., McDonagh, L., Hamilton, F., Atherton, H., Farr, M., Blake, S., Banks, J., Lasseter, G., Ziebland, S., Hyde, E., Powell, J., & Horwood, J. (2022). Unintended consequences of online consultations: A qualitative study in UK primary care. *British Journal of General Practice, 72*(715), e128–e137. https://doi.org/10.3399/BJGP.2021.0426

U.S. Department of Veterans Affairs. (2024). *Mental health and Behavioral therapy apps*. U.S. Department of Veterans Affairs. https://mobile.va.gov/mental-health-and-behavioral-therapy-apps

Young, J. R., Galla, J. T., & Appelbaum, L. G. (2021). Transcranial magnetic stimulation treatment for smoking cessation: An introduction for primary care clinicians. *The American Journal of Medicine, 134*(11), 1339–1343. https://doi.org/10.1016/j.amjmed.2021.06.037

Zhang, T., Schoene, A. M., Ji, S., & Ananiadou, S. (2022). Natural language processing applied to mental illness detection: A narrative review. *npj Digital Medicine, 5*(1), 1–13. https://doi.org/10.1038/s41746-022-00589-7

Index

M. L. C. Williamson and D. L. Terry (eds.), *Essentials for Treating Behavioral Health in Primary Care*, https://doi.org/10.1007/978-3-032-09558-9

MIX
Papier aus verantwortungsvollen Quellen
Paper from responsible sources
FSC® C105338

If you have any concerns about our products,
you can contact us on
ProductSafety@springernature.com

In case Publisher is established outside the EU,
the EU authorized representative is:
Springer Nature Customer Service Center GmbH
Europaplatz 3, 69115 Heidelberg, Germany

Printed by Libri Plureos GmbH
in Hamburg, Germany